The Sanity of Survival

The Sanity of Survival

*Reflections on Community
Mental Health and Wellness*

Carl C. Bell, MD

Third World Press

Chicago

Third World Press
Publishers since 1967
Chicago

First Edition
Printed in the United States of America
Printed by R. R. Donnelley

10 09 08 07 06 05 04   6 5 4 3 2 1

Cover design by Bryant Smith
Inside text layout and design by Kimberly Foote

Library of Congress Cataloging-in-Publication Data

Bell, Carl C.
  The sanity of survival : reflections on community mental health and
    wellness / Carl C. Bell.–1st ed.
    p. ; cm.
  Articles previously published in various sources.
  Includes bibliographical references and index.
  ISBN 0-88378-267-7 (hardcover : alk. paper)–ISBN 0-88378-213-8 (pbk. :
  alk. paper)

1. African Americans–Mental health. 2. African Americans--Mental
health services. 3. Community mental health services--United States. 4.
Community psychiatry–United States.
  [DNLM: 1. Community Psychiatry–Collected Works. 2. African
Americans–psychology–Collected Works. 3. Mental Disorders–
ethnology–Collected Works. WM 30.6 B433s 2004] I. Title.
  RC451.5.N4B45 2004
  362.1'08996073–dc22
                                    2004015267

The Sanity of Survival

Contents

Section Four
States of Consciousness

Section Five
Cultural Sensitivity and Racism

Section Six
Health and Wellbeing

Common abbreviations found in this book:

ACE, Adverse childhood experience
ACTH, Corticotrophin
APA, American Psychiatric Association
AMA, American Medical Association
BPA, Black Psychiatrists of America
CDT, Community Day Treatment Program
CIP, Crisis Intervention Program
CMHC, Community Mental Health Council, Inc./
    Community Mental Health Clinic
DSM, *Diagnostic and Statistic Manual*
EEG, Electroencephalogram
ESA, Emergency Services Affiliates
EMH, Educable mentally handicapped
JAMA, *Journal of the American Medical Association*
JNMA, *Journal of the National Medical Association*
LD, Learning disability
MBD, Minimal brain dysfunction
MED, Medical (patient)
NMA, National Medical Association
OBS, Organic brain syndrome
PES, Psychiatric Emergency Service
PSY, Psychiatric (patient)
PTSD, Post-traumatic stress disorder
SMA, Screening and Medical Assessment Program
TLE, Temporal lobe epilepsy
TMH, Trainable mentally handicapped

Preface

Over the years, many colleagues and friends have suggested that I put into book form all the articles I've written on community psychiatry during the past twenty-five years of my career. I've finally taken their advice, and the result is in your hands. This book will be of special interest to people interested in African-American health and mental health. Profits from the sale of this book will benefit the Community Mental Health Clinic's efforts at further developing our African-American Mental Health Think Tanks, Institute for Managerial and Clinical Consultation, and Institute for Violence Prevention and the Promotion of Wellness.

When reading this book, there may be questions about the relevancy of some of my older work. I have observed that, unfortunately, not a great deal of progress has been made in addressing the health needs of the poor and underserved, many of whom are African Americans. Therefore, most of the observations I made twenty-five years ago still hold true today and are very germane when considering African Americans' health care and mental health care.

It's always been my great concern that as African Americans, we don't know very much about ourselves because we don't spend adequate time looking at ourselves. Instead, we're constantly defined by others and getting wrapped up in European-American culture. I think this is a tragedy. We need to start taking a good, long look at where we are.

My studies have always had this basic focus, which is an essential tenet in public health. These studies have defined health problems from the larger community context, examining large, underserved populations that happened to be poor and black. As a result, the studies have had strong implications in the practice of community psychiatry, which in my mind is a subspecialty of public health. My efforts call for systemic interventions to address problems of the community rather than solving them on a case-by-case, individual basis. Most of the articles found in this book have been published in the *Journal of the National Medical Association* (JNMA). I've intentionally published the bulk of my work in the JNMA, since I've always felt its readership would be the most responsive to my ideas and work.

I've come to realize that all my work has been based on a few common principles, though I wasn't aware of this initially. For one, it's now clear to me that we're all interdependent. This reality demands that we take a systems approach to health and mental health in the United States and on the planet. It is also now apparent to me that aspects of the inner life, such as states of consciousness, play a vital role in health and mental health. This enlightenment occurred after ten years of writing and research. Once I became aware of these concepts, which had always been guiding my scientific inquiry, I saw how my earlier, less planned work fit into a pattern and had been guided by a deeper force. This force is very common and yet indescribable—one we all can access if we only let ourselves experience it.

My research colleagues and I have done a kind of "bent nail" research because we've never really had the types of resources found in academia. By "bent nail," I refer to a concept that came to me growing up on Chicago's Westside. I always wanted to build something but never had the appropriate tools or materials. I learned to use what was available. When I decided to make a bookcase one summer, I found some old wood thrown away in the alley. The nails I used were bent and had to be straightened. The completed bookcase leaned to one side and looked like hell! Yet, it could always hold more than its share of books, and that was all that mattered to me. The quality of the research contained in this book is very much like that bookcase. It may not be airtight scientifically because of limited resources and far-from-perfect methodology. However, our findings have been just as useful as my bookcase was. In many instances, our work has even pointed the more academic social scientists in the right direction and shown them what they should be studying.

I've organized this book in a way for readers to see the basic principles I've followed during my years of service, research, and teaching. The book opens with an overview of the work I've done over the past twenty-five years. Here, I introduce the principles that have produced the seemingly diverse scope of my work. I ultimately hope this overview will help younger, exploring kindred spirits understand and select their paths.

Following this introduction, my articles are arranged in six sections under the following themes: "Public Health and Community Psychiatry," "Intervention Research and Advocacy," "Violence and Victimization," "States of Consciousness," "Cultural Sensitivity and Racism," "Health and Wellbeing." I hope readers will see that these themes are interdependent and interrelated.

Each article is followed by a commentary on my process of producing the work, because I feel the "stories behind the article" are interesting and instructive. I also describe the impact each article has had. This commentary represents my version of the truth, but I want the reader to come away with his/her own truth. However, I do hope that the reader will comprehend not only the science of my work but also the emotion and spirit I've put into it. In understanding the science, one can see the rationale and validity of my beliefs. In understanding the emotion and spirit, one can see the context and meaning of my work.

Acknowledgements

I thank the following journals that have allowed Third World Press to republish articles written by my coworkers and me: *Journal of the National Medical Association* (from which the vast majority of articles in this book come), *Journal of Health Care for the Poor and Underserved*, *Community Mental Health Journal*, and *Psychiatric Annals*. Appreciation is also due to Dr. Calvin Sampson, Editor of the *Journal of the National Medical Association*, for giving me the opportunity to publish in "the Journal."

I am a product of my life's experience, and a great deal of people have helped me on my journey. The work I've done has never been mine alone. I name my supporters throughout this book because I've always felt people should be given legitimate credit for their contributions. I'd like to acknowledge certain people and organizations that have made contributions to my work by assisting me with a project or teaching me a critical life lesson.

I'm grateful for Bert and Geraldine Pratt, who taught me many lessons of leadership. I acknowledge the Meharry Medical College faculty, especially Dr. Henry A. Moses, for giving me the opportunity to perform my first publishable research.

Gratitude is due also to the people and institutions that have helped me produce my articles over the years. I'm grateful to Jackson Park Hospital, the institution that allowed me to develop nearly half the articles in this book. Though the vast majority of the work presented here was accomplished through volunteer effort, the financial support of the United Way of Chicago has helped with the operation of some more recent projects and articles, which I greatly appreciate. I also thank the staffs of the District 14 Pupil Service Center (Chicago Board of Education) and the Chatham-Avalon Mental Health Center (Chicago Bureau of Mental Health) for supporting my clinical work, which led to two articles.

I also give thanks to Dr. Robert A. Washington, my former supervisor at the Community Mental Health Council (CMHC), for allowing me to organize their first African-American Mental Health Think Tank. The think tank led to numerous articles, some of which have been reproduced in this book. I also thank Drs. Esther J. Jenkins and Belinda Thompson at the CMHC for working with me to develop several of the articles. I would be remiss to neglect mentioning the CMHC staff and Board of Directors as well, since they've been supportive of my efforts.

I thank Dora Dixie, MD, for invaluable help with the family studies on isolated sleep paralysis. I am also grateful to Nancy Lance, MD, for translating a French article on the neurology of sleep that helped me understand the neurologic mechanisms behind isolated sleep paralysis. Appreciation is due to George Hu and Paul Hannah, MD, for their internal martial arts instruction. In the area of victimization research, I acknowledge Leatrice Allen, Bambade Shakoor, Debra Chalmers, Andrea Jacobson, and the Near North Health Service Corporation staff in Chicago.

I dedicate "The Need for Psychoanalysis is Alive and Well in Community Psychiatry" to Merton M. Gill, MD, Professor of Psychiatry at Abraham Lincoln School of Medicine, University of Illinois. I thank Merrell-Dow Pharmaceuticals, Inc., for supporting my research for "The Relationship between Isolated Sleep Paralysis, Panic Disorder, and Hypertension."

In addition, I would like to thank my administrative assistant, Bettye White, who has worked with me for nearly twenty years, and Judy L. Woods for typing some of the original article manuscripts for publication. Thanks to Dr. Faith J. Butler of the College of the Bahamas and Ms. Kimberly Foote for editing and proofreading the book. Thanks to Third World Press for keeping its promise to publish my work.

I would especially like to thank my various families for tolerating my drive to follow my calling. They have understood that when the Creator gives you a gift and you do not use it, the Creator takes it out of your hide!

I cannot possibly thank individually all those who have supported me. However, when a pharmaceutical company awarded me for my work in removing stigma and when the American Psychiatric Association let me give a Distinguished Psychiatrist Lecture on community psychiatry, I made a mental list of the following, all of whom I am grateful for (everyone I forgot, please forgive me!):

Meharry Medical College, for teaching me the public health concept of "getting rid of rats."

The patients who (despite their poor judgment of putting themselves under my care!) have taught me a great deal.

The CMHC MBA Senior Vice-Presidents, Juanita Redd and Hayward Suggs, who've shown me the importance of creating a work culture that emphasizes the "ah ha!" experience. I am grateful for the 400 geniuses that work at CMHC, as they allow me to work and think outside the box.

My partners in New York and in Durban, South Africa, who are in CMHC's R-01 National Institute of Mental Health-funded HIV prevention program. I am grateful to Dr. Roberta Paikoff for involving me in this work eight years ago.

All my colleagues who have replicated my "bent nail" research using better science than I could afford and who've found my work "directionally correct."

All my non-white colleagues on the fringe of European-American psychiatry who've been bringing innovation to the field. All my European-American colleagues who've had the courage to listen and have ended up being better psychiatrists because of their openness.

The State of Maine, for putting into place throughout the state CMHC's system of identifying children exposed to domestic violence and other forms of community violence.

My partners at the Illinois Department of Children and Family Services and Urban Services, who helped us reduce the number of African-American children going into child protective services from 35/1,000 in FY00 down to 14/1,000 in FY02 in McLean County, Illinois.

The following at the University of Illinois at Chicago: my partners at the Institute for Juvenile Research, since we are constructing a Conduct Disorders Clinic on Chicago's West and South Side, and for their support in attempting to construct a children's mental health and wellness infrastructure in the schools. My partners at the Health Research and Policy Center, for involving me in my first evidence-based prevention research project, Aban Aya. The Department of Psychiatry Chairman, for making me a part of his inner-circle so we could emphasize community psychiatry and correctional mental health care. The School of Public Health Dean, for making me a Professor of Public Health so we can sit together on the Chicago Board of Health and create early intervention programs.

The Chicago Board of Health and Commissioner, Dr. John Wilhelm, for making me a member so we can create a mental health system that will emphasize early intervention and wellness.

My partners at Morgan State University, for inviting me to be involved with their School of Public Health (emphasizing health behavior change), the first of its kind at a historically black university that will.

My partners at the National Commission on Correctional Health Care, for allowing me to assist with their work enforcing health care standards within correctional facilities around the US.

Mrs. Rosalynn Carter, for making me a member of the Atlanta Carter Center Mental Health Task Force so we can continue the work she began as First Lady.

The African-American research think tank at the CMHC and Drs. Esther Jenkins and Lynne Mock, for providing significant leadership for our think tanks.

Arnie Duncan, CEO of the Chicago Public Schools (CPS), for continuing the CPS Violence Prevention Project that CMHC began with Paul Vallas, former CPS CEO.

The American Academy of Pediatrics, for implementing some of CMHC's violence prevention strategies in their Violence Intervention Prevention Protocol, which pediatricians will have to use in their offices during well-baby visits.

The American Psychiatric Association, for allowing me to join the Work Group for the Practice Guidelines for the Treatment of Patients with Post-traumatic Stress Disorder/Acute Stress Disorder, the steering committee to implement the Surgeon General's report, the editorial board of the American Psychiatric Press, Inc., the Joint Commission on Public Affairs, the Committee on Psychiatric Diagnosis and Assessment, and the editorial board for *Psychiatric Glossary*, 8th edition.

Briatta, for teaching me joy, and William, for having a positive attitude.

Finally, to keep a promise I made to a little girl who is now an accomplished, talented woman, I dedicate this book to Cristin Carole for being my friend, which is no easy task.

Introduction

The Making of a Community Psychiatrist

I've always loved being adventurous and have felt that the greatest adventure is exploring life's mysteries. Such an attitude has been important for me as a healer, researcher, and teacher—jobs that have called for taking risks. I've always, therefore, been interested in research. Nothing turns me on more than having that "ah ha!" experience. I consider it a small part of the "expanded state of consciousness" that I've written about. Through this state of consciousness, we connect and remain attached to our spiritual nature.

My interest in life's mysteries was piqued when I performed one of my first scientific medical studies. It was 1968, and I was in my sophomore year at Meharry Medical College in Nashville, Tennessee. There was an observation in the field that some women on birth control pills seemed to have increased problems from blood clots. Biochemistry professor Henry A. Moses, PhD, who got me started in research, advised me on a project in which I tried to test the hypothesis. Using laboratory rats, I observed how birth control pills affected a rat's blood-clotting and reproductive systems, which would also have implications in humans.

This study was important because it could indicate whether birth control pills cause more infarcts in the human heart or brain (more commonly known as a stroke). Naturally, I was hoping to discover something that no one else had and with my breakthrough, save countless lives. Yet, most of the rats in the experiment showed no ovarian pathology. They didn't have an increase in plasma fibrinogen, which would increase blood clots. A few rats, however, had an abnormally high level of fibrinogen due to the birth control pills I'd given them. Thus, I was able to conclude that due to genetics, some animals might develop increased fibrinogen in response to birth control pills, which might also be true of human females.

My lesson from this study was that life expectancy is based on both individual genetic nature and one's life experiences. I also learned that knowledge in science does not occur in leaps and bounds, but in inches. I was grateful that the study was published in the Meharry Medical College *Journal of Pathology* (January 1969), but I realized that I shouldn't expect the Nobel Prize in science for my research unless I got extremely lucky!

More importantly, I discovered the rigor of hard science and the scientific method. Too frequently, African Americans disrespect the scientific method because they feel it is a European tool that concentrates only on the hard facts. Fortunately, going to a black medical school taught me the African origins of this method. Further, Meharrians learned that it's wise to do good work where it's most needed. We also learned that we're inseparable from our brothers and sisters in the greater community. This gave us a strong spiritual foundation, because it became clear to us that we were only as strong as our weakest link. When the scientific method was properly melded with wisdom and spirituality, we could better determine what to study and how to use the information obtained. Rarely did Meharrians study esoteric issues that would benefit only a small minority. Our research concerns instead focused on numerous and commonplace problems.

One of the most important lessons I learned at Meharry was a paradigm I call "getting rid of rats." I was taught that if a child from the community came into my office with a rat bite and I gave him/her proper medical treatment, I was a good physician. On the other hand, let's say twenty children from the community come into my office with rat bites. If I were to just give them medical treatment, I'd be considered a lousy physician, because I hadn't gone into the community to "get rid of the rats." This perspective of a public health, systems approach to problem solving would show up in my work constantly.

In my sophomore year at Meharry, I designed a study that started me on a trend I've followed since. I was propelled to go into the black community and study the status of its health. My interest was sparked during a microbiology class where Dr. James P. Carter lectured on nutrition and parasitism among rural preschool children in South Carolina. I was appalled at the findings, which revealed that the children were malnourished and that many were infected with various parasitic worms. As the relationship between good nutrition and health and wellbeing became clear to me, I wanted to be part of the exemplary work being done at Meharry.

Because of my interest, two of my professors recommended me for a Goldberger Fellowship. I used it to study nutrition after finishing my sophomore year in 1969. It was decided that I would examine the nutritional status of North Nashville's extremely poor children who were coming to the Children and Youth Center (pediatric clinic at Meharry). I designed an extensive questionnaire on socioeconomic status and diet that included the nutritional measures I planned to study. I developed an informed consent form for the parents to sign granting me permission to study their child and family. Once the study design was approved by Meharry's Biochemistry and Pediatrics Chairs, I went to the Children and Youth Center to enlist volunteers from the patient population. I conducted, in scientific lingo, point-in-time, prevalence, empirically based research—a cornerstone of basic public health research.

The poverty of many of the children's families was profound. During the summer, many of them would build fences from stray wood gathered around their homes. In the winter, they would use those fences as firewood to heat their homes. It wasn't surprising, then, that the study clearly illustrated that many North Nashville children were nutritionally deficient. Fifty percent had low or deficient parameters of nutrition, which also wasn't surprising, considering that the average amount spent on food for six people per week was $28.50. In my study, which made detailed notes about the residents' dietary habits, I found that their meals included many starchy foods like potatoes and corn that were inexpensive and filling but bad for their health in such a large quantity. I suspected that the children who weren't coming to the clinic were much worse off. The study documented that poor, African-American children catch nutritional hell.

RESIDENCY YEARS

After medical school, I combined an internship with a three-year psychiatric residency at the Illinois State Psychiatric Institute in Chicago. A pivotal part of my residency was when I received the American Psychiatric Association's (APA) Falk Fellowship, which allowed me to work with the APA's Task Force on Delivery of Psychiatric Services to Poverty Areas. The task force produced a report in 1973 that matched my desire to take a systems approach to large problems. I wrote the section on training psychiatric residents to deliver psychiatric services to poor areas. Although the report did not get much exposure, a few articles on residency training cited it. It is reassuring to know that my earlier, almost unknown work had an impact somewhere.

The Falk Fellowship more importantly allowed me to continue the professional socialization started at Meharry, where I was taught by Doctors Harold Jordan, Ralph Hines, Henry Tomes, Joseph Phillips, Lloyd Elam, and Jeanne Spurlock. I had a chance to meet with several prominent senior black psychiatrists like Orlando Lightfoot, Douglas Foster, and Rose Jenkins. I was also introduced to the Black Psychiatrists of America (BPA) a few years after it was formed, and met stellar psychiatrists such as Chester M. Pierce, James Comer, Alvin Poussaint, Alfred Cannon, and James Ralph.

My early involvement with the BPA led me to examine leadership and politics, particularly in "Analysis of the Political Sophistication of the Black Psychiatrist," an article I published in 1974 (Bell CC. Analysis of the political sophistication of the black psychiatrist. *Newsletter Black Psychiatrists of Am*. 1974;3). In the article, I criticized black psychiatrists for not having "the cognitive and affective recognition concerning the dynamics of political groups" to make changes in the political system to influence services for black mentally ill and training for black mental health professionals. Further, hoping my lessons wouldn't be ignored, I outlined some leadership principles that could increase the BPA's political clout. Looking back, I realize these were my early efforts at identifying leadership and management skills. This would be necessary to actualize a public health/community psychiatry, systems approach to the very large health and mental health problems facing the African-American community. I believe that if more African-American health and mental health professionals get involved in scientific research on major, real-life problems within the black community and then provide leadership on how to apply the solutions we discover, we'd be further along.

In the early 1970s, I'd begun involving myself with Eastern practices—various forms of exercise and meditation—as a self-improvement effort, because I've always tried to correct my horde of faults. If a physician wants to make a contribution, he or she has to be healthy. It's hard for the physician to tell people to stop smoking if the physician smokes. As a physician, I've been concerned with the other side of illness—wellness. My studying the Eastern practices led me to produce several articles that fit under my "Health and Wellbeing" category (see Section Six). I stressed the various health benefits of Eastern exercises that I thought would be particularly important for the African-American population.

During my last two years of residency, I did some work at Jackson Park Hospital, a general hospital serving Chicago's Southside African-American community. I joined Dr. Leroy Foster, who was developing a comprehensive community mental health center at Jackson Park Hospital. We teamed up with Ruth Williams, State of Illinois Department of Mental Health Administrator, who shared our mission.

After my residency training, my medical career was put on hold for two years because of my time at the Great Lakes Naval Training Center. At Meharry, I'd been pressed into service by an Armed Forces recruiter and had signed up for the Berry Plan, which forestalled drafting until after my residency. The Vietnam War was over by then, but I was asked to honor my commitment because the military was short of physicians. While at Great Lakes, I had a chance to digest my psychiatry education received as a resident. I also experienced and learned from the military's leadership and management techniques, which not surprisingly were based mainly on tradition and bullying.

THE EARLY WORKING YEARS

After leaving the Navy in 1976, I returned to Chicago's Jackson Park Hospital and implemented its Psychiatric Emergency Service, which catered to African Americans with inadequate resources. At the time, the South Side's mental health system infrastructure was extremely underdeveloped, and there were few alternatives to hospitalization in a state hospital. The general hospital had few psychiatric beds, outpatient psychiatric placements were limited, and day treatment or residential placements didn't exist. As a community psychiatrist, I felt it my mission to use our resources—however limited—and develop a system to address the needs of the poor and underserved African-American population. After proving that the service model was efficient and effective, I advocated for the systemic intervention I'd developed in the emergency room to keep psychotic patients out of the hospital. Based on my early experiences with the model, I wrote the first paper I would classify under my "Intervention Research and Advocacy" category (see Chapter 4). Our Crisis Intervention Program was advocated as a method to correct the inadequate health care delivery to the black population.

My efforts were successful at keeping needless admissions out of the hospital—a mandate the hospital informed me the State of Illinois had hired them to do. When the hospital's census began to drop with the state hospital's, though, I got called on the carpet. The hospital management wasn't happy because I'd done my job too well. I was unaware then that the hospital was serving two apparently opposing mandates: they shouldn't have been making unnecessary admissions, but they had to keep psychiatric beds filled. Unfortunately, Jackson Park Hospital's management philosophy was to not share information, so they didn't give me a clear reason why they chewed me out. I knew I was working in the wrong place, so I quit.

After a few months, I had two part-time jobs—one with the Chicago Board of Education (with whom I now consult) and one with the Chicago Department of Mental Health (I now sit on their board). I also got a small job as staff psychiatrist at the newly developed Community Mental Health Council's (CMHC) day treatment center, which Ruth Williams had managed to get funded. Though I was still delivering psychiatric services to a South Side African-American population, I had less control in developing a service system. I decided to do something to change this. As at Meharry, I first performed empirical studies to describe the populations I was serving. Most of the research I'd read about at Meharry and during my psychiatry residency was based on observations of white Americans. Therefore, I wasn't sure if the results would hold true for black Americans for a variety of reasons, ranging from genetics, social class, racism, the environment, and culture. As a result, during this period, I wrote several intervention research and advocacy articles aimed at the black population (see Section Two).

Because the leadership within Jackson Park Hospital's Department of Psychiatry had changed, I became Associate Director of the hospital's Division of Behavioral and Psychodynamic Medicine in 1979. I oversaw the daily operation of their twenty-four-hour Psychiatric Emergency Service, a fourteen-bed psychiatric unit and an outpatient clinic with pre-care, after-care, alcoholism, senior-age, and children's programs.

During this phase of my life, my interest in organized psychiatry reemerged. I reconnected with the BPA, was elected their Vice-President, and edited their quarterly newsletter, *The Bottom Line*, from 1977 to 1982. Each year, I published four substantive issues and mailed them to the 800-plus black psychiatrists around the country. Thanks to Dr. Phyllis Harrison-Ross, the BPA broke all of its ties with its sponsor, the APA. Under the leadership of Andrea Delgado, MD, the BPA began to have its own conferences. While the break from the APA was helpful—it allowed black psychiatrists to function independently, free from the APA's oversight, it was also trying because, like most black not-for-profit organizations, we didn't have any organizational support (e.g., a paid secretary) or infrastructure (e.g., a formal office site).

During the late 1970s, I became interested in issues of cultural sensitivity and racism in the United States and produced two articles on racism (see Chapters 32 and 33). As my diagnostic skills improved and I gained more experience in psychiatry, I made the perplexing observation that black patients didn't receive the same amount of "quality time" spent on their assessments and diagnoses as did whites. This inadequate assessment frequently led to misdiagnosis, which had been a concern of mine working with children and later with adults. My studies on the prevalence of misdiagnosis of African Americans led Dr. Harshad Metha and me to write "The Misdiagnosis of Black Patients with Manic Depressive Illness" (see Chapter 25), which began a trend in the US of finally recognizing that African Americans could have psychotic illness other than schizophrenia.

I was able to apply my knowledge of cultural sensitivity in 1979, when Dr. Jay Chunn, Howard University's School of Social Work Dean, asked me to help train mental health professionals who would work with people of color. My APA Task Force training work begun ten years earlier came in handy and got refined. I helped the professionals develop cultural sensitivity and overcome racism issues to become culturally competent to treat African Americans. There has been considerable debate over which "culturally sensitive" approach is more effective in treating African-American mentally ill patients. My work with Howard University's School of Social Work synergized with most of my prior work examining how public health and community psychiatry principles are included in psychiatric training. In order to know how to accurately address the needs of a large Non-white US population, we must know the major patterns of problems it faces. Leadership was also crucial for actualizing our training curriculum into schools. Importantly, this project revealed the mental health service needs of the black population.

My curriculum development work at Howard was published in my first book chapter in 1983, which was co-authored with Doctors Irma J. Bland, Earline Houston, and Billy E. Jones, who I'd met through the BPA (Curriculum development and implementation: enhancement of knowledge and skills for the psychiatric treatment of black populations. In: Chunn J et al., eds. *Mental Health and People of Color: Curriculum Development and Change*. Washington, DC: Howard University Press; 1983:205–237). We questioned the appropriateness of using Western psychiatric theories in cross-cultural diagnosis and treatment. This line of inquiry would later lead me to conceptualize mental illness and mental health in terms of states of consciousness (see Section Four). We also highlighted the need for more scientific research on black mental health and illness. Specifically, we wanted to find out more about how socio-cultural factors affect mental illness within the black community and especially how racism takes its toll on African Americans. I haven't since spent a great deal of time writing about training professionals to treat black patients. Mostly, I've been busy writing articles directed toward professionals who want information on mental health issues relevant to black patient care (see Chapters 27 and 28).

One item on the research agenda of my book chapter co-authors' and me was to understand better the influence of increased mortality and morbidity within the African-American community, a gap I hope my better known violence and victimization research has begun to address. We discussed the assessment and diagnosis of black patients and discussed how blacks fare in dynamic psychotherapy. We advocated for a better understanding of child-rearing practices, social forces, and personality development for African Americans. Further, we suggested the need for better mental health measures and for a more accurate assessment of patients from the black community. Lastly, we suggested various leadership/political strategies to get more non-white curriculum content into psychiatric training.

In 1981, I made an attempt to fill knowledge gaps identified in the Howard University chapter—specifically, how increased mortality and morbidity within the black community influences our mental health. I wrote an essay, which the *Chicago Sun Times Views* published in a small column, "How Blacks Can Overcome Combat Fatigue" (November 14, 1981:22). In the article, I highlighted that traumatic stress is usually associated with war conditions and labeled "combat fatigue." The column went on to suggest that because African Americans are under similar levels of inordinate stress (due to social conditions, causing infant mortality and increased mortality in adults from cancer and homicide), they are at risk of developing what I coined "survival fatigue." I noted that drug abuse, black-on-black murder, inappropriate sexual activity, and acceptance of defeat are some of the major negative coping responses to this stress. I also suggested positive coping responses such as expressing stressful feelings, involvement in spirituality, using frustration to generate positive action designed to relieve stress, and being proactive in preventing stress. My colleagues and I would later refine a central underlying theme in this essay: how stress can cause an alteration in one's state of consciousness, with either positive or negative results.

Considering the amount of violence in some black communities, it was impossible to avoid the issue in my work as a community psychiatrist. The first paper I wrote addressing this issue was "Interface between Psychiatry and the Law on the Issue of Murder" (see Chapter 10). Because I'd been addressing the needs of acutely psychotic patients in emergency rooms, safety issues also became a major concern of mine. As a result, Dr. John Palmer (currently the head of Harlem Hospital) and I wrote "Security Procedures in a Psychiatric Emergency Service" (see Chapter 5), complete with pictures on how to handle one's self if attacked. We published more on this issue in "Survey of the Demographic Characteristics of Patients Requiring Restraints in a Psychiatric Emergency Service" (*J Natl Med Assoc.* 1983;75:981–987).

In 1981, I'd been out of medical school for ten years. By then, I'd produced twenty-two articles, the vast majority of which were published in the *Journal of the National Medical Association* (JNMA). The JNMA provides a voice for the health care needs of a poor and underserved population. It was and continues to be a major source of information for health and mental health issues affecting African Americans. Its articles are extremely relevant to public health in the African-American community. "The Journal," as it is affectionately known, provides a forum for professionals to share vital information about African-American health and mental health concerns. In addition, it provides a platform for professionals to affirm or challenge each others' work, a necessary tension to advance science.

I was quite proud to publish in this journal that served the oldest black professional association in the country—the National Medical Association (NMA), established in 1895. Since my work had begun to have some impact, some of my senior colleagues questioned why I seemed to publish most of my work in a black medical journal. One even had the temerity to suggest that I might get more status and have a greater influence if I were to publish in the "white journals," as they had a wider audience. His comments were appreciated, because by publishing in "white journals" my articles would have had more prestige and more influence, which was an accurate assessment of how things work in the US. Since so many people were curious about my decision to publish in the Journal, though, I felt it necessary to write an editorial about it, reprinted at the end of this introduction.

During my early career, I didn't receive any grant money for my research, and all of it was fueled by volunteer effort. For my intervention-focused research, I had the cooperation of the staff in the clinical settings where I was conducting the research. On a couple of occasions, I also had co-authors who helped with data collection and writing. Still, I had to do much of the work by myself. On my time off from work, I would collect data, bring the few supplies necessary to do the research, and calculate the statistics myself. I would type and retype the papers, mail them to the JNMA editor, proofread the galley proofs, and pay for reprints of the articles. It's not that I like hard work. I just didn't have any funds or support to do the work. By "support," I'm referring to what is usually given when one conducts academic research: salaries for researchers, office space, secretarial support, statistical analysis, supplies, and paid time to think, plan, and write the article. I wanted to see the work done, so I just did it. I obtained this attitude from the "bent nail" training I had as a young man.

CONGRESSIONAL ADVOCACY

Since my time at Meharry as a medical student, I've combined congressional advocacy with my medical profession. Meharry always emphasized a public health approach to problems, so my investment in my study on the poor, African-American population of North Nashville didn't end with finding results. I decided to intervene and improve the nutritional status of my study population. I sent a copy of my paper to Richard Fulton, a Tennessee congressman on the Committee of Ways and Means, to let him know of my findings and to suggest that he take action.

Congressman Fulton sent me a nice letter thanking me and agreeing that something needed to be done. He suggested, however, that since I was "far more qualified to suggest what course of action is necessary," he would welcome my suggestions. A few months later, I received a letter also from Marjorie Whiting, Nutrition Advisor for the Emergency Food and Medical Services Division, Office of Health Affairs, Office of Economic Opportunity (OEO). She'd heard about my work from William Boehne of the Food and Drug Administration and was interested in obtaining more information.

I wrote Congressman Fulton again, telling him that Meharry's Children and Youth Center and Meharry's OEO-funded Matthew Walker Community Health Center provided services at no cost to families below a certain income range. I explained that though both clinics allowed poor patients to receive adequate health care, many poor residents were excluded because the government had set its low-income levels according to OEO not low enough. I pointed out that not enough money was spent on individual health centers and that there were too few health centers. Lastly, I noted that while the poor people being served by Meharry had decent health care, their diet and standard of living were poor. I explained that this was due to the "psychological state of the ghetto," to a lack of training for skilled jobs, and to the fact that only a few good jobs were available. Congressman Fulton wrote me back telling me he shared my concerns. He said he would bear my views in mind when Congress considered measures to further benefit low-income families and provide additional assistance in health.

Being young and inexperienced, I assumed that by doing scientific research and discovering a legitimate problem and making Congress aware of it, something would be done. The reality is that my efforts never got any real mileage in Congress. Yet, I felt I'd made a difference. Though Congress may not have taken any action about my findings, the African-American medical community would later address them. In 1976, a Meharry research team led by Dr. Edward G. High published a paper in the JNMA on a project designed to improve the nutritional and health status of a poor population in Nashville, Tennessee. Looking back, I now realize that I was part of a team of African-American health professionals who were deeply committed to the improving the health care status and wellbeing of the "least of us."

Years later, I learned how to make sure that scientific facts got translated into Congressional action. On April 28, 1992, I testified before the congressional Subcommittee on Labor, Health, and Human Services Education and Related Agencies. In my testimony, "Correctional & Community Health Care: A Prescription for a Healthier America," I requested that Medicaid entitlement follow youths placed into juvenile correctional facilities. The current situation was that Medicaid benefits stopped accumulating for such youths. This meant that the county, rather than the state or federal government, was responsible for paying for the youth's health care. The problem was that numerous counties of course had fewer resources than did the state and federal government. County financial resources available for youth health services were slim, and sophisticated health services for them were limited.

The head of the committee gave me fifteen minutes to testify, thanked me, and told me that the committee would consider my request. He said the same thing to the ten other experts advocating for the appropriation of funding for various other legitimate causes. I recall thinking that none of us got very much respect and that the Congress members didn't seem to share our passion for our crusades. When I testified, only two Representatives were present. There were several empty chairs.

When Mary Tyler Moore came into the room to advocate for the allocation of more funds for diabetes research, her response from the committee was very different. A few minutes after she entered, Representatives began to pour out of the back room, and soon the whole committee was present. They hung to her every word. She got 45 minutes to testify. When she finished, each Congress member asked her questions and told her how much each had loved her television show. Afterward, the chairperson assured her that they would seriously consider her request. He then adjourned the committee so they could take a group and individual photos with Moore! She had more presence than any of the scientists present, even with our "expert" status and with all our research and compelling facts.

The lesson wasn't lost to me: it's not the facts you have, but how you market them. Despite all the important research we scientists do, if we don't figure out a catchy way to present it, we'll be wasting much of our time, because very few people will read it. Most people are rarely interested in the rigorous scientific steps we take to make sure our conclusions are valid. They only want to know the bottom line, in a way they can remember.

PROFESSIONAL LIFE AT THE COMMUNITY MENTAL HEALTH COUNCIL

In 1982, I decided once again to leave Jackson Park Hospital. While I'd had some success building a mental health care system there, the hospital's management philosophy was still at odds with mine. Because the administration didn't believe in sharing information or open planning, I frequently found myself in the dark about what to expect. This made my efforts at infrastructure-building a very frustrating experience, as I didn't have any control over the destiny of the Department of Psychiatry.

During my tenure at Jackson Park, I'd supported the growth of the CMHC. By the time I left Jackson Park, it had become a fully funded, comprehensive community mental health center with a mission to deliver outpatient mental health services to Chicago's South Side black population. CMHC Executive Director Dr. Robert Washington offered me the opportunity to join the staff as Medical Director. We'd gone to high school together, and when he'd first came to Chicago after working at the National Institute of Mental Health (NIMH) as a psychologist, I'd helped him secure the job at the CMHC.

In my role as Medical Director, I had to provide quality psychiatric evaluations for CMHC's psychiatric patients and give them medication if they needed it. Since I wanted to develop the agency into a research and training center, I asked for some support for my research. Dr. Washington gladly consented. I thought I'd died and gone to heaven! For the first time since medical school, I was given time to think about and plan research. I wouldn't have to type and retype papers. There would be help in doing the library work required to write an article. Other interested staff could assist with the research as a part of their job. Essentially, I had research support and a research team. Two very bright, African-American, well-trained social psychologists, Dr. Belinda Thompson and Dr. Esther Jenkins, made a critical contribution to my work. Their insight allowed me to tighten the scientific aspects of my work while still maintaining a strong focus on real-life issues for African Americans. Several years of productive research followed, with much of it getting published.

My interest in states of consciousness led me to form a theoretical framework from which the new CMHC research team began research on altered states of consciousness within the African-American community. After some focus-group testing, we planned a study to measure the quality and quantity of each of the seventeen states of consciousness in black patients. Because of this basic empirical research, my colleagues and I published three studies (see Chapters 20, 21, and 24). A few years later, we refined our work on isolated sleep paralysis and wrote two additional articles on the topic (see Chapters 22 and 23). During this period, CMHC formed another research team to study the states of consciousness, intoxication, stupor and coma. We produced the book article, "The Misdiagnosis of Alcohol Related Organic Brain Syndromes and Treatment Issues in Blacks" (In: Brisbane F, Womble M, eds. *Treatment of Black Alcoholics*. New York: Haworth Press; 1985:45–65).

In 1984, James Ralph, MD, (who had been placed in the NIMH by the BPA so he could ensure that research issues concerning African Americans were addressed) invited me to develop a paper on homicide for a second national conference (NIMH) on black-on-black murder. The CMHC research team responded to this challenge in several ways. We'd found that many of our states of consciousness research subjects had experienced some type of coma. As a result, we began to look at the relationship between coma and violence. In 1984, we presented "States of Consciousness: Their Relationship to Black-on-Black Murder," for the Black Homicide Workshop on Mental Health and Prevention, sponsored by the National Association of Social Workers and the NIMH (Office of Prevention and Center for the Study of Minority Group Mental Health). A few years later in 1986 and 1987, I would publish a literature review connecting violence and coma (see Chapters 11 and 12). Also in 1987, my CMHC colleagues and I published a case history of a young woman whose head injury had clearly been the etiology for her later violent and psychotic behavior (see Chapter 13).

Recognizing the importance of the issue of violence within the black community, the CMHC research team approached this issue from various angles. One was to get organized medicine more involved in violence as a public health issue. After two years of planning, I organized a plenary session of the NMA's 1986 annual meeting that focused on the NMA's role in solving this problem.

Shortly after, I made a call to address the issue of violence from a systemic perspective based in public health/community psychiatry (see Chapter 1). These initial suggestions grew, and I was able to publish an article in the *Community Mental Health Journal* presenting a more detailed picture of what I thought should happen (see Chapter 2). The philosophy behind the *Community Mental Health Journal* is very similar to that of JNMA. I felt the publication of my work in this journal was compatible with my public health/community psychiatry principles. In late 1986 and early 1987, I wrote more articles focusing on my category of "Cultural Sensitivity and Racism." The first to appear was "Impaired Black Health Professionals: Vulnerabilities and Treatment Approaches" (see Chapter 29). The second, "Faked Out Again," published by the JNMA (April 1987) as guest editorial, highlighted a trip the BPA had taken to Kenya. There, we discovered that the "traditional" Massai village we visited was actually a African plantation owned by white Kenyans who were profiting from our presence and who weren't encouraging the Masai on their property to attend school. We were reminded that even on the African continent, people of African descent could be exploited and could be unwitting pawns in the degradation of people of color.

Realizing that violence produced victims, CMHC's research team also began to conduct victimization research on CMHC's patient population and the service area youth. Our work with patients produced three articles (see Chapters 14–16). Our work with the youth and their issues of victimization began in 1985, when we conducted a survey that highlighted the exorbitant amount of violence some African-American children witnessed (see Chapter 3). Our research began a national trend in this area. The Select Committee on Children, Youth, and Family of the House of Representatives invited me to give the testimony, "Children and Violence," on May 15, 1989. In October 1992, we were presented the APA Hospital and Community Psychiatry's Gold Achievement Award for the CMHC's Victim's Services Program's outstanding contributions in understanding, treating, and advocating for victims of violence at both the community and national level.

After the prestigious *Journal of the American Medical Association* (JAMA) published an abstract of "The Need for Victimization Screening in a Poor Outpatient Medical Population" (see Chapter 15), Dr. Ezra Griffith from Yale suggested that he and I write an article on suicide and homicide trends among blacks for JAMA. He felt the topic needed a wider audience. Further, because the peer review standards for the American Medical Association's journal were higher than the JNMA's, our work would have more clout. I reluctantly agreed, and in late 1988 and early 1989, we began to work on the article, with Dr. Griffith focusing on suicide and me on homicide.

Articles submitted to very prestigious journals are given to reviewers who are familiar with the topic so they can decide the appropriateness of the article and the quality of its theories and science. The names of the articles' authors are withheld from the reviewer in an attempt to keep reviewer bias out of the evaluation process. The reviewers' identities are likewise kept from the submitting authors to prevent an undue influence or animosity, depending on the reviewers' assessment of the work. Unfortunately, the problem with this attempt to ensure a measure of fairness is that there are only a few experts in any given area of study. Usually, they can identify each other's work by how it's written.

The article Dr. Griffith and I wrote was rejected. When I read the reviewer's anonymous comments, I had a really good idea who it was. It seemed to me that the reviewer's major problem was that Dr. Griffith and I hadn't cited his work on violence in our paper. We hadn't done so because despite the clear quality of his work, it wasn't at all related to the issue we were addressing in our article.

We revised the article by dropping in a paragraph on the reviewer's work. The paragraph ended with the message that this important work was not much help in trying to address the questions raised in our article. We resubmitted the article to JAMA, and it was published (Griffith E , Bell CC. Recent trends in suicide and homicide among blacks. *J Am Med Assoc.* 1989). So much for the anonymous, high, peer-review standards!

I raise this issue to expose the games some people play. I hope that young authors won't get discouraged by the supposed bias-free peer review process that keeps their work from getting published. It isn't that I don't believe in some quality control, but one thing I've learned in psychiatry is that where there are people, there is feces. Sometimes a process that is supposed to be fair is really quite biased.

Around the early 1990s, I began to receive invites to sit on various journal editorial boards. I was asked to write articles and books chapters on the issues CMHC's research team had been exploring. My colleagues and I would continue conducting research and writing and publishing several articles in the 1990s and beyond.

In terms of the CMHC's latest efforts, I now believe we have a community psychiatry model that will address issues of mental health and mental wellness, and we recently applied it in McLean County, Illinois. With much help from multiple partners in and outside of the county, we've been able to decrease the number of African-American children entering protective services from 35/1,000 in 2000 to 14/1,000 in 2002 (a 61.3% decrease). We've been able to decrease the number of European-American children entering protective services from 3.56/1,000 in 2000 to 1.56/1,000 in 2002 (a 57.2% decrease). However, with the election of a new governor of Illinois, resulting in a change in the head of the Illinois Department of Children and Family Services, I've struggled with how to institutionalize and sustain our intervention.

Being on the Carter Center's Mental Health Task Force has proved to be of enormous benefit in solving this problem, because I've been able to discuss my concerns with much wiser and experienced individuals. One such was with Dr. Julius Richmond, the former Surgeon General under President Carter's administration, who suggested to me that the way to sustain something is to (1) acquire the knowledge that the intervention was efficacious and effective (which I believe is best done using good science), (2) develop the public will (which I believe is best done through public relations and marketing), and (3) develop an implementation system, or as he called it, an "effector limb" (which I believe is best done by developing a business plan or through administrative rule or a plan to pass legislation and appropriations). By using these strategies, we at the CMHC hope to help change how the child welfare system is practiced in Illinois and in the country.

Unfortunately, most psychiatrists and social service professionals believe that all we need to do to make the larger society use our wonderful evidence-based interventions is to hold hands and sing "Kumbaya." What we really need is public relations, marketing, political pressure, and a business plan. The CMHC is using this strategy as well to institutionalize our work in McLean County, Illinois. In terms of marketing, I've come to realize that a painful reality we academic research scientists must come to grips with is that not many people in the general public will read our scholarly works. So, if we don't break down and advertise, our work will go on the shelf, never to be used or implemented. I've been fortunate to make several television appearances, which has helped me advertise my research and findings to the American public. In 1983, I presented my states of consciousness work on WVIT Channel 30 in Hartford, Connecticut. I presented my homicide prevention work on television stations in various cities: ABC affiliate WJRT-TV's local news in Flint, Michigan, WSB-TV's local news in Atlanta, Georgia, and on "America's Black Forum" with Julian Bond in Washington, DC. I've also spoken on homicide prevention on local Chicago television stations such as the local PBS "Chicago Tonight" and local ABC, CBS, NBC and WGN news shows. In addition, I was featured on several of ABC "Nightline" shows, "The Today Show," PBS's "Tony Brown's Journal" and "Bodywatch," "CBS Evening News" with Dan Rather and Connie Chung, CBS's "Nightwatch," PBS's "News Hour" with Jim Leher and "Bill Moyer's Specials," and several cable stations like CNN's "The World Today" with Bernard Shaw and "C-SPAN."

Thanks to the CMHC's MBA Senior Vice-Presidents Juanita Redd and Hayward Suggs, I've also learned that the level of "teamness" within an institution determines how effective that institution will be at getting the job done. For years, I would leave the CMHC, go out into the larger social science arena, and learn about other people's work that could benefit our own. I would return home to the CMHC with methods and models I felt to be efficacious and effective and suggest that my staff use them in their work. But, like at most agencies, my staff listened carefully to my discovery but would go back to doing their business as usual. During one of CMHC's Executive Team Strategy sessions, Redd and Suggs asked me what I could use to help the CMHC's work improve. I told them about my frustration at our staff's lack of welcoming innovations in the field of human services. For years, we'd talked about the need for training CMHC staff to do their jobs in an efficacious, effective manner, but we'd been unsuccessful in obtaining Human Resources support to make such training possible. So, they got the CMHC team together, and we began to develop an in-house training program that would help staff develop several attributes.

We were hoping to cultivate a strong work culture that would welcome new evidence-based developments from the field. We also wanted to train staff in negotiations so we could monitor and supervise each other to ensure that we were true to our mission, "Saving Lives, Making a Difference." We created various teams within the agency to assess, plan, and implement changes in how we did business. I believe that we now have a system that allows us to bring to the African-American community evidence-based interventions that are culturally sensitive as well. Thus, we're far ahead of the curve. Furthermore, I'm convinced that our training methodology can be useful to other organizations trying to provide services to various communities that may or may not be African American. We've found another universal principle of human existence that makes all of our travels less burdensome.

Currently, we're doing HIV prevention work in South Africa, which is going extremely well. We've had the good fortune of finding good partners in Durban who are helping us spread the work we began in the Robert Taylor homes on Chicago's Southside. This work has re-taught me the importance of cultivating community partnerships when an interventionist does community psychiatry work with a culture that is unfamiliar to him/her. While I believe I've come to understand that I have knowledge of some universal principles that can improve the public's health, I'm also clear that in many cultures, I wouldn't be considered sensitive. I don't speak Zulu. While I do plan to study Zulu culture as often as possible, I don't plan on learning the language, since I have too much other work to do. Yet, in developing activities like "Rebuilding the Village," "Providing Access to Health Care," "Improving Connectedness Between People," "Improving and Creating Social Skills," "Improving and Supporting Self Esteem"—all of which create a sense of power, connectedness, models, and uniqueness, as well as activities like "Reestablishing the Adult Protective Shield" and "Minimizing the Effects of Trauma," I've learned the need to be culturally sensitive. However, if I can enlist the support of "cultural bridges," who can get me access to Zulu people and who can extract the universal healing principles in our US-based, evidence-based interventions and apply them to Zulu culture, then I'm doing the Creator's work.

During the CMHC research team's tenure over the past twenty-five years, we've tried to focus on research relevant to the African-American population in the United States, which we view as an underserved, under-researched population. We've since learned that much of our work has been relevant to the country as a whole, and we feel it's been of some benefit, as can be seen in many of the commentaries following the articles in this book. The information we've gathered has been useful in training professionals on what to expect when they serve the African-American population. Thus, it serves to help them be sensitive to African-American health and mental health issues. In keeping with this task, some of our work has also focused on racism.

Our work has also influenced the practice of public health and community psychiatry by calling attention to previously neglected, significant problems within the country, such as violence and victimization. We've suggested models of intervention for these problems and have field-tested them, which has led us to advocate for these models. In addition to concentrating on pathology within the African-American community, we've emphasized strengths and health within our population and have proposed a model for understanding mental illness and positive, coping strategies, based on our understanding of states of consciousness.

Finally, through the production of research from a community-based comprehensive mental health center, we've served as a training ground for young professionals, researchers, and teachers. This has been a strategy to ensure that the dedication, creativity, and service-focus of our work does not get lost with my transition.

WHY THE *JOURNAL OF THE NATIONAL MEDICAL ASSOCIATION**

Because I have published the bulk of my articles in the JNMA, both my black and white colleagues are forever asking, "Why do you keep submitting your articles to the black medical journal?"

Some of the arguments I have heard for not submitting to "the Journal" is that it is less prestigious, that I could receive wider exposure in a journal with a larger circulation, and that my articles would be given more credence if they appear in a better known publication (i.e., a white one). Others claim that by publishing in JNMA, my work is limited to a black readership.

To counter these arguments, I would like to explain my motivations so that my colleagues might follow my lead. Regarding the contention that the JNMA is a less prestigious publication, I would have to answer that this perception depends on one's reference points. My emotional and personal reference point is black. From a professional standpoint, my medical reference point is black patient care, since I was trained at the predominantly black Meharry Medical College. I was once warned to carefully watch my professional career so as not to risk becoming known as a professional who knows only about issues concerning black patients. Actually, I am not seeking a reputation in the white professional community (or the black one, for that matter). My chief priority is to deliver competent medical care to black people. I am convinced that one way to further this aim is promoting medical competence in black medical professionals. In my opinion, there is no better method of achieving this goal than publishing articles that address black medical care in the Journal.

The readership of the JNMA is unique. The Journal is circulated not only to all members of the National Medical Association, but also to physicians, black or white, practicing in inner-city areas in the United States. Therefore, the argument that the information in my articles—relevant to both black and white medical professionals—will be strictly limited to a black readership does not hold.

---

*Originally printed as Bell Carl C. Guest editorial on "Why the *Journal of the National Medical Association.*" *J Natl Med Assoc.* 1981;73:477–478.

I do not judge the Journal as less prestigious than other publications simply because it is a black effort. Rather, I feel that the very fact that it is a black effort makes it all the more important and all the more integral to the improvement of health care delivery to minorities. Further, I have received requests for reprints of my JNMA articles from Germany, Spain, France, Romania, England, Italy, Canada, Mexico, Israel, China, and India, as well as from all fifty states. This tells me that medical professionals from many areas find articles of interest in the Journal. I have also found that JNMA articles are mentioned, cited, or abstracted in many other journals with a larger circulation. Although the JNMA may not have as wide an audience as other publications, it has an unmistakably discernible impact and—as far as I am concerned—reaches the readership who will be most responsive to its content.

Finally, the most important reason why I publish in the JNMA is to stimulate my colleagues to develop empirical data that can be used to treat the minority populations of the world. We must begin to define for ourselves our major problems and determine the best ways for us, as professionals treating blacks, to address them. For too long, we have believed what we learned from the various studies others have conducted on us. We must begin to study and help ourselves. The Journal is an excellent vehicle for aiding us in this process. It offers role models, substantive data, treatment methods valid for the black population, and studies relevant to specific black health needs. It deals with the context in which most blacks find themselves; as this is different, by necessity, from that experienced by most whites, the treatment modalities for blacks cannot be the same as those geared to whites.

So, I ask my medical colleagues: do you take the time to write an article on how you deliver health care to your minority practice? Do you take the time to compile empirical research to find out where we are and what needs to be researched further? It may help your brother and sister medical professionals to know that you and they face similar problems or have found similar solutions. You may hold the key to questions that, if answered, would improve the health care of the black population of the world. Therefore, your input into the Journal is essential. Please take the time to record it so that we may share and lighten our loads, as I have attempted to do by publishing my work in the JNMA.

Section One

PUBLIC HEALTH

AND

COMMUNITY PSYCHIATRY

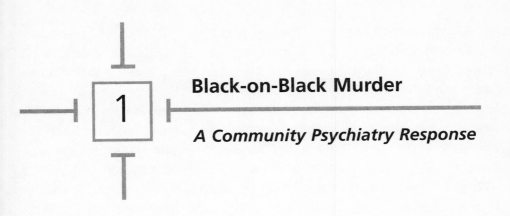

Black-on-Black Murder

A Community Psychiatry Response

BLACK-ON-BLACK HOMICIDE: THE NATIONAL MEDICAL ASSOCIATION'S RESPONSIBILITIES*

During the 1986 National Medical Association's (NMA) 91st Annual Convention and Scientific Assembly Plenary Session, the NMA's responsibilities in preventing black-on-black murder were discussed. The discussion was timely because a *Journal of the National Medical Association* report has just clearly stated that homicide accounts for 38 percent of the "excess deaths" of black men younger than 45.[1] At the plenary session, it was pointed out that a national public awareness campaign could be mounted. Because NMA physicians are often on the front line caring for blacks involved in interpersonal violence (the end point of which is often homicide), they have a responsibility to raise the black community's consciousness about the problem. The black community must be made to realize that the leading cause of death of black men aged 15–44 years is black-on-black homicide, and that there are at least 100 assaults for each homicide.[2]

*Originally printed as Bell Carl C, Prothrow-Stith Deborah, Smallwood-Murchison Catherine. Guest editorial on black-on-black homicide: the National Medical Association's responsibilities. *J Natl Med Assoc.* 1986;78:1139–1141.

An example of how to exercise this responsibility is the role taken by the Community Mental Health Council, Inc. (CMHC). They designed a "Stop Black-on-Black Murder" t-shirt for the Black-on-Black Love Campaign's "No Crime Day" in Chicago. The CMHC urged several groups to wear the t-shirts to raise consciousness about how blacks can be their own worst enemy by killing one another. As a result, on June 20, 1986, numerous individuals throughout Chicago, including black physicians of the Cook County Physician's Association and members and staff of the National Association of Black Social Workers (Chicago chapter), Cabrini Green Public Housing North Tactical Unit (Chicago Police Department), Anchor-Coleman Health Center, Near North Health Service Corporation, Jackson Park Hospital, black pharmacies, and CMHC, wore the t-shirts. The entire Jackson Park Hospital emergency room staff wore the t-shirts and even handed out fact sheets on black-on-black murder to everyone who visited the emergency room. These efforts were well received by the black community.

During the plenary session, internist Dr. Prothrow-Stith noted that because emergency rooms are places of repetitive contact with victims and perpetrators of interpersonal violence, they are ideal settings for the early identification of individual in risk for such violence. The emergency room is also a good setting to investigate the biological, interpersonal, and social causes of black-on-black homicide, from which interventions can be framed.

Dr. Prothrow-Smith also presented her prevention efforts designed to stem the rise of the black-on-black murder epidemic. She modeled a health education curriculum consisting of ten sessions on anger and violence prevention, and used it on a Boston public high school tenth-grade class. Initial research on the pre- and post-study of attitudes and knowledge about black-on-black violence indicates this effort is effective in decreasing attitudes promoting violence and increasing knowledge about violence.

Speakers for the Cindy Smallwood Medical Education Foundation, Inc., added an essential part to the discussion by saying that the NMA had a responsibility to assist in prevention of black-on-black crime by taking political action to reverse the cycle. Doctors Smallwood-Murchison and Hare of the Foundation remarked that establishing centers in high-risk areas designed to assist people with "quasi-morticide" (a newly recognized phenomenon encompassing homicide, sub-intentional suicide, suicide, and all other self-destructive behaviors in the black community) would be effective in decreasing the number of victims. Consequently, any such decrease would be reflected in a concomitant decrease in correction and health care institutional expenditures. A tertiary prevention approach requiring political action and policy change was recently suggested in a JNMA guest editorial. The author, Dr. M. L. Walker, noted that "A strong case is being made for regionalization of care, for preparation of guidelines for acceptable trauma management, and for specialized centers prepared for handling around-the-clock trauma patients." [3]

From the Foundation's contribution to the NMA's plenary session, it became apparent that the National Medical Political Action Committee (NMPAC)[4] needs to become involved in shaping the political decisions and legislation that could reduce black-on-black violence. For example, NMPAC could implement some of the Attorney General's Task Force on Family Violence report recommendations that have shown to reduce family violence.[5]

The plenary session focused on other new trends in research, procedures, and policy on the problem of black-on-black homicide. Neuropsychiatric correlates associated with "pathological aggressiveness" (e.g., electroencephalogram abnormalities, minimal brain dysfunction, history of coma—traumatic and non-traumatic, history of seizures, non-schizophrenic intermittent psychotic symptoms, pathological intoxication, and neurologic impairment) were outlined as possible acquired biologic causes of violence that NMA physicians need to study further.[6] In addition, once such an etiology was suspected, treatment with carbamazepine, lithium, propranolol, or trazodone was highlighted as a possible answer to the dilemma of treating some subjects with acquired biological predisposition to violence. It should be understood that this focus on acquired biologic causes of black-on-black murder does not negate the intrapsychic, interpersonal, and social causes of the problem. All black health and allied health professionals must address the issue from their own area of professional expertise.

Because of the new emphasis on providing services to victims, not mentioning the victims and their relatives would have been remiss. All of the black physicians encouraged the standard use of a brief victim-perpe-trator screening form to create an assault or victimization history invento-ry. This would provide a quick, easy case-finding tool to identify patients at risk for interpersonal violence that may result in murder. Such skills need to be taught as standard curriculum in all continuing medical educa-tion courses involving the care of black patients and in all black medical schools.

The plenary session concluded by pointing out that these new pro-posed directions to solve the problem of black-on-black murder should focus on places with a high concentration of violent subjects, such as emergency rooms. Other likely settings are the nation's correctional facil-ities. With the NMA's representation on the National Commission on Correctional Health Care, the issue of identifying and appropriately treat-ing "pathological aggressiveness" has been raised in formulating standards to improve health care quality in this nation's jails, prisons, and juvenile detention centers.[7] It is sincerely hoped that the NMA will meet its respon-sibilities regarding black-on-black homicide.

LETTER TO THE EDITOR ON BLACK-ON-BLACK MURDER*

To the Editor:

On a recent trip to Flint, Michigan, I was gratified to see a media initiative to reduce the extraordinary levels of "black-on-black" murder. Barbara Schroder, a reporter with WJRT Channel 12 (an affiliate of ABC), decided to look at the problem as a responsible journalist (i.e., not as a sensationalistic-minded, "our job is to sell air time" type of reporter). She researched the problem for several months and even went so far as to attend the national conference, "Crime and the Black Community: Causes, Effects, and Remedial Approaches," sponsored by the National Organization of Black Law Enforcement Executives and the National Black

---

*Originally printed as Bell Carl C. Letter to the editor on black-on-black murder. *J Natl Med Assoc*. 1987;79:471–472.

Police Association. I feel that Barbara Schroder and WJRT-TV should be commended for taking action aimed at the community's basic problems instead of simply pumping out sensationalistic coverage of rare problems.

Ms. Schroder did five brief stories on black-on-black murder Monday through Friday and a one-hour live special on Saturday evening. The city council head, the police chief, and I were available to give technical information, answer questions, and pose solutions. In the audience were community members such as relatives of murdered victims, ministers who had begun youth programs, victim assistance advocates, members of Flint's Human Services Department, and so forth. It will be interesting to see whether this media-initiated action will help mobilize Flint's black community to start the self-help initiatives suggested at the National Medical Association's (NMA) plenary session last July.

At the request of the Richmond city council, I went to Richmond, Virginia, after leaving Flint, as Richmond (like Flint) has been experiencing record homicides (mostly black-on-black). In Richmond, I met with Mayor Roy A. West, the chief of police, the superintendent of schools, a representative of the Virginia chapter of the National Association of Blacks in Criminal Justice, the vice-president of Family & Children's Services, Inc., a representative of the Black Ministers Conference, and several councilmen, who were clearly committed to resolving the problem of black-on-black murder. Richmond's city council is working actively to support a group called BMAC (Blacks Mobilizing Against Crime) with combating the problem of black-on-black murder. Thus, I have seen a unique city council-initiated action, which will help Richmond's black community start the self-help initiatives suggested at the NMA's plenary session.

I continue to watch the development of the black-business-initiated action to fight black-on-black crime. One example is the Black-on-Black Love Campaign, sponsored by the American Health and Beauty Aids Institute (spearheaded by Ed Gardner of Soft Sheen Products). They have tried to mobilize the black community to reduce crime. In the Baltimore area, the effort to reduce black-on-black murder is being led by a group of black ministers, the Urban League, and the Black Alliance for Mental Health (in conjunction with Baltimore's Black Psychiatrists of America).

Having been involved with all of these efforts, I am very interested in seeing which approach will succeed. It seems that different segments of the black community are starting self-help initiatives that hopefully will involve other segments. The media, police departments, city councils, business community, ministers, civic organizations, and health care professionals must work to combat the problem of black-on-black murder.

I am very pleased with the support I have gotten from black physicians who have written to me asking how they might impact the problem, or sharing their own successes at attacking the problem. If we continue to pull together, we can take even more ground.

> ### COMMENTARY

There is a long story behind the short editorial and letter reprinted here. In 1972, while I was doing my psychiatric residency, I met with the leadership of the Black Psychiatrists of America (BPA), an association that had begun in 1969. Because the group was interested in mental health issues facing African Americans, one of its agenda items was violence in the black community. In 1984, BPA Director Dr. James Ralph convened the second national meeting about black-on-black violence, where several substantive papers were presented. I was interested in that area and was working on a related paper, so I attended. I presented my preliminary states of consciousness studies on the relationship between head injury and violence (see Chapter 24). At the BPA conference, I met Dr. Deborah Prothrow-Stith, one of the current experts on the violence problem in America. After sharing our current efforts on alleviating this problem, I enlisted her aid to bring the issue to the NMA to make a difference.

I had my chance at the 1986 NMA convention when I organized the plenary scientific session and planned black-on-black homicide for its focus. I had already invited Dr. Prothrow-Stith to help me. Dr. Smallwood-Murchison, who had heard of my work and contacted me because of our similar interests, was also willing to participate. Thus, the plenary panel had perspectives from the East and West coasts and the Midwest.

Once the NMA leadership realized what I was doing, they became a bit concerned for three reasons. The first involved the release of the Secretary of Health, Education, and Welfare's Task Force Report on Black and Minority Health in 1985. This report noted five reasons in addition to homicide for "excess deaths" in blacks: infant mortality, cancer, cirrhosis of the liver, cardiovascular disease and stroke, and diabetes. Accordingly, the NMA leadership was concerned that having a plenary session on homicide would reduce the importance of the other health problems. Secondly, the NMA leadership was not clear on the association's role in addressing the homicide problem; taking a public health approach to violence was brand new and had not been fully embraced. Finally, they feared that by focusing on homicide as an African-American problem, the plenary session would be used as a weapon against blacks. As a result, they decided to hold five concurrent plenary sessions focusing on the other causes of excess mortality.

Though the session probably had the lowest attendance of any other in NMA history, a friend of mine fortunately brought a *New York Times* reporter there. As a result, the session was covered in "Black Doctors told to Screen Patients for Violent Feelings," which appeared on the front page (July 23, 1986). Not having read the paper, I had no idea of the frenzy I would face the next day at the conference. I was besieged by every major television station, radio station, and newspaper in the country. I spent the next ten hours answering media questions about the black-on-black homicide and about my work. The session even made international news!

Naturally, the NMA leadership was quite pleased, as this was probably the largest press coverage they'd received for a convention. I was happy because the reduction of the problem of black-on-black homicide had picked up considerable speed and support.

A year after we wrote the guest editorial, I wrote the letter to JNMA Editor Dr. Sampson updating him on my efforts to eradicate black-on-black murder. I was hoping that by my example, I could provide examples of what other physicians can achieve working with the media, politicians, businesses, and social service providers. Since writing this letter, Dr. Prothrow-Stith and I have become national experts on the question of violence in America and have worked very hard to combat it. In addition, Dr. Prothrow-Smith has continued to develop violence prevention efforts, has written a book on it, and has worked with victims of violence. I have continued to explore the severity of the problem as it affects children (see Chapter 17).

More importantly, Dr. Prothrow-Stith and I have managed to work in accord all these years. Frequently when two experts work in the same arena, petty bickering over differences in philosophy does not allow them to work harmoniously. I suspect the main reason for our compatibility is our understanding of the main purpose of our work. I believe our mission is not to feed our narcissism, but to do something about the violence in our community. My advice to others trying to make a difference is to realize that one cannot do it alone. You will probably need all the help you can get. Therefore, always put the mission before your "ego."

I am very happy that the NMA has continued to work on solving the problem of violence in the African-American community. In 1994, the NMA and the National Institute of Mental Health held the workshop, "Violence and the Conduct of Research." The NMA is making a difference in our lives and our children's lives.

The impetus to tackle the large community problem of violence did not happen overnight, nor was the effort the result of one person. This is important to keep in mind when embarking on any crusade.

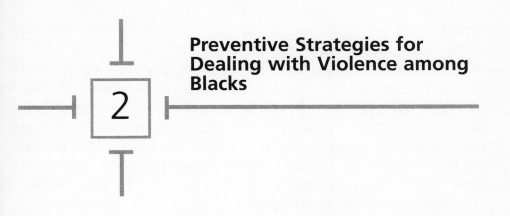

Preventive Strategies for Dealing with Violence among Blacks

2

In general medicine, if a patient goes to a doctor to be treated for a rat bite, the physician will clean and dress the bite and then administer antibiotics and a tetanus shot. The physician practicing social medicine would go a step further and arrange for someone to set rat traps in the patient's community. A similar distinction is made between general and community psychiatry. This highlights one of the main principles of the community psychiatrist's mission: community development, the art of helping a community achieve a social and interpersonal milieu that promotes an optimum level of mental health.[1,2] This aspect takes on even greater significance when the community being served is a lower socioeconomic, minority one, because conditions found in such communities can impair the overall mental health of its individuals, families, and groups. This article will illustrate the principle of community development and its importance to deprived minority communities by describing a community psychiatry approach to the problem of black-on-black homicide. This article will also discuss one psychiatrist's role in community development.

Originally printed as Bell Carl C. Preventive strategies for dealing with violence among blacks. *Community Mental Health J.* 1987;23:217–228.

THE PROBLEM

Black-on-black homicide is the leading cause of death for black males aged 15–34 years old. The majority of black-on-black murder occurs in the interpersonal context. Two-thirds to three-fourths of victims know their murderer as a family member, friend, or acquaintance. Since there are an estimated one hundred assaults per murder,[3] it is apparent that there is a significant amount of violence in black interpersonal relationships, with murder being a mere measurable tip.

The focus on black-on-black murder should not be taken as a denial of murder in general society. It is noted that although black males experience the highest rate of homicide and have the greatest absolute increase in homicide, homicide rates have been increasing more dramatically for Hispanic males than for black males.[4] In addition, in the greater society, husbands give their wives injuries requiring medical treatment more than car accidents, rapes, and muggings combined. Yet, statistics show that black males have a chance of being murdered ten times that of white males, and black females have a chance of being murdered five times that of white females. More specifically, the chance of becoming homicide victims for black males is 1:21 as opposed to 1:131 for white males, and 1:104 for black females as opposed to 1:369 for white females. The black-on-black murder problem is a discrete, epidemiological phenomenon that allows itself to be addressed by a community much like Tay-Sachs disease.

Violence in the black community, viewed from several different perspectives, can have detrimental affects on mental health. Individuals assaulted in the family context like child abuse or spousal abuse are likely to develop a variety of psychiatric symptoms including suicide attempts, psycho-physiologic disorders, anxiety disorders, and interpersonal difficulties.[5,6] We see the majority of black-on-black offenders committing murder in the context of "crimes of passion" or rage as opposed to felony homicides (i.e., homicides that occur during a felony like armed robbery). Such out-of-control emotional states are often at the base of domestic violence that occurs prior to homicide. A study of family homicide in Kansas City in 1977 found that in 85% of the cases, the police had been called to the victim's residence at least once before the murder, and in 50% had been called five times or more.[7] Often, the abuser's rage-filled behavior is regretted after the violent episode. Because this causes psychic pain, the abuser might engage in batterer's counseling, which may have a positive outcome.[6]

If a child witnesses his/her parent being murdered, he/she will undergo major psychic trauma that will seriously impact his mental health. If a parent is informed of the grisly death of his/her offspring, he/she will have to mourn the loss in addition to coping with the stress of knowing the horrendous details of the death. This combination can lead to symptoms of depression and post-traumatic stress disorder.[8]

I recall the case of an elderly black woman patient of mine at the Community Mental Health Council, Inc., (CMHC) whose daughter had been killed. The daughter's boyfriend, in a state of rage, had repeatedly stabbed and killed her in front of their seven-year-old child during a domestic quarrel. My patient complained of prolonged grief over the loss of her daughter, which had developed into a major depressive disorder. She also had signs and symptoms of post-traumatic stress disorder, characterized by intrusive fantasized thoughts of the horrible scene of the killing, sleep-onset insomnia, irritability, an exaggerated startled response, withdrawal from her usual activities, and panic attack symptoms. Further, the patient was saddled with her grandson's care, an issue of great psychological ambivalence, since she had raised nine children and had looked forward to her "golden years" being a time for herself. Yet, at the same time, she felt a great deal of responsibility for her grandson. The case was also complicated from the patient and her grandson both suffering the loss. In one way, this allowed the patient to identify with her grandson and be more responsive to him. Yet, she directed a significant amount of anger at him since he resembled his father, the murderer. The grandson had problems of school failure, nightmares, and excessively aggressive behavior, which indicated that he was also having difficulties adjusting to his mother's death (as well as the loss of his father due to incarceration) and that he needed treatment.

The etiology of black-on-black murder can be approached from at least three different but credible manners: psychological, sociologic, and biologic. Psychological issues, such as stress caused by inadequate socioeconomic milieus and self-depreciation because of racist attitudes in the majority culture, play a role in generating violence among blacks.

Sociologic factors such as the establishment of a gang amongst idle youth can also encourage violence. Literature on the etiology of violence tends to emphasize psychological and sociological as opposed to biologic factors factors, because the medical profession has not considered the issue of violence as something they could prevent. I have been trying to correct this error.

From a biologic perspective, it is suspected that a diagnosis of intermittent explosive disorder, a significant predisposing factor for acquired central nervous system damage (perinatal trauma, head trauma, infection, etc.), is at the base of many interpersonal violent episodes.[9] Epidemiologic studies show clearly that lower socioeconomic groups are more predisposed to having head injuries[10] due to freefalls[11] or auto accidents,[12] with blacks having more occurrences than whites. D. O. Lewis et al.,[13] who outlined the bio-psychosocial characteristics of children who would later commit murder, found that head injury caused by falls from roofs and car accidents was present in two-thirds of their sample. In another study, Lewis et al.[14] found that the 15 death row murderers they studied for psychiatric, neurological, and psycho-educational characteristics all had extensive histories and evidence of head injury. These findings, along with the high prevalence of coma in black subjects,[15] suggest acquired (as opposed to genetic) biological factors as a contributor to the disproportion in high number of black-on-black murder. More research in this area needs to be done to support this preliminary hypothesis. Other acquired biologic factors have been linked to alcohol abuse, which has shown to deplete serotonin levels in the brain (serotonin being an important regulator of aggression in animals). One study also found low levels of serotonin's major metabolite in the cerebrospinal fluid of impulsive violent offenders with antisocial or intermittent explosive personality disorders and impulsive arsonists.[16]

TAKING ACTION: CONSCIOUSNESS RAISING

Community psychiatrists seeking to alleviate the pathogenic phenomenon of black-on-black violence can do so from several preventive medicine standpoints—namely primary, secondary, and tertiary intervention.[17] However, in order to intervene on these levels, much community development groundwork must be made. Services are often unavailable.

Established black institutions such as black churches and colleges, civil rights organizations, and beauty parlor/barber shops also may need some support and guidance to adequately address the issue. There must be a great deal of public awareness and education in order to develop community institutions and support systems into vehicles that will prevent black-on-black murder.

In Chicago, the CMHC got involved with black-on-black murder at my request. I had felt that such a mental health agency serving a black community would be remiss for not dealing with the psychic impact of the problem. I had also felt the CMHC had an obligation to prevent this source of stress amongst blacks. My personal experience growing up black in an inner city and witnessing violence among blacks strengthened my convictions. The CMHC began a weekly series of twelve call-in radio programs featuring an array of professionals with expertise in murder, interpersonal violence, rape, child abuse, suicide, spousal abuse, violence portrayed in the media, etc. I was responsible for three shows: one on black-on-black murder; one regarding biological, psychological, and sociological causes of violence; and one on violence prevention.

The response from the community was good, although opinions about black-on-black violence varied. There were many misconceptions about the sources of violence. A number of callers thought police, for example, caused most black homicide victims. Some callers advocated a "head in the sand" approach, as they believed that focusing on the issue would only cast blacks in a bad light. One caller felt that attributing murders to perpetrators' head injuries could bring up the old racist argument that blacks are biologically inferior. Others felt it would also fuel the racist stereotype that most blacks are violent.

I responded that some—not all—murderers' head injuries might have played a role in their murderous rage. I also stated that because head injury was an acquired—not inherited—biologic factor in violence, there were no grounds to support racial predisposition to violence. I also noted that because black-on-black violence statistics are easily accessible from various public sources, we were not really exposing a well-hidden secret. Furthermore, if blacks did not do something about the problem, no one else would. The important thing was that we raised the issue, that people in the black community discussed it, and that we involved a number of black professionals. The program guests formed a CMHC advisory board to address violence in the black community. The board continues to function.

The CMHC also became involved with the Black-on-Black Love Campaign, designed to fight black-on-black crime. The campaign was sponsored by the American Health and Beauty Aids Institute, a consortium of black hair care products companies. As campaign advisor, I focused on two types of black-on-black crime: murder and theft. Murder was a more important topic to the black health professionals. Black-on-black robbery, burglary, felony homicide, etc.—a great deal of which is committed by strangers who are habitually criminal types, garnered major concern from the business people, law enforcement officials, ex-offender representatives, and so forth. For strangers committing crimes, we needed to address education, employment, the criminal justice system, neighborhood watch programs, and so forth. For "family" crimes, we needed to address violent interpersonal episodes like spousal abuse and child abuse. The campaign motto, "replace black-on-black crime with black-on-black love," was directed to foci and to emphasize respect, discipline, and self-esteem.[18]

The campaign's major public education activity was "No Crime Day," a citywide effort in Chicago. Chicago's media, politicians, police department, judicial officials, business leaders, clergy, hair care establishments, health care professionals, and many more have been involved in making the "No Crime Day" a reality. The event has been successful. Each year, more leaders with influence in the black community support it, and media cover increases. More advantages will be realized as "No Crime Day" establishes a track record of influence and accomplishment.

Another CMHC effort to raise consciousness about black-on-black murder was the creation of "Stop Black-on-Black Murder" t-shirts. Using a crude drawing done by a public aid volunteer for the CMHC's radio series, I developed and refined the concept into the t-shirt design. The shirts were given away in exchange for a five-dollar donation to the CMHC to cover the cost of the shirts and mailing. Within three months, I had personally given over 1,000 t-shirts to physicians, congressmen, celebrities, mayors of major cities, and so forth. This effort received national attention, including in the American Medical Association's (AMA) national newspaper.[19] A picture of me selling the t-shirts also appeared on the front page of the *New York Times*, which resulted in national electronic media coverage of black-on-black crime and its solutions.

As the CMHC's executive/medical director, I continue to bring the issue into public awareness by making presentations to professional organizations and giving lectures around the country. These efforts have been helpful, as several of my black psychiatric and non-psychiatric physician colleagues have heard my message and begun to engage in activities designed to prevent the problem.

All of these consciousness-raising efforts have enlightened the public to interpersonal violence in the black community. More importantly, it has helped the black community become receptive to intervening in the problem. This has made community development work preventing the problem easier.

PRIMARY PREVENTION STRATEGIES

In looking to prevent all violent behaviors, the CMHC surveyed 538 second-, fourth-, sixth-, and eighth-graders in three of its catchment area schools, regarding children's attitudes about and experience with violence. Though about one sixth of the children had seen parents and relatives fighting, a striking number had witnessed extreme violence: 31% had seen someone shot, 34% had seen a person stabbed, and 84% had seen someone "beaten-up." There were indications that families with frequent violence in the home had children with violent attitudes and behaviors. Armed with this knowledge, the CMHC arranged for about 70 children and their parents to go on a retreat to discuss violence and its prevention to develop strategies for reducing family violence. It was found that several of the children knew of a murder that had occurred in an interpersonal context. Several of the mothers had been abused, either as children or spouses. Most left the retreat better understanding the problem and knowing some strategies to avoid violence. With the aid of a CMHC facilitator, the women formed a support group for victims of violence. The establishment of such a social network for families at risk for violence has been shown to reduce isolation and lack of support and thus reduce those families' abusive potential.

The Surgeon General's *Source Book on Violence* points to the growing problem of elderly abuse occurring in this country.[3] Depending on the support system, caring for the elderly can be quite taxing. With this in mind, the CMHC established the Alzheimer's Disease Family Support Group. In addition, the Elderly Respite Care Service was established, obtaining its manpower from volunteers. These two support networks educate families about elderly care and let them take a break from elderly care. This is a useful strategy in preventing elderly abuse. Similarly, the CMHC's Family Systems Program outreaches in its catchment area to troubled families that may be at risk for interpersonal violence resulting in murder. Parenting classes, family orientation to community support services, and individual and group family therapy can all help prevent family violence.

Other primary intervention strategies include vocational programs that help patients start patient businesses and activities for community residents that offer an alternative to gangs or illegal activities that lead to violence. A center that develops a boys' club, such as a self-defense sport team or Boy Scout troop, will develop its community by offering an alternative to gangs. I managed to constructively influence young black males more during my 15 years as a karate instructor rather than as a psychotherapist.

Since it has been suggested that central nervous system damage may predispose some individuals to violence, it is vital to lobby for better health care and housing to improve infant care and prevent children from falling from windows by advocating for mandatory screens in windows.[1,2,20]

SECONDARY PREVENTION

The secondary prevention of black-on-black murder is the identification and treatment of perpetrators or victims of violence not leading to murder. This can be done with an existing patient population of a community mental health center. Several studies have noted the frequency that general medical practitioners do not attend to abused women, who as a result often end up in the mental health care system.[5] It has also been pointed out that many women who murder their husbands do so in self-defense to prevent another beating.

I directed the development of a screening form at the CMHC to identify potential future victims or perpetrators of violence that could escalate and result in murder. This form is now given to all CMHC patients. Once identified, victims can turn to the CMHC's Victims Assistance Service for help in preventing continued abuse through the criminal justice system. Others[21,22] have advocated this approach to violence intervention by community mental health centers, which has shown to get results.

Counseling can also help victims of spousal or child abuse. A liaison relationship between community mental health centers and women's shelters aids in placing at-risk women in a safe environment. Through the CMHC's work with the community's clergy, a number of ministers have become more sensitive to the issue of family violence and have also sought to provide services such as shelter and counseling.

Community hospital emergency rooms are excellent places for finding cases. In the CMHC's catchment area, Jackson Park Hospital's emergency room staff participated in Chicago's "No Crime Day" by the whole staff wearing "Stop Black-on-Black Murder" t-shirts for 24 hours and handing out fact sheets on black-on-black murder to all of their patients and their families. This effort was well received by the black community and the patients who visited the emergency room that day. In educating the community, the emergency room staff at Jackson Park Hospital was also enlightened.

As a result, it was easier for me to request that the emergency room staff familiarize themselves with the acquired biologic causes of violence[23,24] and that they begin looking for situations like those Lion et al.[25,26] found in their emergency room work. Staff could also screen for Lewis et al.'s[13] five criteria for potentially differentiating homicidal from non-homicidal adolescents (neuropychiatric impairment, non-schizophrenic psychotic symptoms that occur intermittently, a history of extreme violent behavior, family members who have had psychotic symptoms, and being a witness or victim of violence in their families). High-risk patients could be offered counseling similar to the therapy Lion et al.[27] offered their cohort. In addition, newer pharmacologic agents such as propranolol, carbamazepine, trazodone, and lithium have been shown to have some value in reducing explosively violent behavior in some patients.[24] Armed with the new information that medically treatable acquired biologic factors may predispose an individual to violence, Jackson Park physicians were more willing to intervene by identifying and treating potential perpetrators of violence. The Jackson Park Hospital emergency room staff, in addition to the now accepted role of emergency room physicians identifying and intervening in child abuse cases, are learning to perform a similar function for spouse abuse and habitual victims and perpetrators of fighting, which has been shown to be associated with a greater chance of being either a victim or perpetrator of murder.[28,29] Finally, by realizing a connection between head injury and potential for future violence, prospective studies can be designed to provide follow-up for head injury victims presenting to the emergency room for treatment to determine if a relationship exists between head injury and violence.

The community psychiatrist can contribute to secondary prevention of black-on-black murder by becoming involved in community groups, state legislative action, and policy-making institutions. When I first began to do this, I was received with skepticism. When I received publicity for my efforts, however, people began to take interest and listen to the common sense in my thoughts. By securing a position of the board of the National Commission on Correctional Health Care, for example, I can advocate for national correctional health care standards that seek to reduce black-on-black violence by taking a public health approach to the problem. Since it is apparent that individuals with intermittent explosive disorder may be prone to being arrested for interpersonal violence, it would make sense for correctional health care professionals to screen for this disorder on a regular basis. Such an argument has been made for tuberculosis, and regular screening has increased the finding of tuberculosis cases fourfold. Since tuberculosis kills fewer black males than black-on-black murder, a policy to routinely ask jail inmates about symptoms of intermittent explosive disorder is in order, and with treatment and a treatment referral upon release from the correctional facility, there might well be a reduction in black murders. The National Commission's Correctional Health Care Standard suggests that inmates be educated about diabetes, hypertension, etc. It seems that education about black-on-black murder, child abuse, spouse abuse, etc., could be equally useful to help inmates understand other factors that cause morbidity and mortality.

Lastly, community psychiatrists can support legislative action and criminal justice policy such as that outlined in the Attorney General's *Task Force Report on Family Violence.*[21] When the Congressional Black Caucus invited me to their annual meeting in Washington, DC, I went and did just that. Pilot projects in cities where the police can arrest men if they see evidence of a wife having been assaulted (e.g., a fresh black eye in the midst of a domestic violence call), where the state's attorney presses charges, and where the witness (victim) is subpoenaed for testimony have been shown to reduce the reoccurrence of family violence.[21,22]

TERTIARY PREVENTION

This type of prevention would unfortunately occur after a black-on-black murder has been committed. Although a black life would be unchangeably lost, however, reducing the sequelae from the murder is still in order. Mention has been made of the stress and separation dynamics that occur in a murder victim's relatives. A survey of a community mental health center's patient population will usually reveal a startling number of black patients who have lost relatives or friends as a result of black-on-black murder. Being a family member of a homicide victim is an issue that psychotherapy should look for and address.

Although counter-transference problems, such as revulsion, anger, over-identification, etc.,[14] often preclude appropriate services for black-on-black murderers on death row, this population, Lewis aptly points out, has a significant occurrence of neuropsychiatric impairment, which was never considered when sentencing the inmate to death. Lewis' work, while considered by some as being outside the community psychiatrist's purview (due to the mistaken notion that a correctional facility does not constitute a type of community), yields significant clues valuable for the primary and secondary prevention of black-on-black murder and is worthy of consideration. In addition, the study of people who have murdered yields important diagnostic and treatment issues for dealing with the released offender. Closer to home for the traditional community psychiatrist is the release of inmates who have committed murder, who have served their time or were found "not guilty by reason of insanity," and who were returned to the community. Often, these patients need aid in adjusting back into society or need treatment for chronic mental illness.

CONCLUSIONS

Work as a community psychiatrist can be rewarding for a psychiatrist who has an interest in practicing social medicine and improving a community's milieu to promote optimum mental health for the community's residents. This approach can be especially rewarding in lower socioeconomic, minority communities that are either underserved or not served at all. By using the principle of community development, the community psychiatrist can help the community mature in such a way that necessary primary, secondary, and tertiary preventive medicine interventions can be established to meet specific problems. While this paper describes the experience of working in a black community, the principles can be generalized to other minorities. For instance, a community psychiatrist can become involved in inhalant abuse in the Mexican-American community or in the adaptation of refugees or in a multiethnic setting. Practicing community psychiatry in this fashion, one man can make a significant difference.

COMMENTARY

Dr. David Cutler, editor of *Community Mental Health Journal*, helped me get this article published. I met him when I was Secretary-Treasurer of the National Council of Community Mental Health Centers and actively involved with the American Association of Community Psychiatrists. He'd heard about my community psychiatry work that was grappling with violence among blacks. It was the first publication in which I discussed how violence affects African-American children.

In republishing this article ten years after its first appearance in print, I realize how it documents the early phases of an initiative that would make a great impact. At the time I wrote this article, the nation was very confused about physical violence. Most people—professionals and nonprofessionals alike—thought of it as a "stranger danger" problem.

Similarly, strangers were once seen as the main perpetrators of rape and child sexual molestation, until the women's liberation movement allowed women to voice their experiences. When it became apparent that friends and family members were more often the aggressors, programs preventing sexual violence against women began to re-shift their focus. It was also once believed that violence in general occurred more frequently amongst strangers. Currently, this misconception is less prevalent in the professional community. As in the case of violence against women, it has since been revealed that violence happens more frequently between family and friends. The "consciousness-raising" initiative described in the article has helped to advertise this information the public.

This article helped me crystallize plans for future endeavors that have since occurred. When I went to the Congressional Black Caucus and advocated for legislative action to address domestic violence, I impressed Ohio Congressman Louis Stokes. As a result, in 1989 I was invited to the 21st Congressional District Caucus in Ohio to present "Preventing Black Homicide." During the 21st Annual Congressional Black Caucus Legislative Weekend in Washington, DC, in 1991, I made another presentation at the Health Braintrust, chaired by Congressman Stokes. During a keynote address, Congressman Stokes credited me as being one of the first to tell Congress about violence and the type of leadership needed in the country. He noted that at that time, he knew this health problem would spread like an infectious disease and destroy communities nationwide without appropriate attention.

My ongoing advocacy for legislative bore fruit. It turned out that Congressman Stokes, a member of the House Subcommittee on Labor, Health, and Human Services, helped to provide funding for the Minority Male Consortium, an initiative still in place. In 1994, the Office of Minority Health awarded over four million dollars to Central State University. Central State, in collaboration with 18 other historically black colleges and universities, began the Minority Male Consortium to showcase their Family Life Centers, designed to prevent minority male violence. I was invited to be a keynote speaker at the consortium's first national conference, "Collaborating for Family and Community Violence Prevention," in 1995. There, I learned that the conference got started partly because of my earlier advocacy.

I feel like I helped plant the seed of taking the initiative to reduce violence in the African-American community. This is a concrete example of community development discussed in this article.

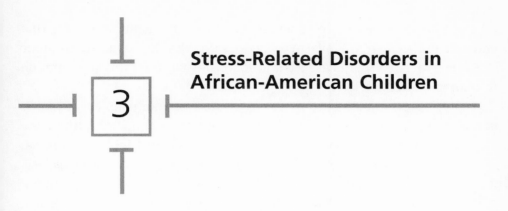

Stress-Related Disorders in African-American Children

3

Children exposed to traumatic stress are vulnerable to a variety of stress-related disorders other than classical post-traumatic stress disorder (PTSD). Several case histories are presented to illustrate some of the diversity in how traumatic stress may manifest in children. African-American children are the main focus of this article, as political, economic, social, and morbidity and mortality indicators suggest that African-American children are at high risk for exposure to potentially traumatic stressors. Different presentations of traumatic stress are discussed in an effort to broaden our understanding of the outcome of traumatic stress and to fully help traumatized children.

INTRODUCTION

In 1984, the CMHC began work that focused on the agency's catchment area children and their exposure to violence. This effort revealed that a significant number of poor, African American, elementary-school-aged children had been exposed to serious violence; 26% reported they had seen a person get shot and 29% reported having seen an actual stabbing.[1]

Originally printed as Bell Carl C. Stress-related disorders in African-American children. *J Natl Med Assoc.* 1997;89:335–340. Presented at the Second Annual Community Mental Health Council Conference, School of Medicine and the School of Public Health, University of Illinois, Chicago, IL, May 29, 1996.

As the CMHC gained more experience in this area, it became clear that children exposed to violence were at risk for developing post-traumatic stress disorder (PTSD). We began to focus our work on this presentation of trauma-related stress.[2,3]

PTSD is characterized by an exposure to a traumatic event that is persistently experienced as unwanted recollections. In addition, there are symptoms of persistent avoidance of stimuli associated with the trauma, along with persistent symptoms of increased arousal. The disturbance lasts more than a month and causes clinically significant distress or impairment in social, occupational, or other important areas of functioning.[4] Currently, there are no epidemiological studies on the incidence or prevalence of PTSD affecting children and adolescents in the general population, but smaller studies on PTSD in youth reveal it is a significant problem in some populations.[5]

Other research groups studying the incidence and prevalence of exposure to violence in poor, African-American children found results similar to those the CMHC's found earlier in the African-American community.[6-9] The CMHC's most recent work in this area revealed that almost two thirds of an inner-city high school student sample reported having seen a shooting, and 45% indicated having seen someone killed. This study illustrated that in addition to classical symptoms of PTSD, exposure to severe violence was correlated with drinking, drug use, fighting, gun carrying, knife carrying, and trouble in school[10]—behaviors that are likely to generate an administrative or criminal justice response rather than a treatment response. By continuing to refine our research, we have learned that focusing on PTSD as the only sequelae to traumatic stress is a mistake.

This article introduces the factor of stress-related disorders in an effort to move away from the concept that exposure to traumatic stress may cause only PTSD. Case histories are presented of children exposed to traumatic stress who do not have PTSD, but who do have other trauma-related disorders.

CASE HISTORIES

The following case histories are given as examples of how children, particularly African-American children, exposed to traumatic stress can manifest various symptoms other than classical PTSD.

Traumatic Stress Resulting in Somatization

A ten-year-old African-American male was referred for having problems with academic performance in school. For more than a year, his grades had been dropping from Bs to Cs and were currently down to Ds. The patient and his mother were at a loss about why he had begun to do poorly in school, as he had always been a B student. He reported he had not been able to concentrate on his homework due to frequently feeling sick to his stomach while studying. When asked what he thought was helping him keep a B average when he had one, he revealed his father used to help him with his homework, and now his father was dead.

When asked about his father's death, the patient reported that he had been with his father when his father died. They had been getting on the elevator when two men began to argue over something, and one of the men began shooting at the other. The patient's father was shot in the stomach before the elevator doors closed. His father was dead before they reached the sixth floor where they lived. He reported the smell had made him sick and made him threw up.

This patient's current symptom of nausea during his study time was connected to the nausea and vomiting he experienced during his father's death. Studying was a trigger that evoked intolerable, unpleasant memories of his father's death that were not directly recognized but rather indirectly experienced through the symptom of nausea. Thus, the focus of therapy was to allow the patient, in a supportive relationship, to re-experience the death of his father and grieve his loss, something he had been unable to do at the time of his father's death because of his mother's inability to tolerate his grief. With this grief work done, it was suggested to the patient that rather than become nauseous at the memory of his father's death, a more apt memorial for his father would be to take those feelings of remorse and transform them into some efforts at getting better grades. Gradually, the patient's grades improved substantially.

Traumatic Stress Resulting in Learning Disorder Not Otherwise Specified

A thirteen-year-old black female was referred due to a drop in her grades. Two years prior, she had been a straight-A student, but she had been getting Ds for the past two years. When the patient did not get any results after following her school counselor's suggestion that she devote an additional two hours a night to studying, the counselor referred the patient to the CMHC for treatment.

Relevant past history revealed that when she was six years old, she had been sexually assaulted by her father on two occasions. He had been placed in prison and she had received therapy for her stressful encounter for about two years. Apparently, the therapy worked, as the patient did not show any lingering behavioral problems and was an outstanding student who consistently got As. Because the patient had been successfully treated for her stress, neither the mother nor the school counselor thought too much of the patient's sexual assault.

The interview with the patient was unremarkable, and she was free from any overt symptoms of anxiety or depression. She reported that she had tried studying for two extra hours but still was not able to get good grades. When asked to describe what happened upon sitting down to study, she said she would be attending to the material for a few minutes before her mind would go blank. When pressed for what she was thinking about, she admitted she would think about what her father had done to her. She reported that when she became eleven years old, she "really understood" what her father had done to her. As a result of her new-found meaning of sexuality, what had happened to her began to really "bother" her to the point that she could not concentrate on her studies. She was provided a supportive relationship with a counselor, and after retelling the story of the abuse and grieving her loss, she began to do well in school again.[11]

Traumatic Stress Resulting in Dream Anxiety Disorder

A twelve-year-old white male was referred because he had been fighting daily in school since more than a year of being in his current foster placement. In addition, despite having had decent grades and decent reading and math scores, he was currently failing in school. The patient had been removed from his mother's home after it was discovered that his stepfather had been beating the patient and making him kneel naked in a closet for several hours during the early morning. The patient was placed with his loving grandmother, who died after the patient had been with her for a year. The patient was then placed with an African-American foster family who were kind and supportive.

The patient did not have a good reason for his fighting behavior and denied any symptoms of PTSD. He seemed to have grieved the loss of his family and the death of his grandmother, and he seemed to be happy that he was in a safe, nurturing environment. He denied any significant impact from his stepfather's torture, except that he was only getting two to three hours of sleep a night due to his having nightmares about how his stepfather used to beat him. He was prescribed 25 mg of doxepin at bedtime in an effort to sleep a little better. At his return appointment, the patient was sleeping eight hours a night, and he reported that he was no longer as irritable as he had been. He stopped fighting in school and had begun to pay more attention to his schoolwork, resulting in better grades.

Traumatic Stress Resulting in Brief Reactive Psychosis

A 25-year-old Latino male was referred after a hospitalization during which he was diagnosed with schizophrenia. He was discharged on haloperidol 20 mg and benzotropine 2 mg at bedtime. He reported that on the day prior to his hospitalization, he had begun to get extremely upset and hear voices. As a result, he became suspicious that someone was going to harm him, and he became combative at home. This was his third hospitalization. His two previous episodes requiring hospitalization had been similar in nature, with the first one occurring when he was about 19 years old.

He reported the voices he heard were repeating what Charlie had said before he blew his friend John's head off with a shotgun. Apparently, when the patient was about 17 years old, he and his friend John were walking down the street and met Charlie, who had a grudge against John because of an argument over a girl they were both interested in dating. Charlie saw John and decided to shoot him. The patient vividly described feeling the heat and shockwave from the shotgun blast. He talked about the smell of gunpowder and said that some of the flesh from John's head got on his face and flew into his mouth. He reported frequent flashbacks of the incident, triggered by witnessing violence such as that he saw in violent movies.

Because he reported feeling drowsy on the medication, the patient was taken off the haloperidol and started taking a tricyclic antidepressant with much better results. He felt less lethargic, resulting in more compliance with the medication. He also had a better response to psychotherapy, which focused on helping the patient tolerate his experience with traumatic stress. Compared with the chemotherapy, supportive psychotherapy, and psychosocial rehabilitation he had received before being properly diagnosed, an insightful psychotherapeutic approach was helpful to this patient.

Traumatic Stress Resulting in Depressive Disorder Not Otherwise Specified

A 17-year-old black male was referred because of a "hostile attitude." He was residing in a foster home and had recently dropped out of high school. He was an angry young man who did not seem receptive to the idea of being interviewed. When asked why he had been referred, he angrily replied, "They sent me." When asked who "they" were, he bitterly mentioned his foster family. When asked about his family of origin, he reported he had been in a stable family environment with his father, mother, and three siblings, but that when the patient was nine years old, his father lost his job and began to sell drugs to support his family. Unfortunately, the patient's mother began to use the drugs his father was selling, and she became unable to properly care for her children.

When the patient was eleven years old, he and his siblings were placed in separate foster homes due to his mother's neglect. Over the next six years, he reported being in five different foster homes, causing him to miss a lot of time in school, thus resulting in poor grades. Because his Department of Children and Family Services case worker refused to let him visit his siblings until he got his GED, he had not seen any of his three siblings in nearly a year and did not know their whereabouts. He had no information either about the whereabouts or health of his father and mother. He had never been exposed to or victimized by serious violence.

Initially, he presented as a surly, angry, irritable teen. As he began to describe what had happened to him, however, his affect became more one of sadness. When he talked about having no idea how his family was doing, he began to cry. He talked about his frustration with his academic performance; he wanted to do well in school but with the exception of his two years in a "good foster home," his multiple placements had interfered with his getting a decent education. He was clear that the events in his life had been extremely stressful, resulting in him having twice weekly hour-long crying spells before sleeping during the past year. He realized he was like this because the stress and hurt he had experienced in his life was beneath the "attitude," but not having anyone to talk to about his pain had turned it into anger.

Traumatic Stress Resulting in Anxiety Disorder Not Otherwise Specified (Excessively Dutiful and Conscientious)

An eleven-year-old black female was referred from the Department of Children and Family Services to get therapy on the assumption that she might need some emotional support. When the patient was seven years old, she had been taken from her mother due to charges of neglect and was placed with her aunt for several years. After the mother had been drug-free for two years, the patient was returned to the mother's care. In addition to being separated from her mother, the patient had witnessed her mother being battered frequently by the patient's stepfather, who was also a drug user.

The patient seemed to be a dutiful and conscientious eleven-year-old child and appeared extremely mature for her age. She was a B+ student and reported never giving her mother any trouble. She denied any anger or upset feelings toward her mother for her abandonment, and when asked about how she had felt when seeing her mother get beaten, she reported that this was not a major concern for her. She reported that a greater concern for her was her fear that her mother would go back on drugs. In fact, this particular worry would keep her up at night, causing her to have sleep-onset insomnia. She was afraid that if she was "bad," her mother would go back to using drugs and she would be separated from her again. She thought her original separation from her mother was due to the patient's having been "bad," and she felt unreasonably guilty. The task of therapy for her was to get her to give up her pseudo-maturity—which was secondary to guilt and fear, but to still have her be a reasonably well-behaved child getting good grades.

DISCUSSION

Recently, in the *Diagnostic and Statistical Manual*, 4th edition (DSM-IV),[4] the American Psychiatric Association took a major step by providing criteria for an acute stress disorder characterized by exposure to a traumatic event that causes the individual to experience three or more dissociative symptoms during or after the event. In addition, the traumatic event is persistently relived, and there is a marked avoidance of stimuli that arouse recollections of the trauma along with marked symptoms of anxiety or increased arousal. Like in PTSD, the disturbance causes clinically significant distress or impairment in social, occupational, or other important areas of functioning. It lasts for a minimum of two days and a maximum of four weeks. The disorder occurs within four weeks of the trauma and is not due to direct physiological effects of a substance or general medical condition, a brief psychotic disorder, or an exacerbation of preexisting Axis I or Axis II disorder. Hopefully, this new category will improve the identification of stress-related disorders.

Despite the inclusion of this new diagnostic entity in the DSM-IV, however, clinical experience with children who have been exposed to traumatic stress reveals their traumatic stress may cause them to suffer from a variety of psychiatric disorders found in the DSM-IV. The cases presented provide an example of how the sequelae of traumatic stress can present as the following: somatization disorder, learning disorder not otherwise specified, dream anxiety disorder, brief reactive psychosis, depressive disorder not otherwise specified, anxiety disorder not otherwise specified. In addition, exposure to traumatic stress also may present as multiple personality disorder,[12] dissociative fugue, dissociative amnesia, panic disorder, generalized anxiety disorder,[13] conversion disorder, depersonalization disorder, borderline personality disorder, antisocial personality disorder, conduct disorder,[14] oppositional defiant disorder, impulse control disorder not otherwise specified, attachment disorders of infancy, separation anxiety disorder,[15] adjustment disorders, sexual dysfunctions, paraphillias, communication disorder not otherwise specified, selective mutism,[16] and disruptive behavior disorder not otherwise specified.

Disorders of extreme stress not otherwise specified have also been proposed[17] and include symptoms (somatization, dissociation, and affective symptoms), personality changes (pathological relationships and changes in identity), and harm-seeking and re-victimization behavior as constellations of the disorder. In addition, cormobidity is associated with PTSD and may include imbedding of the traumatic response into the personality, substance abuse,[18] eating disorders, depression, suicidal behavior, and vocational impairment, all of which may obscure the etiology of traumatic stress.

CONCLUSION

The case histories described here illustrate some of the various forms that stress-related disorders may take in children and illustrate the complexity of how exposure to traumatic stress may manifest. As Pynoos[19] points out, issues of development make understanding traumatic stress in children a particularly difficult subject to fully understand. Despite these difficulties, health professionals must realize the myriad presentations of exposure to traumatic stress in order to appropriately identify and intervene in these cases. Accordingly, we must broaden our case-finding activities to identify traumatized children not only in mental health settings, but also in correctional facilities, special education settings, drug abuse populations, and general medical settings. Further, we need to develop systems of care and intervention for these children as early as possible, as waiting only increases morbidity and mortality.[20]

COMMENTARY

This article was written to give some clarity to how traumatic stress affects children. Since it addresses an issue of victimization, it might properly belong in this book's third section, Violence and Victimization. However, I've included it here in the section on Public Health and

Community Psychiatry because it raises more than the problem of victimization. It also raises a systems issue on how the field of public health and community psychiatry conceptualizes the outcome of traumatic stress. It's according for it, then, to be in this section, which contains my articles exploring patterns of needs.

The "Traumatic Stress and Children" article Dr. Jenkins and I did first outlined our work on children who were exposed to traumatic stress such as from witnessing a murder (see Chapter 17). In that article, we also asserted that exposure to violence could have serious consequences for a child's mental health and could result in PTSD. We made this observation from the research we'd been doing at the CMHC since 1984. Our original ideas about how children could develop PTSD were accurate. However, as we got more experience with children exposed to violence, we learned they could develop other types of stress-related disorders as well.

In many ways, this recent article took me back full circle. In April 1979, the JNMA published "The Need for Psychoanalysis is Alive and Well in Community Psychiatry" (see Chapter 6), which was written to advocate for use of psychoanalytic theory to understand and alleviate traumatic stress often experienced by lower socioeconomic individuals because of their social environment. At the time, I had no idea that 18 years later, I'd write another article addressing traumatic stress, only this time in children. This article is important because it appropriately expands the outcome of exposure to traumatic stress in children from PTSD to a variety of other problems. By being aware of traumatic stress as the underlying cause for various behaviors, a person trying to provide a "corrective emotional experience" for a "problem child" will be better equipped to get to the root of the problem and relieve the difficulty.

Section Two

INTERVENTION RESEARCH

AND

ADVOCACY

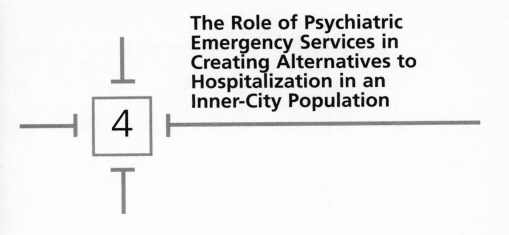

The Role of Psychiatric Emergency Services in Creating Alternatives to Hospitalization in an Inner-City Population

4

In the proper political/economic environment, crisis intervention programs can reduce the recidivism rate of patients who suffer from recurrent intermittent acute psychotic episodes. The author seeks to outline such a program and demonstrate its effectiveness in providing an alternative to brief hospitalization. It is believed that this form of management of the psychiatric emergency aids the practice of community psychiatry and supports the use of day treatment facilities, outpatient clinics, emergency housing, family therapy, and other community support systems.

INTRODUCTION

In recent years there has been an ever-growing trend to shorten hospitalization for mentally ill patients. This has been fostered by the advent of psychotrophic medication, the community mental health movement, and the rising cost of hospitalization. It is for these reasons that there has been an attempt to go a step further and circumvent inpatient hospitalization altogether by offering alternatives to hospitalization. These

Originally printed as Bell Carl C. The role of psychiatric emergency services in aiding community alternatives to hospitalization in an inner city population. *J Natl Med Assoc*. 1978;70:931–935. Presented at the 55th Annual Meeting of the American Orthopsychiatric Association as part of the workshop, "Community Alternatives to Hospitalization for an Inner City Population," Chicago, IL, March 1978.

include day treatment facilities, temporary housing, halfway houses, boarding homes, family therapy, crisis intervention, and various workshops and rehabilitation programs/services that were historically provided via inpatient hospitalization.[1] It is clear that alternatives to hospitalization will not have significant impact if the management of the psychiatric emergency is not handled in a manner drastically different than admission to the inpatient ward.[2] This paper seeks to give guidelines and clinical support of the type of psychiatric emergency management that aids alternatives to hospitalization and that is ethically, morally, and therapeutically sound.

CHICAGO'S MENTAL HEALTH SERVICES

In order to understand the setting in which the clinical work was done, it is necessary to briefly sketch the delivery system of mental health services of Southside Chicago.[3] Illinois was one of the first states to regionalize, i.e., set up specific target areas to be serviced by specific state institutions. Region 2 is one such region, composed of Chicago and several surrounding counties. Region 2 is divided into 53 planning areas, with one or more making up one of nine sub-regions. This paper concentrates on Sub-region 12, which comprises a target population of 700,000 and is located on the Southside of Chicago.

Sub-region 12 is composed of six planning areas: South Shore, Chatham-Avalon, Roseland, Southwest, Southeast, Beverly-Morgan.[4] The first four areas are inhabited primarily by black residents, with 25% percent of the population on welfare in each area. The latter two planning areas are predominately white, with a low enough rate of welfare recipients (10.6% and 3.7%, respectively) to produce a total welfare recipient rate of only 17% for Sub-region 12. Sub-region 12 patients are served by Tinley Park Hospital, which has a total of 290 adult beds. Tinley Park serves two additional sub-regions; as a result, 290 psychiatric beds serve a target population of three million. Fortunately, the other two sub-regions have available several private and university-affiliated psychiatric inpatient services. As a result, beds utilized by Sub-region 12 patients ranged from 110 to 140 of the 290 "first come-first served" state hospital beds. 86% of patients at Tinley Park are black and come from four predominately black planning areas. Residents of the other two areas have lower utilization rates, not due to less mental illness, but rather to the use of private, predominantly white hospitals. Blacks are not as welcome at "other than Subregion 12 facilities" due to the Department of Public Aid's untimely and inadequate payment of bills for services rendered. The result is that white-owned hospitals limit their welfare patients to about 20%. Black-run hospitals (e.g., Provident, Meharry, Homer G. Phillips, etc.) usually do not refuse welfare patients and therefore have financial difficulty.

In terms of other than State resources, Sub-region 12 has six outpatient psychiatric clinics whose target population is the six planning areas comprising Sub-region 12. Five are operated by Chicago's Department of Mental Health and one by Jackson Park Hospital, a private, predominantly white, general medical hospital. There is no CMHC in the area, so federal funds are not available. The State funds some aspects of outpatient services. In addition, the State aids Jackson Park Hospital in maintaining a "fourteen twenty-one-day stay" unit with 14 beds and provides for patient overflow with backup hospitalization at Tinley Park. There are two entrance points to the State Mental Hospital, one being Tinley Park's intake system, which is not located in the city (public transportation to the hospital is poor). The other is Jackson Park, which is in the sub-region and is easily accessible. Thirty percent of Sub-region 12 patients hospitalized at Tinley Park were first seen at Jackson Park Hospital.

The intake system for Jackson Park's inpatient unit was simply a 24-hour service that determined whether the patient needed hospitalization or referral to an outpatient clinic. The State was constantly at odds with Jackson Park because of the overflow of patients from Jackson Park into its system. The overflow was eased to a degree by an agreement with Garfield Park Hospital, on the West Side, to hospitalize patients referred from Jackson Park. However, in spite of this agreement, Jackson Park's referrals to the state hospital were, in the state's estimation, too high (30% of the Sub-region 12 admission rate). This resulted in overcrowding (patients sleeping on couches); therefore, the State gave Jackson Park Hospital additional funds to add a Crisis Intervention Program (CIP) to the standard emergency intake services.

CRISIS INTERVENTION PROGRAM

Illinois statistics for Sub-region 12 showed a clear drop in admissions to Tinley Park six months before and after the start of the CIP (see Table 1).

TABLE 4.1. Comparison of Admission Rates Before and After CIP

	Six Months Prior to CIP	**Six Months After CIP**
Average total admissions	126.1	106.1
Average readmissions	78.0	63.3
Average first admissions	47.0	40.3

During the first two weeks of the program, utilization of Jackson Park's fourteen-bed brief-stay unit dropped from full to two or three patients. Only two patients were sent to Tinley Park for committal, as opposed to the usual 15–20 patients. This brought quite a reaction from the economic/administrative faction of the private hospital's Department of Psychiatry—as the CIP was obviously not keeping the beds full, questions were raised about its quality, and the aggressiveness of the CIP was therefore to be hampered. It is the author's contention, however, that such a program is valid and important in this setting.[5] A description of the CIP follows, along with follow-up data for a random sample of treated patients to substantiate that the program is clinically and ethically sound.

Aside from the function of making admissions to either Jackson Park or Tinley Park Hospitals, the CIP practiced aggressive crisis intervention to deal with certain psychiatric emergencies. The aggressiveness of the intervention techniques depended on the training of the staff involved. At night, the staff consisted of a medical resident and a psychiatric nurse, who were responsible for the inpatient unit and (when emergencies presented) the emergency room. In the evenings, a trained psychiatric nurse (assigned only to the emergency program) and a medical resident were available. During both the evening and night shifts, one of three psychiatrists was available for phone consultation. If possible, the night and evening teams medicated the patients, when necessary, and referred them to the day shift the next morning. In more serious cases, voluntary hospitalization was attempted, but if the patient refused and was felt to be of harm to self or others based on prior behavior or verbalized intent, he was admitted to Tinley Park via certificate. During the day shift, a board-certified psychiatrist, a psychiatric nurse, a social worker, and a patient aide were available, along with a driver to transport patients to Tinley Park. There was additional support from other day staff at the outpatient clinic. Linkage to the CMHCs or Jackson Park's outpatient clinic was accomplished during day shifts, while the patient was available.

Families and patients were seen during diagnostic interviews done by either the psychiatric nurse or social worker; however, during the day, all patients seen had contact with the psychiatrist, and supervision was thereby provided to other primary care team members.[6] Every patient was used as a teaching case. It was felt that evening and night personnel could rotate through days and enhance their skills. As this was an emergency service, the first questions cleared were legal ones: the patient was asked to sign a voluntary emergency service treatment form. If he agreed, as soon as he was medically cleared by a physician, the emergency was evaluated and handled by the use of physical restraints (if needed), intramuscular medication (if needed), and counseling as ordered by the physician in charge. Once patient combativeness, agitation, excitement, panic, and overwhelming anxiety or fear had been "cooled out," a more extensive interview was performed, focusing on precipitating events leading to the crisis. A past history of previous psychiatric treatment was elicited. From this evaluation, a determination of need for referral, hospitalization, or crisis intervention was made. If crisis intervention was deemed appropriate, the patient was adequately medicated and given an appointment to return to the CIP.

If hospitalization was determined to be needed, the patient was asked to sign voluntary admission forms. If the patient refused hospitalization, he was evaluated for the probability that he would harm himself or others. If that probability could not be documented on the basis of verbal declaration, recent history of such behavior, or goal-directed behavior towards that end, the patient was released with an explanation that he needed treatment but was not "crazy" enough to be legally forced to accept treatment. All patients in this category were offered services of the CIP, provided that they would agree to a treatment contract of cooperation that included taking medication, if needed.[7] The patient who refused voluntary hospitalization and who was deemed to be of harm to self or others was certified and sent to Tinley Park.

Finally, if the patient refused to sign the initial voluntary emergency treatment form, he was evaluated from the standpoint of being dangerous to himself or others. If he was not found to be harmful, he was told to either sign or remove himself (or be escorted) from the premises. If certification was deemed appropriate, he was taken into custody against his will, certified, and sent to Tinley Park. Patients who presented violently were not asked questions; they were quickly put into restraints as a self-defense measure to protect staff and medical equipment. If the patient could not be reasoned with when calm, he would be certified and sent to Tinley Park on the basis of presenting behavior. The importance of organic factors causing such behavior was clearly shown, and several clinical examples (delirium tremens, phencyclidine overdose, and hyperthyroidism) were available to make clear the differences in management of organic as opposed to mood or cognitive agitation.

The following intramuscular medications were given: haloperidol 5–10 mg every one-half hour with a second dose being rarely necessary; diazepam 5–10 mg every one-half hour up to two doses, or benzotropine mesylate, 1–2 mg. Use of haloperidol or diazepam depended on whether the anxiety was primarily, respectively, psychotic or stress-related.[8,9] Benzotropine mesylate was administered to patients with acute dystonic reactions secondary to neuroleptic medication. In addition to these short-term intramuscular medications, fluphenazine decanoate, 25 mg, was given intramuscularly to patients who presented with (1) symptoms of an acute psychotic episode (confusion, auditory hallucinations, no history of drug abuse, sleep loss, incoherence, bizarre behavior, flat or agitated affect, disheveled appearance, etc.); (2) a clear history of previous psychiatric hospitalizations due to acute psychotic episodes that benefited from neuroleptic medication; (3) a history that they had discontinued outpatient clinic visits or psychotrophic medications.[10] These patients were referred to the CIP five days after they received the fluphenazine injection and were given a three-day supply of chlorpromazine, 200 mg, twice a day until the medicine could take effect. They were also given a two-week supply of 2 mg tablets of benzotropine mesylate to take at bedtime. Although less than one third would have neuroleptic side effects, it was best to "over-prevent" any reactions that might give patients further negative feelings towards medication. Families were invited to bring the patient back in three days if they did not see improvement. Patients rarely returned before their "five days after initial contact" appointment. Those few who did were usually hospitalized, because the family could not tolerate the patient's psychotic behavior, even with CIP support.

Patients were able to receive three crisis sessions in addition to the initial contact; however, two crisis sessions per patient were rare. This was primarily due to the fact that a number of patients referred to the CIP had acute psychotic episodes. They responded to medication and to the aggressive linkage with local outpatient clinics. It was primarily the social worker's function to see patients after their initial visit and attempt to perform linkage. In addition, the social worker often called or wrote patients who did not return for their first crisis visit.

During the initial interview and subsequent crisis sessions (if indicated), patients were confronted point-blank with their behavior, intrapsychic dynamics, familial pathology, and strengths. It was felt that the defenses had broken down (producing a crisis) and that the underlying dynamics, thus exposed, were to be handled directly. Before this direct rapid-interpretation technique was used, the staff person had established a firm empathetic rapport with the patient.[11] Problems were clearly identified "out loud" for all persons concerned and it was made clear that the staff would without hesitation take total control to ensure a calm "working through" of the crisis.[12,13] There was a clear distinction made between understanding the "whys" of behavior and the acceptance of that behavior. Patients and family were essentially told that they were in "our house" and that we respected them but also expected them to respect us. Everything done to the patient was explained simply, and an attempt was made to answer all questions (except personal ones). In short, the milieu was down-to-earth and directive, with the staff maintaining a warm but no-nonsense attitude.

A total of 70 patients were studied retrospectively during the first two weeks of August 1976. Most patients were placed into one of four categories, depending on the clinical pictures during the intake interview. These were acute psychotic episode, character disorder in crisis (usually due to pressure from social forces), substance abuse with intoxication, and acute transient situational stress with or without previous psychiatric illness (see Table 2).

TABLE 4.2. Diagnostic Categories of Patients Seen the First Two Weeks in August

	Treated by Standard Emergency Psychiatric Procedures	Treated by CIP	Total
Acute psychotic episode			
N	13	20	33**
%	28	83	46
Acute transient stress			
N	10	3	13
%	22	12	19
Substance abuse+			
N	13	—	13
%	28	—	19
Character disorder			
N	4	—	4
%	9	—	5
Total			
N	46*	24*	70*
%	100*	100*	100*

N=Number of patients.
*Totals do not add up evenly because of seven miscellaneous diagnoses.
**Only three were without previous histories of such episodes.
+2/3 were alcohol abuse.

Six percent were certified and sent to Tinley Park. Of 94% who were not dangerous, only four percent refused treatment. Of 70 patients, 24 (34%) were referred to the CIP, with two thirds of that number returning to the program for their first crisis appointment. On return, they were substantially improved, and follow-up revealed that half of them were successfully linked to their local mental clinics.

Of the 46 patients (66%) who were not referred to the CIP, one fourth were hospitalized (half certified and half voluntary); one fourth were successfully linked to their local mental health clinics; one eighth refused referral or were not referred; one eighth were lost to follow-up because they did not belong to Sub-region 12; and one fourth were given appointments to their local mental health clinics, but did not show for their initial appointment.

CASE REPORTS

Examples of management of typical emergency psychiatric treatment cases are presented. Patient A, a 32-year-old black male was brought to the emergency psychiatric service by his family with a complaint that he was "acting peculiar again." The patient acted in an agitated, bizarre, and combative fashion. It was necessary to restrain the patient to a cart in four-way leather restraints and give him an injection of haloperidol, 10 mg, intramuscularly. As the patient calmed, a history was obtained from the family in the same room. He had been in the hospital five times previously for the same reason. Upon feeling that he was better, he had stopped going to his local mental health clinic and had stopped taking his medication. Although the family was familiar with this pattern, they had again allowed him to discontinue his clinic visits and had been well aware of his regressive behavior five weeks before they brought him to be hospitalized.

At that point, the patient was calm enough to be removed from restraints and was allowed to join the family discussion. The family and patient were advised that they had acted unwisely by allowing the patient to discontinue treatment and for their lack of early intervention. It was explained that if the family had spent five weeks tolerating regressive behavior, they could wait three days with the support of the CIP. It was further explained that the patient would be given a "two-week" injection (fluphenazine decanoate, 25 mg). Chlorpromazine, 200 mg, was prescribed, one in the morning and one at bedtime, for three days until the injection had its full effect. The family members were visibly angry but said they were willing to try.[14]

They did have concerns about what should be done if the patient became violent again. It was suggested that they call the police and have the patient brought back to the emergency service. He would be re-evaluated for possible hospitalization and would probably be admitted. Since he was on welfare, it was likely that during hospitalization, he would be dropped, requiring at least two months for him to be restored. They agreed to try to keep the patient out of the hospital. It was requested that the patient return in five days to check for improvement and to reconnect him to his clinic.

Five days later, the patient returned unescorted. He expressed gratitude that hospitalization had been avoided, since he had recently obtained a job. During this first crisis visit, he was given a clear understanding of the importance of taking his medication and that even if he felt he was better, he should remain in contact with his clinic "just in case." Finally, the patient was linked to his former outpatient clinic; since they were unable to see him before his medication would be due, he was seen one more time. He kept his appointment.

Patient B, a 17-year-old black female, was brought in by the police because she had attempted suicide by drug overdose. Although it was reported that the patient had regurgitated most of the capsules she did not digest, her stomach was pumped. The examiner found her to be an upset, angry, arrogant adolescent who gave a history of breaking up with her boyfriend and deciding she would overdose. It was revealed that she had called police but no longer cared to discuss the matter because she had to keep a date to go shopping with her girlfriend. From her mental status examination, it was determined that the patient was not psychotic. She had poor impulse control. She was devoid of neither hope nor the capacity for humor and had good judgment when not upset. However, the examiner felt that she needed to be apprised of the consequences for her behavior. He informed her that on the basis of her recent suicidal behavior, he would have to certify her to a state hospital for the mentally ill. She balked, became extremely angry, and stated that such a thing was outside the examiner's jurisdiction. The seriousness of her act and the examiner's concern for her life were impressed upon her. She was reassured that it probably would not be as bad as she thought and that if she cooperated with the in-patient evaluation, she might be discharged in two to three weeks. At this point, she dropped her arrogance and said she had "really gone too far this time." She went on to talk about how "silly and immature" she felt when she let her emotions carry her thinking away. In talking, she gave assurances that she would seek treatment regardless if she was hospitalized. She said she had not dealt with the fact that she had a problem and said she could deny it no longer because of "the way it was brought to me." She was linked to her local mental health center instead of being certified and on follow-up she had made the connection.[15]

Patient C was a 29-year-old black male who was brought in by the police because he was involved in a robbery. Because of a previous psychiatric history, he was brought for hospitalization instead of being taken to jail. Upon examination, it was determined that the patient was not psychotic, neurotic, homicidal, or suicidal. His prior hospitalizations had been secondary to drug abuse, and episodes of anger were secondary to conflict with persons in authority. He was able to tell right from wrong and cooperate with a lawyer defending him. He had not engaged in treatment for two years but had wondered if he could be. He was hospitalized for several days at Tinley Park, where he was given diazepam, 10 mg. He was returned to the custody of the police.

Patient D was a 78-year-old black male who was brought to the emergency service by his wife because of growing confusion. The wife wanted him "committed to an old folks home because of his senility." The patient denied all of his wife's complaints, but he did show signs of disturbance in recent memory and orientation. He was given haloperidol, 1 milligram, three times a day, and told to return to the clinic in five days. His wife returned with the patient in three days. This time she brought papers requesting she be made executor of his estate and a request from their lawyer that the psychiatrist document his mental incompetence. The patient seemed improved at this visit. On calling the lawyer, it was determined that although he did not feel the patient was incompetent, he had given the wife the papers because of the wife's insistence. The papers were not filled out and the patient's medication was increased to haloperidol, 2 mg, three times a day. On the patient's last visit before linkage to his local outpatient clinic, he appeared to be much improved though still dependent on his wife for care. On follow-up, he had not returned to the clinic.

DISCUSSION

The difference between the total number of patients admitted six months prior to and six months after the CIP started had a Student t-test probability value between 0.1 and 0.2. The average total number of admissions per month dropped to 20 patients after initiation of the program. The percentage of total admissions to Tinley Park from Jackson Park dropped from an average of 30% per month to an average of 20% per month. In addition, the total number of patients readmitted dropped to 15 patients per month when comparing rates of readmission six months before and six months after beginning the program. The drop in first admissions between the two samples per month was only seven patients. This was probably due to the focus of the program, which was to maintain previously admitted patients with clear histories in the community and to circumvent rehospitalization. Patients referred to the CIP had hospitalization rates of 12.5%; ordinarily, the majority would have been hospitalized, owing to their diagnosis of "acute psychotic episode."[16] Patients with first episodes of psychiatric difficulties were likely to have been managed in the standard fashion, due to a lack of thorough inpatient diagnostic evaluation. As a result, the rate of hospitalization for patients not referred to the CIP was 21.7% during the two-week sample. These results concur with the observation of a greater impact readmission rate in Sub-region 12 at the start of the program; although there was a drop in first admissions, it was not so large. In addition to the fact that patients referred to the crisis program were clearly less likely to be hospitalized, they were also more likely to be successfully linked to their local mental health clinics than were patients managed by standard emergency psychiatric techniques.

Finally, in terms of patients' reasons for not seeking hospitalization, it is probable that patients with a prior high readmission rate were able to learn they could get relief from the chaos of an acute psychotic episode on an outpatient basis, rather than through hospitalization. In addition, the technique used increased the families' awareness of their role and responsibility in keeping the patient out of the hospital. One parent told me, "I've been lackadaisical in seeing that my son got to the clinic, but after all this trouble, he'll go from now on." By enlisting the aid of the family in the treatment, the family members, rather than the treating agency, put pressure on the patient to conform to standard codes of behavior. The patient and family became responsible for determining how to act, which allows for a more cooperative type of treatment contract to be formed between the patient and therapist. One woman (whose son insisted on opening the bathroom door while she was using the toilet but was not, in the author's opinion, dangerous) was advised to either put a lock on the door, put her son out, or see that he got proper treatment for his "nerves." As she was afraid of what he might do in a locked bathroom and could not put her 26-year-old "baby" out, she agreed to see that he got to the clinic regularly for his "three week shot" (fluphenazine decanoate). Although her new attitude was in the best interest of both her son and her, she left the service angry because he had not been hospitalized, as on six previous times.

SUMMARY AND CONCLUSIONS

In summary, the following are to be learned from this experience:

1. Clinicians must take into account political, administrative, and economic factors when introducing a program that will cause a shift in patient flow. This is an especially important factor to consider when there is a conflict of interest in the facility that is delivering the service. These factors are probably the main reasons that day treatment centers, crisis intervention programs, emergency housing, etc., are not gaining more popularity in treating psychiatric patients.

2. Crisis intervention techniques, described herein, will reduce the total admission rate at state hospitals, with a greater impact being seen on readmissions rather than first admission. First admission rates will also decrease.

3. Crisis intervention techniques used for patients falling into the category of acute psychotic episode, who have had previous hospitalizations, will probably be more successful than those who are having an acute psychotic episode for the first time.

4. Psychiatric emergency intervention is best done with an attitude of interest in the patients' wellbeing and an attempt to "hookup" with the patient, while at the same time being clear that no foolishness will be tolerated.

Follow-up data supports the contention that the program described is just as effective as most brief hospitalization units. Crisis intervention programs put into effect statewide would change the manner of managing psychiatric emergencies and would greatly benefit the practice of community psychiatry. The decrease in hospitalization, resulting from the use of this program, would allow for better utilization of day treatment programs, emergency housing, outpatient clinic involvement in early intervention, and sheltered living facilities.

┌─────────────────────────┐
│   COMMENTARY   │
└─────────────────────────┘

As an African-American physician, I've always had a very different mission from most European-American physicians. European-American physicians are often concerned with trying to improve the "quality of life" of their mainly European-American patients. Since leaving medical school, one of my major missions has been to *save* lives of my mainly African-American patients. Although I'm interested in their "wellness," until African-American life expectancy reaches that of European-Americans, I feel obligated to spend more time on "saving lives—making a difference," the CMHC's mission. Achieving this mission as an African-American community psychiatrist has always been a challenge. There are very few people who value poor, mentally ill black people. As a result, resources allocated to help this population are scarce. This reality has always demanded the need to develop creative and innovative ways of effectively and efficiently serving the poor and underserved. Unfortunately, resources to develop such imaginative and resourceful ways and to prove their usefulness are also sparse. Accordingly, much of my professional life has involved developing interventions that adequately serve patients in a cost-effective manner. In addition, since I've always felt it important to know if my interventions are efficient, I've always reviewed my efforts by evaluating their outcome. Toward achieving this goal, I always do outcome research on the interventions I develop or investigate.

When I left the Navy and went to the Southside of Chicago to practice community psychiatry, it was immediately clear to me that the state hospital that served our patients was overcrowded. This overcrowding was causing a negative ripple effect throughout the Southside care system. Patients needing admission were sometimes turned away, and patients needing to stay in the hospital longer were released too soon. This placed additional unnecessary burdens on the psychiatric emergency service and outpatient clinics. Their response was to send more patients to the hospital. Although I wasn't a state hospital employee, I felt (because of my understanding of ecology and my efforts to see the larger picture systemically) the need to initiate an intervention to help solve the problem for the whole system. This article describes that intervention. It was my first major systemic contribution to the mental health care of the mentally ill African-American population in Southside Chicago.

Despite the benefits, the Psychiatric Emergency Service/CIP was dismantled several years after its start because of the cost. With the help of the Chicago Medical School Department of Psychiatry residents, I rebuilt the service in the late 1980s. Despite losing the residents from Chicago Medical School in the early 1990s, we were able to recruit Dr. Theodur Ranganathan (a former Chicago Medical School psychiatric resident) and Verbie Jones, an outstanding manager, which has enabled the service to still exist. In 1995, the CMHC, in partnership with Jackson Park Hospital and several other community mental health providers, began the Emergency Services Affiliates (ESA). Our intent was to provide 24-hour psychiatric emergency and crisis intervention services from Jackson Park Hospital to four Chicago Southside communities.

ESA represents an improvement in the Psychiatric Emergency Service I first conceptualized over 20 years ago. Although I was writing about alternatives to hospitalization such as day treatment, emergency housing, and other community support systems, the reality then was that there were very few such services on Chicago's Southside. Currently, because of agencies like the Beverly-Morgan Mental Health Center, the CMHC, the Human Resources Development Institute, Metropolitan Family Services, and the Roseland Mental Health Center, there are many more alternatives to hospitalization. Now we have assertive community treatment, case management, crisis beds, day treatment facilities, a mobile assessment team, residential beds, and services for the substance-abusing mentally ill. In 1996, the Illinois Department of Mental Health awarded the CMHC nearly a million dollars to support the ESA. While we still need more community support systems for our patients, we are farther along than we were in 1978. When I got busy with other projects and had to pull away from Jackson Park Hospital, the hospital closed the Psychiatric Emergency Service for about three years. This was a huge tragedy because the program monthly saw 400 patients, who now had nowhere to go except the state hospital. The state hospital's location is inconvenient, since it is about 30 miles from the patients' homes and since the public transportation is poor. Fortunately, we were able to get the program restarted, and it has been going well ever since.

Recently, the CMHC, Inc., was given the responsibility of providing psychiatric services to Chicago's Englewood community and has been able to set up a similar Psychiatric Emergency Program there at St. Bernard Hospital. The program has worked out quite well because we used a template based on the Jackson Park Hospital model.

Not long ago, I was the subject of a *Nightline* interview, where I had the opportunity to share with a broad audience how psychiatric services can be delivered to an African-American community to benefit this underserved population. I hope my suggestions will serve as an example for others.

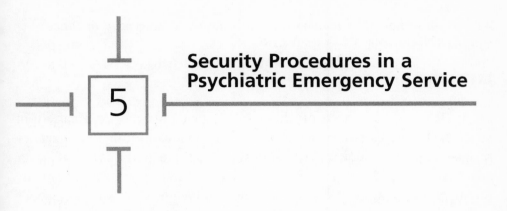

Security Procedures in a Psychiatric Emergency Service

The issue of violence in the mental health setting has recently begun to gain attention in the literature. As there is not enough research on this issue to draw conclusions as to the frequency of violence in mental health settings, there is a need to gather empirical data on the frequency of violence in various settings and to investigate the causes and management of this phenomenon. This article seeks to assess the prevalence of violence and potential violence in an inner-city psychiatric emergency service using several parameters as indicators. In addition, the article seeks to outline skills necessary for the management of violent patients, which includes the recognition of potentially violent behavior, a hierarchy of management techniques to prevent the occurrence of violence, and techniques specifically designed to stop violence without causing patient or staff harm. Various etiologies of violence in mental health settings are discussed and a cognitive hierarchy of aggression is presented. Legal and ethical issues surrounding the concept of forcing patients to accept treatment on the basis of their dangerousness are discussed. Finally, the question of a difference in the prevalence of violence between ethnically different patient populations is raised, along with the possible implications of such a dif-

Originally printed as Bell Carl C, Palmer John M. Security procedures in a psychiatric emergency service. *J Natl Med Assoc*. 1981;73:835–842. Presented at the 134th Annual Meeting of the APA, New Orleans, LA, May 1981.

ference. Recommendations are made for the management of the
violent or potentially violent patient.

INTRODUCTION

Patients come to a psychiatric emergency service for a variety of reasons. Lazare et al.[1] catalogued what patients want from an emergency service into the following categories: (1) administrative (I need your administrative or legal power); (2) advice (tell me what to do about my problems); (3) clarification (help me sort out my ideas or feelings so that I can put things in perspective); (4) community triage (tell me where I can get the help I need); (5) confession (please let me assuage my guilt); (6) control (please take over and protect me from myself); (7) medical (be a doctor, diagnose and treat my problem); (8) psychological expertise (use your special knowledge to explain why I feel or act the way I do); (9) psychodynamic insight (please help me understand myself better); (10) reality contact (please help me know that I am real and not losing my mind); (11) succorance (please be warm and caring to help fill the void); (12) ventilation (I have some things I need to get off my chest); (13) nothing (I don't want anything from the service). Of all these, the hardest one to deal with is control (please take over and protect me from myself), because this request implies a loss of control, with a strong possibility of violence.

Violence is an integral part of our environment. It appears out of nowhere and invades public and private sectors with no regard to those persons it affects; it then disappears, only to recur at an unexpected place and time. Violence that occurs in the mental health setting has this same will-o'-the-wisp quality. While the prevalence of serious violence appears to be greater in persons not thought to be suffering from psychiatric disorders,[2-4] violence in a mental health setting is just as terrifying and destructive.

Statistics on violence in the mental health setting[5] are not numerous, but a number of studies has been done attempting to define the parameters of this phenomenon. Whitman, Armao, and Dent[6] surveyed 101 therapists and found of all patients seen in one year (6,720), 9.2% presented a threat to others, 11.9% posed a physical threat to a therapist, and 0.63% actually assaulted a therapist. The overall data indicated that one of every eleven patients presented an assaultive threat to others in their environment. They found that 24% of the 101 therapists were attacked by at least one patient during the year. A ten-year study reviewed 476,152 admissions and found that six percent were involved in assaultive acts two weeks prior to entry into treatment.[7] Madden, Lion, and Penna surveyed 115 psychiatrists regarding assaults by patients.[5] Forty-eight (42%) of 115 psychiatrists reported that they had been assaulted. In all, 68 assaults were reported. With the data on violence in mental health settings being as sparse and diverse as it is, any analysis along hypothetical lines would be very difficult. Despite this problem, certain valuable evidence can be gleaned from the available information: (1) there is a substantial level of violence in the mental health setting; (2) the level of violence varies across facilities and populations; (3) the effectiveness of violence management varies across facilities; (4) research on violence in the mental health setting lacks effective congruence and organization.

Beyond measuring the frequency of violence in a mental health setting, the causes and management of this phenomenon need careful assessment. This article involves attitudes, values, and techniques used to prevent or manage violence in a psychiatric setting.

BACKGROUND

During the past year, the authors have worked with the staff of a psychiatric emergency service provided by an inner-city general medical hospital on the Southside of Chicago (Jackson Park Hospital) in an attempt to formulate a comprehensive program for the safe management of violent patients. The service was responsible for providing psychiatric emergency services (crisis intervention, rape counseling, referral for inpatient hospitalization, and certification for involuntary hospitalization) to a population of 700,000 in an area known as Sub-region 12. Sub-region 12 consists of six city planning areas: South Shore, Chatham-Avalon, Roseland, Southwest, Southeast, and Beverly-Morgan. The first four areas are primarily inhabited by black residents, with 25% of the population on welfare.[8]

In August 1976, the number of patients seen was approximately 140,[8] compared with 293 patients (neither number counting return visits) seen in August 1979. Thus, it is clear that the utilization of the psychiatric emergency service has increased over a three-year period. In looking at a three-month sample (August, September, and October 1979), in which a total of 687 patients was seen, 140 (20%) presented in an agitated manner, and 106 among the agitated group (15.6% of the total sample) were so out of control that they had to be physically restrained by four-way leather restraints. With this patient load and with the prevalence of agitation among them, it was the goal of the authors to systematically interweave specific interpersonal communicative modes, behavioral structuring, and martial art techniques with the established policies and procedures of the psychiatric emergency service[8] in an attempt to adequately manage patients whose out of control behavior is harmful to themselves or others.

MANAGEMENT OF VIOLENT PATIENTS

The first step in managing violent patients was to educate the staff about the ideas and concepts necessary to successfully interact with hostile, agitated, psychotic, and combative patients. Five two-hour in-service educational seminars were presented to introduce and reinforce the necessary core material for increasing staff confidence and efficiency in this area. In addition, weekly group and individual training sessions were held throughout the year as patient load and activity permitted.

The next step was the systems analysis and the interweaving process, which were necessary for incorporating the core material into the psychiatric emergency service treatment procedures. The systems analysis consisted of isolating each step of the patient-staff interaction patterns that characterized the routine service procedures and interweaving specific communicative modes, appropriate behavioral structuring procedures, and martial arts techniques to secure patients and staff from milieu violence.

Each patient entering the emergency psychiatric service interacts with at least three of the four crisis intervention team members. The nurse performs the triage: taking the patient's temperature, blood pressure, pulse rate, respiration rate, and immediate medical history and evaluating the patient's general physical condition. Next, a technician completes an intake interview and turns the patient over to the psychiatrist. At this point, the patient is evaluated and a disposition is made. If the patient has to be transported to another facility, he will then come into contact with the fourth member of the core crisis intervention team—the driver. At each of the interaction points mentioned above, two communicative modes dominate. First, the staff intervenes in the patient's crisis to help him maintain use of appropriate defense mechanisms and coping strategies. Staff members then communicate amongst themselves to evaluate the patient's behavior and potential behavior.

The third communicative mode used at the entry point to the psychiatric emergency service system conveys the milieu values and attitudes of the service and people who staff it. The search of the patient's person prior to triage communicates a number of crucial realities to staff and patient: (1) this is a controlled environment; (2) no one is allowed to hurt himself or others; (3) although we are strangers, a certain amount of intimacy is necessary. The search has the very practical value of relieving staff anxiety when dealing with patients who evidence violence potential. The value of the search should not be underestimated, as more than one thousand contraband items confiscated from patients in one year's time consisted of over 150 knives, one gun, and numerous razors and other sharp instruments, as well as marijuana, cocaine, phencyclidine (angel dust), and other illicit drugs. In a service where 35–40% of the 350–400 monthly referrals come from the Chicago Police Department, the search has proven its value.

Each point of staff-patient interaction requires specific communicative modes as well as a certain level of behavioral structuring. For 70% to 80% of patients seen in the psychiatric emergency service, behavioral structuring consists of nothing more than an adequately calming interview (succorance, clarification, advice, reality contact, ventilation, community triage, psychological expertise, and psychodynamic expertise). For the remaining 20–30% of the patient load, however, a calming interview was only the first in a series of attempts to help the patient structure his behavior in an appropriate manner. Characteristically, this 20–30% were the violent, destructive, agitated, hostile, combative, homicidal, suicidal, and occasionally psychotic patients. The lack of limits inherent in using a calming interview to help these patients hold together may actually lead to an increase in decompensation. In these cases, the staff would escalate the behavioral structuring procedure using contractual and limit-setting techniques, respectively. Half of these patients could respond to the contractual techniques, but the other half required limit-setting, usually in the form of physical restraints.

In the patients requiring physical restraints, the authors recommend the use of specially selected and developed martial art techniques for the safe controlling and restraining of violent patients. The authors hold advanced degrees in karate, with 18 years of combined experience in various martial arts, and were able to draw directly from this knowledge to adapt the appropriate techniques. Since the restraining of patients is at best a risky business, the chief fear being injury of the patient or staff, the martial arts techniques were welcomed as a safeguard for all those involved in the restraint process. The techniques taught to the staff were designed strictly for defensive use (see Figures 1 through 5). They enabled the staff to more effectively control the most violent of patients, as well as to defend against the attacks of the combative ones. Results from the training in martial arts restraint techniques were seen on practical and psychological levels. Injuries to patients being restrained were cut to almost nil, paralleling the reduction (though not the extinction) of staff injuries. Psychologically,

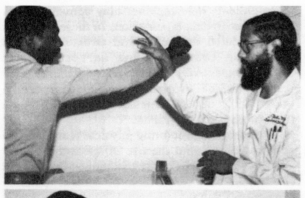

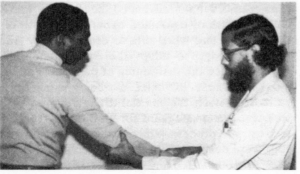

FIGURE 5.1. Mock patient throws right jab at staff member, who steps and blocks with the right hand (top). Staff member grabs mock patient's right wrist with his right hand and grabs mock patient's right elbow at the distal end of the humerous bone, just above the epicondyles, with his left hand (bottom).

the staff commented on having increased feelings of confidence in dealing with violent patients. This feeling of staff security also seems to help patients feel safe in the milieu.

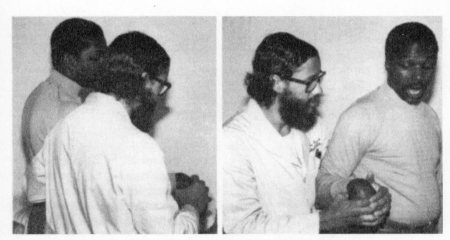

FIGURE 5.2. Staff member circles to right of mock patient while flexing patient's right wrist, still maintaining a grip on patient's right elbow (left). Staff member tucks mock patient's right elbow into crook of his own left elbow and uses both hands to hyperflex mock patient's right wrist (right). This "come along" does not produce permanent damage or pain, but causes pain only when patient struggles to free himself from staff member's control.

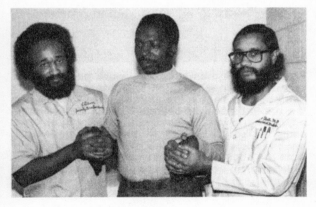

FIGURE 5.3. Two staff members apply "come along" to mock patient to ensure complete control over the violent patient.

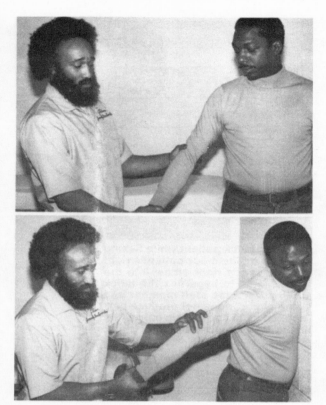

FIGURE 5.4. Staff member grabs mock patient's right arm in the proper fashion to apply an "arm bar," enabling staff member control over mock patient's body movement (top). Applying "arm bar" to mock patient's right arm, staff member uses his body weight to force mock patient against the wall, where patient is immobilized. Note the hyperflexed right wrist of mock patient, which aids in controlling patient (bottom).

DISCUSSION

Examination of the causes of violence in the mental health setting tends to focus on the violent patient or the provocative environment (i.e., staff transactions), as a means of explaining its occurrence. The description of the violent patient's personality constellation varies because of the unpredictability of the phenomenon, but some useful, albeit general, observations can be submitted. A patient suffering from an acute psychotic episode can be so out of control that he must be restrained for his own safety and to prevent him from leaving in such a fragmented state[9] that he is unable to care for himself. Borderline and alcoholic patients in crisis can present very explosive and combative behaviors. Patients with developmental disabilities often present as a "time bomb" that can enter a state of frenzy[9] at any time. Some patients, fearing their impulses to hurt them-

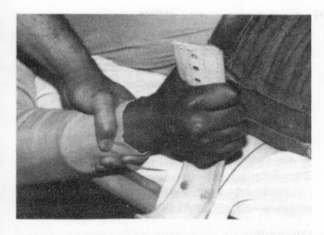

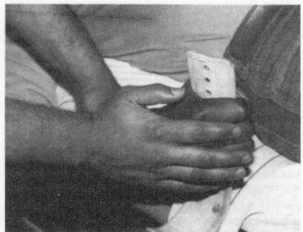

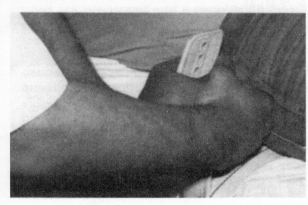

FIGURE 5.5. Mock patient being placed into four-way leather restraints grabs restraint cuff to thwart the procedure (top). Staff member applies pressure to mock patient's hand while holding the wrist, attempting to cause flexion of the wrist (center). Flexion of mock patient's wrist is accomplished with patient's attending inability to securely grip any object, which will allow staff member to continue restraining patient (bottom).

selves or others, act out in a manner to attract external controls or limits, and may occasionally request restraints.

In addition to individual patient dynamics, the mental health setting has an overlapping effect on patient violence. In fact, the treatment environment—principally the staff—seems to play more of an integral role in the provocation of violence than first suspected. Madden et al.[5] reported that many of the 115 psychiatrists they interviewed thought they might have had a role in provoking an assault on themselves. Others point to problems in patient/staff communication prior to, during, and subsequent to patient violence as being the key to violence in the mental health setting. Prior to patient violence, the inattention of the staff to early warning signals can begin a distortion of communication patterns between staff and patients, and amongst staff members. Prior to and during patient violence, the communication patterns of patients and staff are maximally strained, which possibly further increases the patient's anxiety, lessens his control over violent impulses, and leads to an incident in which he could injure staff and/or the patient.[10] Staff "splitting" is another problem frequently linked to patient dissention and epidemic violence. When poor morale or staff conflict issues are passed on to the patients, the therapeutic milieu is destroyed. Violent patients are not controlled effectively and other patients may resort to violence to protect their territorial integrity.[11] Cornfield et al.[10] surmise that the threatening patient provokes a counter-transference from the staff, resulting in staff reactions that encompass improper therapeutic distance, denial, and over-intellectualization. These intrapsychic defenses can impede efficient handling of violent and potentially violent situations. On the other side of the coin is the belief that the expectation of and preparation for violence may represent a self-fulfilling prophecy and thus lead to the violence sought to be prevented.[12]

It was the authors' experience that agitated and possibly imminently violent patients were best handled by the anticipation and prevention of violence before it occurred. Violence was anticipated with help from the cognitive hierarchy of aggression, which was developed from martial arts experiences and psychiatric/psychological training. Aggression was conceived as a general term covering all forms of behavior aimed at exerting control or mastery over objects, self, or situations, and was not viewed either as a positive or negative phenomenon. Lowest in the aggression hierarchy are activities involving alertness, curiosity, attentiveness, and explorative behavior. Next comes self-assertion, which is the attempt to establish, maintain, and expand one's boundaries or integrity while not intruding into another's territory. The next level of aggression is the expression of dominance, which implies the capacity to exert influence over the behavior of other people or groups in an intended direction (power). The foundation of this dominance tends to be grounded in coercion, with the expectation of great rewards or great punishments for certain kinds of behavior, and the ability and readiness to exert this power. When this dominance is legitimatized by legal, professional, or social mandates, it is known as authority.[13] Finally, towards the top of the hierarchy is hostility, which implies behavior or attitudes intending to hurt or destroy an object or the self. The etiology of hostility may come from either the need to obtain a goal (e.g., pleasure, as in sadism, or war to gain survival needs); the need to hurt or destroy whatever frustrates a goal-directed activity such as self-assertion, exploration, dominance; or the need to protect oneself from a threat or actual trauma. Finally, when the injury or destruction of an object, self, or situation is the end rather than the means to an end, the type of aggression expressed is hatred. This cognitive hierarchy[14] was taught both in a theoretical framework through the use of didactic lectures and from an experiential framework through the use of martial arts training and on-the-job experience with patients exhibiting the range of aggressive behaviors. Once the range of aggressive behaviors could be accurately identified without either under- or overreacting, it was then possible for the staff to attempt to prevent violence using a hierarchy of management techniques ranging from the use of a calming interview (providing empathy, giving the patient some distance between himself and the examiner, giving reassurance, and having an attitude of helpfulness and calmness); psychotrophic medication (pleasant-tasting liquid concentrates); contractual and limit-setting techniques; relative seclusion; and finally physical restraints.

All patients entering the psychiatric emergency service were requested to sign a written consent to psychiatric emergency room treatment. If the patient refused to sign, an immediate evaluation of the patient's danger to self or others was made, and if found not to be harmful to self or others, was asked to leave. If the patient was found to be overtly dangerous to self or others or in such a state that he cannot provide for basic physical needs to guard himself from serious harm, a psychiatrist certified him and forced him to comply with psychiatric emergency service intervention. This culminated in transferring the patient to a state hospital, where the certificate was used to initiate the legal process of commitment. For patients who signed the voluntary psychiatric emergency room treatment form, the authors contend that forcing a patient to comply with psychiatric emergency service intervention is justified only when a patient must be prevented from physically harming himself or others, or when a patient is in such a state that he cannot provide for basic physical needs to guard himself from serious harm. This meant that all patients forced not only agreed to treatment, but were also certifiable by Illinois standards. This is a subjective clinical evaluation subject to over- or under-reactions and is therefore the subject of great controversy.[15-17]

It is the authors' belief that mentally ill patients should not be allowed to directly or indirectly cause physical harm to themselves or others in an attempt to preserve patients' legal rights. While the removal of these rights is subject to court decision, not psychiatric judgment, the first step in the removal is a psychiatric decision. It is within the clinical purview of psychiatrists to initiate the necessary steps without incurring legal action against themselves while they act in good faith. Fortunately, the law concurs. It must be emphasized that it is the psychiatrist who is responsible for beginning the process of legally forcing patients to accept treatment to prevent them from harming themselves or others. The psychiatrist must also monitor of services delivered in order to prevent staff from inappropriately using power, authority, or restraining techniques that meet staff needs, rather than treating psychiatric patients. This is best accomplished by the establishment of strong leadership in the staff group. A professional hierarchy must exist, in which there is demonstration of respect for authority and employee rights. Since the interpersonal milieu between director and line staff will be transferred to the analogous milieu between line staff and patient, the care of staff interpersonal milieu cannot be overemphasized if the staff is to appropriately deal with anxiety-provoking issues like hostility and violence. Despite a concerted effort to ensure that a patient's rights and dignity are respected regardless of his or her psychiatric condition, however, certain individual incidents involving patients or staff were unavoidable and cannot be legislated or influenced. Among such were the accusation of rape made by an acutely psychotic patient while she was in restraints and the staff's documentation that an elderly confused patient came to the service with $200 (his life's savings) but discovered it missing upon his arrival at the state facility for hospitalization his money was missing. These occurrences, whether shown to have been the responsibility of an individual staff member or the product of a psychotic patient's confusion, have an extremely demoralizing effect on the staff and are best turned over to legal authorities for investigation.

It has been reported that the prevalence of violence (e.g., the homicide rate for non-whites) is eight to fifteen times greater than that for whites[18] and is even higher for blacks,[4] and the question remains whether there is a greater prevalence of violence in inner-city psychiatric emergency services serving blacks. This study found empirical evidence that 15.6% of patients seen in a three-month sample had to be restrained and that during the year, over 150 knives, one gun, and numerous razors and other sharp instruments were confiscated from a predominately black patient population. While the authors believe the majority of patients seen were not dangerous[19] and decry acting like policemen by searching patients, the fact that approximately one sixth of the patients seen needed restraint and that a dangerous weapon appeared at least once every other day emphasizes the need of a search. In an attempt to preserve respect for patients' privacy, patients were told that everyone seeking service must be searched. If the patient refused but did not appear to be certifiable, he was invited to leave the area and return after a few minutes to be searched. Since a predominately black staff was treating a black patient population, there seemed to be no problem in establishing and maintaining good patient-staff rapport, despite the fact that the staff employed police-like techniques. Searching is clearly a sensitive issue for inner-city residents. The authors suspect that results would have been different if the staff had been white, due to the racism that is sometimes present in an interracial staff/patient mixture.

Thus, the issue of whether or not there is a higher prevalence of violence in a black psychiatric patient group is a very delicate one; if it turns out there is a higher incidence, there could be several disturbing ramifications: (1) the idea that it is dangerous to treat black patients, which might make some treatment facilities exclude black patients from their facility; (2) since it is already a racist expectation that black patients are more violent, this attitude is may be communicated to the patient with attending avoiding doing anything (such as exerting limits) to make the patient "go off," thus perpetuating a pattern of violence; (3) the idea that black psychiatric patients are more dangerous, which makes treatment facilities decide they must employ severe, police-like treatment techniques to adequately deal with the problem; (4) the idea that black psychiatric patients are more dangerous but, with mental illness is seen to be a myth, should be jailed rather than treated; (5) the idea that black patients are more dangerous and that the etiology of this dangerousness needs to be investigated and prevented. If this dangerousness is related to a lability of affect and impulse controls secondary to a type of "combat fatigue," perhaps it could be better thought of as "survival fatigue" in inner-city black psychiatric patients.

RECOMMENDATIONS

By way of summation, the authors would like to share some of the concepts learned from research and experience, which may serve as successful focusing points for the management of violent patients:

1. Mental health professionals may be familiar with theories concerning aggression and violence, but few have adequate training or expertise in predicting and managing the overt expression of hostility-violence. Clinicians need to learn techniques to specifically manage violent patients and protect themselves from harm. Martial arts training in the use of specific defensive and controlling techniques is helpful in obtaining these goals.

2. Empathy plus observation leads to anticipation, the most important concept one can learn in controlling patient violence.

3. Do not be afraid to manipulate the environment to help a patient maintain use of appropriate defensive mechanisms and coping strategies. If necessary, ask a provocative family to leave the area, place the patient in a quieter area where the phenomenon of aggression contagion is less likely, or transfer

provocative staff members who consistently approach patients with an "edge" (which incites an escalation in aggression) to a less sensitive area.

4. If you are afraid of a patient, do not pretend not to be. Instead, let the patient know you will control yourself and the patient if necessary.

5. Violent patients want limits (no one likes being out of control).

6. Violent patients should never be left alone with only one staff member.

7. Do not threaten a patient with restraints, but when restraint is needed, use maximum force necessary rather than being ambivalent about the process.

8. At all times, tell the patient in a fashion clear and understandable to the patient what you are doing and why. He may not always like your actions or the reasons for your actions, but he will accept them.

9. Treat your violent patients as you yourself would like to be treated were you out of control, i.e., with respect and dignity. This gives one a firm foundation in respecting patients, which is communicated and engenders rapport.

10. Never place a potentially violent patient in a position that would give him the feeling of being trapped. While you might feel more comfortable closer to the door in order to make a quick exit in case of trouble, it is actually better to give the patient a way out rather than have his back to the wall.

11. When setting limits on a patient, give him some room to cooperate while at the same time "saving face."

12. Restraints should be used only to teach a patient a lesson, never to punish.

COMMENTARY

John Palmer and I wrote this article to describe efforts in managing actual violence as it occurred in the Psychiatric Emergency Service at Jackson Park Hospital. At the end of our discussion, we advocated for violence prevention in the black mentally ill population, a line of thought we wanted to expand into the black community as a whole (see Chapter 1). At that time, I didn't realize that my personal experiences in managing real-life violence while growing up would come in handy later when doing my public health work in violence prevention. I still draw on this earlier work, and did so especially when I was a faculty member for the APA's Continuing Medical Education Conference, "Violence: Implications for Clinical Practice," which has been held regionally in New Orleans and New York.

I thank University of California at Davis professor of psychiatry Dr. Joe Tupin, who has helped me clarify my thoughts on various aspects of this early paper. Dr. Tupin made it clear to me that the most important factor in managing violence is the amount of time you have to respond to violence. Accordingly, when you know that "potential" violence can occur, you'll have a lot of time to plan and practice what to do should violence actually occur. In many ways, our writing this article was a part of prevention planning: what to do if violence should occur in the emergency room. It continues to act as an orientation guide for new emergency room staff. Searching patients is another one such example of managing "potential" violence. In "urgent" situations where violence is on the verge of occurring and there is not a great deal of time to plan, there is time to try to de-escalate the situation with verbal and behavioral techniques. The "calming interview" we wrote about fits into this category. Finally, the martial arts techniques we recommended are designed to manage "emergent" violence, which is when violence starts to occur, and the time for physical action is needed.

This article became useful in April 1990 when I presented on homicide prevention at Wright State University in Dayton and met Dr. Rodney Hammond. Dr. Hammond was at the time Assistant Dean for Student Affairs and Associate Professor at Wright State University's School of

Professional Psychology. He had recently begun working on a violence prevention project aimed to help African-American youth, and he asked me for my assistance. I told him the nature of the "calming interview" techniques we had always used in managing violent patients in Jackson Park Hospital's emergency room. Being a good psychologist, he took my clinical experience and organized it into steps that could be used in a violence prevention program. He and his colleagues went on to develop the Positive Adolescent Choices Training Program, which serves as a model for violence prevention groups comprising African-American youth. They have continued to refine their work and have produced several useful violence prevention/intervention strategies. In addition, they are training others how to intervene. I'm proud to have been associated with their work. It is good work. This serves as another example of how African-American professionals from different disciplines can work together in harmony to benefit our community.

This work finally culminated in the first book I've ever edited, *Psychiatric Aspects on Violence: Understanding Causes and Issues in Prevention and Treatment* (Jossey-Bass: San Francisco; 2000). The chapter that Dr. Berg, Dr. Tupin, and I wrote was selected by the series editor, Dr. Richard Lamb, as one of the "Best of New Directions for Mental Health Services" during the series, which ran from 1979 to 2001.

After Dr. Palmer and I published the article reprinted in this chapter, we revisited our efforts and published "Survey of the Demographic Characteristics of Patients Requiring Restraints in a Psychiatric Emergency Service" (*J Natl Med Assoc.* 1983;75:981–987.), which focused on the characteristics of the patients we restrained during our initial work. One main finding was that 23.9% of the patients had returned for services in the psychiatric emergency service within the one and a half years between the two studies. This finding was significant. It meant that nearly a quarter of the patients we saw in Jackson Park's Psychiatric Emergency Service didn't find a stable placement and treatment alternative in the community, indicating that more community support systems needed to be in place for severely mentally ill African Americans to remain in their community. Another major finding came from our comparison of how the police functioned in an affluent, white community verses a poor, African-American community. In the affluent, white community study, the police referred assaultive patients to the hospital six times more likely than they did non-assaultive patients. In our study, however, restrained patients were only twice as likely as non-restrained patients to have been referred to the hospital by the police. In the affluent, white community, the police acted as police. When they brought a patient to the emergency room, the patient would frequently be restrained because the police had detained the patient for behaving violently. In our context, a poor, African-American community, the police acted more like social service outreach workers. When they brought a patient to our emergency room, the patient would frequently not need to be placed in restraints. The police had picked the patient up for being homeless or acting bizarrely in the street. This finding made it clear that the context in which social services function frequently decides their roles. Research findings cannot be separated from the context in which they were made.

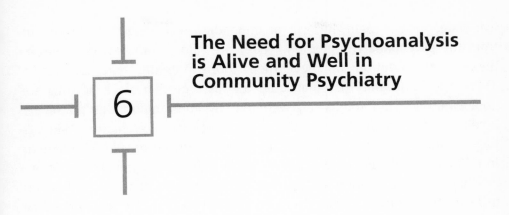

The Need for Psychoanalysis is Alive and Well in Community Psychiatry

6

While the author recognizes the positive impact community psychiatry has had on post-psychotic patients with the use of medical management and environmental manipulation, he demonstrates that there is a deficiency in the treatment of lower socioeconomic patients with neurotic illnesses. Specifically, neurotic patients tend to be given supportive therapy and psychopharmacotherapy when a form of psychoanalytic psychotherapy would be more appropriate. The author supports these contentions by presenting three cases that have a diagnosis of hysterical neurosis and which clearly demonstrate the economic, topographical, structural, dynamic, and genetic components of the psychoanalytic theory. Finally, as psychoanalytic psychotherapy is too time-consuming, the author suggests that Freud's early psychoanalytic technique of symptom removal by memory recovery be used when appropriate.

INTRODUCTION

Community psychiatry is often associated with the medical management of psychiatric patients who are usually psychotic and from lower socioeconomic classes. Lower socioeconomic patients are said to be too bound up in external stimuli stemming from "an acute extraordinary phys-

Originally printed as Bell Carl C. The need for psychoanalysis is alive and well in community psychiatry. *J Natl Med Assoc.* 1979;71:361–368.

ical state, such as pain, hunger, or impending real danger..."[1] to benefit from the psychoanalytic method. They are said to rather need environmental manipulation to meet their more pressing external needs. Therefore, community psychiatric clinics "assume that black persons are poor candidates for intensive psychotherapy and support this notion by invoking psychoanalytic theory."[2] A group of black psychiatric residents have pointed out, however, "This theory stresses that people who benefit from intensive psychotherapy are those whose ego strengths of motivation, intelligence, introspection, delay of gratification, and repudiation of action in favor of thinking are rated highly. Invariably a black person is rated as having few of the desired ego strengths and is therefore not a good candidate for anything more than the supportive therapies."[3]

The purpose of this paper is to demonstrate that a wealth of sophisticated psychoanalytic psychotherapeutic treatment cases are available through the practice of clinical community psychiatry. The author hopes to demonstrate that while the community psychiatry movement has admirable qualities, the tendency toward environmental management and pharmacotherapy tends to cause what Freud termed a psychoneurosis, to be overlooked. This leads to inappropriate somatic and sociologic treatment methods and tends to minimize the use of psychoanalytic psychotherapy as an appropriate treatment modality.

CASE REPORTS

Case 1

A 35-year-old, married black mother of three initially presented with a complaint of being nervous and tense for several months. She reported that she was upwardly mobile and that the stress of her success was causing her tension. Other reported symptoms were throat constriction, occasional anxiety attacks, and headaches. In addition, she complained of insomnia, secondary to being tense and fidgety. The initial diagnosis was anxiety neurosis. In an attempt to break the sleep loss/anxiety cycle and to relieve the patient's symptoms in a "typical public clinic" fashion, flurazepam 15 mg at bedtime was prescribed. She was given an appointment to return in two weeks and was asked to see her clinical therapist to receive supportive therapy, which hopefully would alleviate her stress and thus her symptoms. The patient returned in two weeks and was feeling better. At this time, the etiology of her tension was explored. The tension stemmed from a conflict: she wished to be dependent but viewed dependent characteristics as disgusting, so even just the thought of such a position was extremely anxiety-provoking.

Before the third two-week visit, she had been seen by a neurologist who had (in view of her unilateral attacks of nausea, visual phenomena, and throbbing pain) diagnosed her as having classical migraine headaches. She had been taking ergotamine and caffeine tablets, but as they did not bring relief, she was changed to a combination of phenobarbital, ergotamine, and alkaloids of belladonna, which decreased her headache frequency. Apparently, the headaches were triggered by anger and frustration that had their root in her task at work. As she was the supervisor on her job, she had to discipline her staff, which directly conflicted with her need to be liked (the boss is, by definition, a job involving unpopularity with the staff). With a supportive reality explanation of the difficulty inherent in her role as supervisor, the patient returned in two weeks having handled her job responsibilities a bit better and feeling proud of her more assertive manner.

She returned in two weeks to report she had been chronically angry with her husband for about five years but had never expressed it. She was angry with him because he had not lived up to her belief that by marrying him her wish to be "fulfilled" would come true. After realizing this dream was impossible, she struggled with what she felt to be her only alternative—to leave him as she had done her first husband after ten years of marriage and two children. She apparently had married the first time for similar reasons and obtained her first divorce when she realized her error. Her dilemma resulted from her belief that divorce was immoral and disgusting; since she had suffered enormous guilt from the first divorce, she did not know if a second divorce would be worth such self-reproaching. Because her headaches had decreased to tolerable frequency and because a two-week medication appointment and supportive therapy had been unable to soothe her stirred-up feelings, she fled from treatment.

The patient returned after seven months of absence because her headaches returned. She was back on medication but without relief. She reported she was having a splitting migraine headache during this return interview; yet, because of her infective laughter and good mood, it was concluded that the "migraine headaches" had a hysterical base. Her reason for fleeing treatment was discovered at this time. She reported that she left because although the initial therapy had improved her marriage, enabled her to function better at work, and allowed her to become more independent, she was afraid that if she grew too much, she would outgrow her husband and stop loving him. She returned in two weeks and reported her headaches were better. Furthermore, she was able to give a clearer picture of her intrapsychic conflicts. Essentially, she reported she maintained a "front" of being the competent, well-balanced, omni-giving mother; adequate work supervisor; perfect wife; and total woman. This was the initial image she had projected and that had been accepted; therefore, her tension was attributed to environmental stress that would probably yield to supportive treatment and pharmacotherapy. On the inside, she felt afraid, alone, empty, helpless, and unacceptable. She told of her mother who had died after giving everything to her kids and leaving nothing for herself. The patient's greatest fear was that she would end up in a similar fashion. She hated to admit that she was so tense and unable to cope, since that was an indication of weak character. She was also concerned about what others thought about her, as well as what she thought of herself. At this point, it was clear that supportive management and pharmacotherapy were not the treatments of choice. With special permission from the clinic director, the clinical community psychiatrist's role was changed from the usual "evaluator and medicator" to psychotherapist. Thus, she began to be seen for thirty minutes per week.

In the first session, collection of some historical information about her earlier life was initiated. She was raised by her moralistic paternal grandparents for reasons unclear to her but which had something to do with her mother's inability to care for her. She was the eldest of three children and was the first to be cared for by this extended family system. Apparently, her father and mother had been separated, owing to her father's vagabond nature. She reported that her grandparents were very giving of material things but that their idea of giving emotionally constituted a very moral upbringing. She lived with her father for three years from ages nine to twelve and thereafter lived with her mother. She described her father as a "happy-go-lucky" guy and reported that her time with him was the happiest in her life. She was disappointed in her mother because her grandparents had told her that her mother was inadequate. She went to college, but after pressure from her boyfriend to have sexual relations, she dropped out and married him. The upshot of this decision was that while she had married to legitimatize sexual relations, she remained frigid for the ten years of their marriage. She reported that she felt she had to submerge herself for ten years in order to try to make her marriage work, as "divorce was a sin." Her grandparents apparently drummed into her head that a woman unable to keep her marriage afloat was clearly inadequate—case in point, her mother, and she believed them. She remarried two years after her divorce but still bore guilt from her first and unforgivable failure. It became clear that she was operating on an all-good or all-bad philosophy, characteristic of a conscience that "becomes pathological when it functions in too rigid or too automatic a manner, so that realistic judgment about the actual outcome of intended actions is disturbed ('archaic superego')."[1]

During the next visit, the patient was reluctant to talk and told of the difficulty she had in revealing her "ugliness" to another person. She felt it was shameful that she had reported her grandparents had a low opinion of her mother, considering all they had given the patient. Her resistance to examine her difficulty in seeing shades of gray was interpreted, and a repressed memory that she had not thought of for a long time surfaced, just popping into her head. She said that her grandmother was a light-skinned woman who could pass for white and as a result, get a seat on the bus in Mississippi, where she had been raised. One day the patient asked if she could accompany her grandmother shopping. She was told no. It was explained to her that her grandmother would be burdened with packages and that because of the patient's darker color, if she went along, her grandmother would be unable to get a bus seat. Although the patient realized the difficult time her grandmother would have had, being loaded with bundles, she felt extremely rejected and unacceptable, even though she was a little girl. Since then, she became very color-conscious and felt dark, although her color could be described as "peanut butter." It is significant that this was her earliest memory and that it represented a screen memory. During the next session, the patient appeared quite defensive due to her need to appear well put-together. When told that her need to be free of all problems and weaknesses was based on a myth and that she was just as plagued as everyone else, she interpreted this to mean she was unimportant. She talked of feeling betrayed, especially after she had trusted and shown all of her ugliness. I apologized for having hurt her, as that was not my intention. I stated that it should be clear to her that if she only presented her "mask," no one would be able to understand how she truly felt.

The next session provided another thread in her repeated experience that her natural drives and biological status were unacceptable and thus had to be warded off by psychic defense maneuvers. She reported that she feared her husband would abandon her because she was unacceptable. This was traced back to the onset of her menses, when she was living with her father. During that time, her father took her to her mother under the guise of a summer visit, only to leave her there for the rest of her unmarried life. She remembered how she had worn summer clothes until the first snow, when her mother made her wear winter clothes. She apparently had attempted to deny that summer was over and thereby deny that her father had abandoned her. She stated that this circumstance caused her to lose her bad temper and become a straight-A student, as well as become a very compulsive and clean child at age 13. We have evidence of the two points by which Freud characterized Frau von N's psychical situation: (1) "The distressing affects attaching to her traumatic experiences had remained unresolved..."[4] and (2) "Her memory exhibited a lively activity which sometimes spontaneously, sometimes in response to a contemporary stimulus, brought her traumas with their accompanying affects bit by bit into her present-day consciousness."[4] Clearly, in this instance, the patient had felt herself unacceptable ("good girls don't show temper") and dirty (possibly from her onset of puberty and thus acquisition of genital primacy, not to mention with a bloody discharge) and used defenses of denial, reaction formation, and repression.[1] At this point in treatment, the patient "acted out" (this was due to the lack of frequent visits, which are designed to soothe the patient from the intensity of emotions stirred up) and bought a new car without telling her husband. This was apparently done to bolster her low self-esteem. It was at this point that she was urged to undertake formal analysis. However, owing to her attachment to the therapist, she declined. Since she took the suggestion as a rejection, she was not pressed on this issue. In addition, the likelihood of such a possibility was beyond her reach, due to environmental and socioeconomic factors.

The next session revealed the patient's fear of the dark, which had persisted since age seven and caused her to need to sleep with the lights on. Her fear was not felt when with another person. Her fear would not have been present had her husband not been absent from home due to the nature of his work. She was able to recognize that when he left, she felt hurt and abandoned. She was convinced he would never return, although she knew better. Yet, when he did return, rather than being happy, she was angry with him. It was pointed out that separation brought up issues of self-worth. These dynamics apparently stem from primitive methods involved in the regulation of self-esteem. Specifically, the first need for a relationship stems from the need to remove disturbing displeasure; therefore, external supplies determine the self-satisfaction or self-esteem. "It is the 'fear over loss of love' or rather loss of help and protection. This fear is more intense than it would be if it represented only a rational judgment about real danger because the early self-esteem is regulated by means of external supplies, so that a loss of help and protection means also a loss of self-esteem."[1]

During a later session, the patient's infective laughter was noted to be associated with her explaining how unacceptable she felt. Her humorous recounting of her believed being was designed to tell of her ugliness yet make its recognition so pleasant (by virtue of the humor she injected) that she would not be rejected. Her gregarious, active, dependent behavior was interpreted to her by telling her that she seduced people into liking and caring for her. Her response to the interpretation was that while she admitted it was accurate, she felt "clubbed."

At the next session, we discussed the colitis attack she suffered during the week after she was told she was sneaking dependency. She was able to recognize that her interpretation had caused her symptoms; she further realized that reacting to the interpretations as criticisms made it all the more difficult for interpretations to be made. Again, had there been more time to see her, the "acting out" behavior would not have needed to be as severe. She returned determined to come to grips with her dependency needs; yet, her revulsion for this trait served as a roadblock. During the session, an old memory resurfaced. Her grandparents had turned her against her mother by telling her that her mother was an inadequate, dependent person. This memory was followed by her sadness at having believed them and never having been able to relax her "critical faculty" and give her mother a fair chance. Tremendous anger at her grandparents for having told her such things about her mother also followed. The connection was made that she and her mother were said to be made from the same mold. This had always disturbed her; she knew that if she were dependent like her mother, she would be found similarly unacceptable.

The next session centered on her anger from feeling she had never been truly loved or accepted. She recognized that this feeling was so strong that when people (husband and children) told her they loved her, she did not believe they were sincere. The next visit saw the patient trying to structure the session in a defensive maneuver to avoid the painful feeling of "never having been loved," which would have led to her lack of self-esteem, i.e., a disturbance in her narcissistic development. "In persons whose self-esteem is regulated by the anxiety over loss of love, secondary anxieties and guilt feelings may be aroused if they try to enforce the necessary supplies by objectional means. Particularly unfortunate are persons who need narcissistic supplies but who at the same time unconsciously are afraid of receiving them."[1] In this case, "enforcing the necessary supplies by objectional means" consisted of using dependency. It is interesting to note that "guilt feelings are connected with oral sensations, or rather with intestinal sensations,"[1] and that the patient had colitis for one week after feeling guilty due to recognition of her use of active dependence to gain approval. Furthermore, it was later learned she had been a thumb-sucker. This session was also one in which she related being unable to comfort herself during the week when she did not see the therapist. The issue was raised of her dependency on the therapist and how disappointing that had been for her. Her response to this was to talk of her lack of closeness to anyone except her father. She said that when she was with her father, she had had fun, but that fun had somehow seemed sinful.

At the next session, she revealed her fear that her dependency would show up in sexual behavior. In addition, she wished her husband would be more affectionate than sexual, but she had to engage in sex with him to receive affection from him. The patient during her next visit spoke quite intellectually about the link between intimacy and sexuality. She seemed to be quite resistive to experiencing the feelings associated with her words (isolation of affect). She returned in a week with a great deal of sexual inhibition and guilt. When asked about masturbation, she practically had to be scraped off the ceiling. Her grandmother had told her masturbation would cause a person to go crazy. She reported that though she did not masturbate, she felt the urge, which made her feel "dirty."

From her presentation in the following session, it was evident that she had managed to scare herself at the preceding one. She arrived very upset over the previous session and refused to deal with any issues of sexuality, dependency, or aggression, as those were unacceptable impulses that made her ugly. The patient came in a week later and was quite on edge. Apparently, she had been harassing her husband to prove he loved her. She "knows" this is related to her feeling inadequate and "unloved," yet she cannot control it. She reported recurrent dreams of her sitting in my lap and my simply holding and comforting her. She admitted that she feared that I might interpret this dream as a sexual one and reassured me that it was not! She further felt ashamed of having traded sex for affection; even when she got affection (which she would not allow herself to believe as sincere), she changed it into sexual feelings. She also admitted that she was starting to feel I was genuinely concerned about her.

The next session, the patient returned with a horrible headache that had started the day before her visit. It was surmised that she had again scared herself; yet, apparently having once tried to scare herself out of treatment and having had that fail (she returned several months later), her treatment contract and therapeutic bond were strong enough to combat her fear. At any rate, it was decided to attempt tracing the psychic origin of her headaches. Her first memory of having the headaches was when she had decided to return to therapy. She told me that she had gotten some pictures of her deceased mother restored. They cost more than she had anticipated, and when she told her husband, he chastised her for being too extravagant. She developed a headache and was bedridden for one week. During this time, she lost her sight and feeling on the left side of her body; however, she was not concerned enough to call for a physician (la belle indifference).

She said the next memory seemed to be "in the back of my head but there seems to be some sort of veil in front of it." She was asked to close her eyes and take ten deep abdominal breaths. Suddenly, she explained it was as though a screen had been lifted, and she was able to remember her first episode of headaches. It was right after she and her family had buried her mother. She proceeded to tell me that her mother had had breast cancer that had metastasized to the brain and as a result had to be hospitalized for seven months. The patient visited her mother every day and would frequently spend the night on weekends to aid in her care. During this time, her mother had developed (based on what was described) an organic brain syndrome, and apparently along with headaches, had difficulty recognizing her daughter. With the resurfacing of these memories, the patient's headaches abated, and she left the office in as unburdened and carefree a state as had ever been observed in her. Freud and Breuer state, "…in the anamnesis of hysteria we so often come across the two great pathogenic factors of being in love and sick-nursing."[4] The etiology of her symptom of "migraine headaches" was due to multiple experiences as was with the case of Frau Emmy, and as Freud stated, "Almost invariably when I have investigated the determinants of such conditions what I have come upon has not been a single traumatic cause but a group of similar ones."[4]

The patient returned a week later to report she had not experienced any headaches. She could feel a sensation in her head, but it was not painful. Instead, the pain was in her neck, and she insisted I stop trying to "talk away" her symptoms (although she acknowledged they were psychological in nature) and give her some medication. Her general practitioner had already given her chlorzoxazone 500 mg and acetaminophen 600 mg four times a day. She was told that while my talking her headache away had relieved her symptoms, there were some emotions she did not want to deal with that had been stirred up. As Freud and Breuer reported, "each individual hysterical symptom immediately and permanently disappeared when we had succeeded in bringing clearly to light the memory of the event by which it was provoked and in arousing its accompanying affect, and when the patient had described that event in the greatest possible detail and had put the affect into words."[4] Freud later points out the existence of a resistance to recollecting these painful, traumatic memories, which thus risks possibly overwhelming the ego. Again, the frequency of this patient's visits did not allow for the therapist to sit with her through the pain that was uncovered; this may have caused her to reconvert her memories into fresh symptoms. This patient's treatment continues.

Case 2

A 35-year-old black, unmarried, childless female who was first seen five years ago as an inpatient, came to the clinic after having been recently discharged from a local general hospital. She had been hospitalized in the psychiatric unit because of "insomnia and depression." She had been receiving imipramine 50 mg three times a day. She came to report that while her medication allowed her to sleep, she had begun to have acute anxiety attacks characterized by palpitations, hyperventilation, muscular spasms, blackouts, paresthesias, and an overwhelming fear of death. She reported that she was also quite phobic of open spaces. She was appropriately dressed and behaved normally, with the exception of seeming quite tense. Her associations were intact and she denied having hallucinations, thought broadcasting, insomnia (while medicated), suicidal or homicidal ideation, or a pervasive depressive mood. She had the capacity for humor and hope for the future. Her main preoccupation was the overwhelming anxiety she experienced without warning. She was well oriented to person, time, and place.

The author decided to continue her on her discharge medication until a review of her past history and the initial impression of her five years prior could be performed. The patient returned in two weeks for a medication review and reported that the imipramine "really knocks me out at night," but that she was doing well. The patient returned in one month for another review and again reported she was well. In three weeks, the patient returned to report that she had had four anxiety attacks since the last visit. As the attacks may have been a reaction to the antidepressant, her dose was decreased to imipramine 50 mg at bedtime and thioridazine 100 mg once or twice at bedtime. The patient returned in two weeks to report that she had continued to have anxiety attacks. She complained of numbness, chills, and headaches. The interesting feature was that while she was out of the country for one week, the attacks stopped but had resumed when she returned (she had lost her fear of open spaces just long enough to go on vacation). As my suspicions about the hysterical nature of her symptoms increased with this report, she was asked about her first fainting spell. She reported that it had occurred when she was twelve and had been informed that her mother needed surgery. Upon asking why she was so easily upset, she reported that she grew up afraid. Apparently, she had been molested by an uncle at age three and again by her brother and stepfather when she was eleven and thirteen. The patient, on being asked about a gynecological history, reported she had experienced two episodes of pseudocyesis. Apparently, she had aborted her first pregnancy and subsequent to this, her periods had stopped on two occasions. Both times, she presented to a clinic and was informed she was pregnant. She reports that during both of the episodes, she regularly visited the clinic for about six months and even began "showing." Her first anxiety attack without fainting occurred about six years ago when she went to the funeral of the uncle who had molested her. She told me of another traumatic life event—her mother would often start beating her while she was asleep, apparently without warning or cause. "In discussing the traumatic neurosis, it was noted that the state of being flooded with excitation gave rise to the need for blocking acceptance of further stimulation; perception and other ego functions were blocked or diminished by forceful countercathexes. These types of "defenses," especially their climax—fainting, may be regarded as the pattern according to which all other pathogenic defenses are formed; fainting is a complete cessation of certain functions of the ego."[1]

The patient returned in two weeks to report that she had had only a few mild attacks. Apparently, she had been able to identify some of the reasons for her attacks and was able to calm herself down. Thus, again, we have evidence that "if a hysterical subject seeks intentionally to forget an experience or forcibly repudiates, inhibits, and suppresses an intention or an idea, these Psychical acts, as a consequence, enter the second state of consciousness; from there they produce their permanent effects and the memory of them returns as a hysterical attack."[5] The patient continued to do well over the next three months despite my having discontinued the antipsychotic and antidepressant medication she was taking. She was seen about once every three weeks during this period and received a prescription for diazepam 5 mg every six hours if needed.

The patient was not seen again until after six months of absence. She returned to report that while she had done well during that time, she had recently begun to again experience anxiety attacks characterized by fear of death, wanting to run, feeling hollow inside, and losing her capacity to taste. Apparently, her stepfather had recently died, which was causing the recent exacerbation of her symptoms. She reported that she was under the care of a physician who thought she had pituitary disease and that she had begun to get special tests. The patient returned in one month's time to report her tests were all normal and that she had been doing well on the clorazepate 15 mg, which had been prescribed if she needed it, at bedtime. As her case was replete with somatic symptoms, it was decided to schedule some special time with her in an attempt to clearly identify what had heretofore presented as an endogenous depression, an anxiety neurosis, a psychophysiologic reaction, and a borderline syndrome childhood history. I used the term "special time" because my ordinary role had been to assess the patient for psychopharmacotherapy and initiate the treatment with medication reviews spaced about three weeks to one month apart.

The initial interview was usually about 30–45 minutes, focusing on symptom assessment, some early history, a history of past hospitalizations, and possibly some diagnostic and dynamic formulations. There was also an attempt to perform an adequate mental status and to rule out organicity as well. The focus of the 15-minute medication review was primarily medication management. Thus, an in-depth symptom review that might take an hour had to be regarded as special time.

The patient reported that her medical history began when she was about 15 years old, when she became pregnant and her mother forced her to have an abortion. She further reported that she had felt sickly for most of her life. She had had fainting spells, loss of control of her left arm and leg, loss of speech, hyperventilation, fatigue, a lump in her throat, dysuria, chest pain, dizziness, palpitations, breathing difficulty, nausea, frequent constipation, occasional anorexia, occasional vomiting, dysmenorrhea for longer than two months, dyspareunia, pseudocyesis, vomiting during pregnancy (she had never successfully delivered), back pain, joint pain, breast pain, nervousness, fearfulness, and depression. Hospital records revealed her first hospitalization was six years prior to my first time seeing her at the clinic. At that time, she was diagnosed as having a depressive neurosis. She was reported to be suicidal with dizziness, blackouts, and nervousness. She was discharged on chlorpromazine 50 mg three times a day and thiothixene 2 mg three times a day.

The next hospitalization occurred a year later, which was when I first saw her as an inpatient. I had diagnosed her as having an acute transient stress reaction, ruling out hysteria. She had been having side reactions on the chlorpromazine and thiothixene. When they were discontinued, she improved. At that time, her medical history revealed she had had five dilatations and curettages, a history of gall bladder disease, ulcers, hyperventilation, stiffness, anxiety, agitation, and blackouts. She was put on diazepam and showed further improvement. At that time, upper and lower GI series as was her gall bladder series were negative. The next year, she had undergone a laparotomy because of unexplainable lower abdominal pain upon urination, defecation, and intercourse. The only report of pathological findings was a "borderline infantile uterus." Her appendix was also removed during this surgery. Methylene blue dye test for tubal patency was normal, as were her electroencephalogram, intravenous pyelogram, chest x-ray, and upper and lower GI and gall bladder series. The final hospitalization was the one she had told of during her first clinic visit. During this hospitalization, she was found to be depressed, with premature menopause and trichomonas vaginitis. Neurologic evaluation and brain scan were normal. She had complained of numbness of her left leg and arm, for which she was checked. Electrocardiogram was normal.

Finally, armed with enough history to make a clear diagnosis of hysterical neurosis, it was learned that the patient would not be returning. She apparently had approached her mental health worker with a complaint that she had a conflict with me, and had requested a change in her doctor. This request was fulfilled. She began to see another physician who although recognizing the hysterical component to the patient's illness, continued her on clorazepate 15 mg at bedtime as needed and was to see her every three to four weeks for medication review. It was later learned that the conflict arose because I would not call in her prescription for clorazepate when she failed to show up for an appointment.

Case 3

A 38-year-old black, divorced female, who during the first interview was so agitated, anxious, tense, and "choked up," she was unable to tolerate more than five minutes of the session. I reviewed her record and discovered that she had been seen by another clinic psychiatrist prior to seeing me. The first psychiatrist had found it equally difficult to obtain information. She recorded a history of "migraine headaches" and while she felt the patient had a schizoid personality or depression, she was not sure because she lacked an adequate history. At any rate, she placed the patient on amitriptyline 75 mg at bedtime. The woman returned in two weeks much improved. She spoke spontaneously, smiled, laughed, and seemed capable of interpersonal interaction. She was seen again one month later and at that time was placed on amitriptyline 100 mg at bedtime and was given an appointment to return in three months (with enough medication for the duration). The patient returned in three months to report she had stopped taking the medication one month before and had begun experiencing insomnia. In addition, she reported memory gaps during which she forgot whole days. She was then placed on perphenazine 2 mg and amitriptyline 25 mg, three at bedtime. The patient returned in one week and, since she had begun to improve, was given a three-week supply of medication and an appointment for when her medication ran out. She returned and again reported that she was losing "big chunks of my days." The patient's psychiatrist then advised her to get an organic work-up and return in one week. At that time, I inherited her case (after the first psychiatrist resigned). All that resulted from her first session with me was her denial of suicidal or homicidal ideation, and the information that both the amitriptyline and an amitriptyline and perphenazine combination had "knocked her out." She was found to be quite easily upset and dramatic.

She was seen one month later (there is sometimes a month lag between when a patient first presents and the first diagnostic session with a psychiatrist). While she was able to complete the interview, she remained very easily upset and quite dramatic. She demonstrated an irregular breathing pattern, alternating between small bouts of hyperventilation, breath-holding, and sighing. As she also demonstrated globus hystericus, she was asked if she ever became so upset that she lost track of time. She seemed almost panic-stricken but said yes. When asked if she had another person inside her, she replied, "How could that be possible?" Her therapist, who had worked with her for one year (and who was sitting in to reassure the patient), asked, "What about Ms. B?" to the patient (Ms.

A). The patient was asked to close her eyes, take ten deep breaths, and let Ms. B out. On doing so, Ms. B emerged a warm, relaxed, even-breathing, "mellow" woman. We talked a bit about how she had managed to get out more recently and how Ms. A was an "old stick in the mud and an old fogy." When her therapist asked Ms. B whether she was as religious as Ms. A (who was of the Church of God religion), the patient painfully grabbed her head, and Ms. A returned with a splitting "migraine headache." Her pleasant smile returned to the grimace that had been apparent before her other personality (Ms. B) had emerged.

When she was seen one month later, she revealed that she had fainted the previous week. She reported she had been doing well otherwise and was placed on diazepam 5 mg twice a day. Ms. B was called forth since Ms. A was unable to say how long she had been split into two personalities. Ms. B told me that her first memory was when she was four years old and she and her cousin took their clothes off and "played with one another." Ms. B apparently had a greater knowledge of Ms. A than Ms. A had of her, and she told me that Ms. A could not "get away with what I do." She also told of how, on a church-arranged date, Ms. A had gone into the bathroom and Ms. B had come out. She reported that she and Ms. A's date had a wild time and that Ms. A woke up the next morning feeling guilty but not knowing why. Ms. B stated that Ms. A hated to be touched. When asked why, she reported she did not know. When asked if Ms. A had ever been raped, Ms. B got angry and stated she did not know everything about Ms. A. She said Ms. A should be asked, and in a flash, Ms. A was back with a mild headache and just as anxious as ever. Ms. A's earliest memory was of her stepfather and how greatly she hated him. She did remember the episode with her cousin and the small town scandal it produced when they were caught. When asked if she had ever been molested, she reported that at age 18 she had been grabbed, but did not go into details.

On her next visit two weeks later, she was questioned further about her relationship with her stepfather. He apparently had undressed her when she was ten years old and had tried to molest her. He had made this a habit whenever he could get her alone. She reported that when she was 14, she became Ms. A, and that prior to that, she had been that "sweet Ms. C child." She showed me a birth certificate she said was hers but which had Ms. C's name on it. She had had her first sexual experience at the age of 14 with an older man who told her "that was what she needed." Apparently, her first sexual experience had revolted her so much that she changed her identity. Shortly thereafter, she left home and moved to Chicago (possibly in a fugue state?). When asked more about Ms. C, her arm began to hurt, and she (Ms. A) wondered if Ms. B was just another name for Ms. C, who Ms. A had tried to "kill" because she (Ms. C) was a "tramp." Apparently, this patient, like Breuer's patient Anna O., had several "distinct states of consciousness."[4] As with fainting and other ego mechanisms of defense, "Dissociative reactions are attempts to escape from excessive tension and anxiety by separating off some parts of personality function from the rest."[6]

Further information was gathered to obtain a complete symptom history to establish a Feighner, Robins, Guze, et al.[7] research diagnosis of hysteria, as was done in the other two cases. The patient indeed had a complicated medical history prior to age 35. She reported a history of dysmenorrhea, stomach pains, headaches, temporary blindness, paralysis, fainting, fatigue, a lump in throat, breathing difficulties, palpitations, dizziness, anxiety attacks, nausea, anorexia, abdominal pain, sexual indifference, dyspareunia, back pain, joint pain, amnesia, depression, and nervousness. She reported that she had had a total hysterectomy about eight years prior to her visit to the clinic and had received hormones for a short period of time. Thus, a clear diagnosis of hysteria (dissociative and conversion type) was made.

During her next visit, her fainting spells were traced to her first menstruation, which started at age 17. She reported that when she looked down and saw that she had stained her dress, she fainted. She refused to go into further details. Just getting her to talk about the incident was quite difficult. Her treatment continues. Despite massive resistance, she has been gradually improving.

DISCUSSION

Often in clinical community psychiatry, the physician's time is so valuable that most of it is spent during non-psychotherapeutic time, during which medication is prescribed. The psychotherapy is left to the psychologists, social workers, and community mental health workers. While they do admirable work with family therapy, group psychotherapy, counseling, and management, it is rare to find one of their number who has been adequately trained and supervised in psychoanalytic psychotherapy. "The development of community mental health centers and the use of therapies other than long-term, analytically oriented approaches were in direct response to the need of providing psychiatric services to the entire spectrum of the American public."[8]

Thus, while the present clinical community system does an excellent job in caring for "after-care" patients who primarily need medication and management, there is a clear deficiency in provision of appropriate treatment modalities to patients whose illness is more neurotic than psychotic. This lack of service is justified with the myth that lower socioeconomic patients are too poor to have a need for psychoanalysis. If you are poor, then by definition you are seen to somehow lack "ego strength," or you would otherwise better your situation. Since you cannot do so, you are seen to be not that sophisticated, and certainly not sophisticated enough to benefit from psychoanalytic psychotherapy. The belief is that the poor for the most part, are not suffering as much from neurotic illnesses as they are from poverty, so an attempt is made to relieve their plight by strengthening their social services and advocacy. Though this is true, we overlook that group of people who, because they have neurotic conflicts, tend to be ineffective at achieving their goals in life and are thus poor.

The three cases documented here have clearly demonstrated that lower socioeconomic patients can suffer from a classical neurosis and do in fact clearly show the topographical, dynamic, economic, genetic, and structural components of Freud's work on hysteria. Case 1 demonstrates not only the role of repression in neurotic symptom formation but also that neurotic patients do not quite fit into plans for using valuable psychiatric time. You may tell a patient whose emotions and memories you are uncovering, "Do not let your emotions drag you into something you should not be doing; just sit and watch them. We know they are rooted in the past and as a result, may not fit into your present-day life, so please be careful." Regardless of how many times you say this, however, the patient may still need more than one session a week to be soothed. Yet, what is the physician to do? Oftentimes in clinical community psychiatry, the necessities for doing an adequate job are too few and too far apart. As a result, one may try a variation of standard psychoanalytic psychotherapy in the belief that it will do more good than harm.

Case 2 demonstrates that there is a lack of understanding of physician-patient relationships, types of resistances, and transference and counter-transference phenomena that occur in a treatment setting involving uncovering repressed memories. This author suspected that the patient had been symptom-free for eight months after her original psychic trauma had been explored precisely because those memories had been made conscious. Furthermore, she realized that controlled drug prescriptions could not be refilled by phone; thus, her desire for a change in psychiatrist was likely motivated by other reasons. As Freud and Breuer noted, "A good number of the patients who would be suitable for this form of treatment abandon the doctor as soon as the suspicion begins to dawn on them of the direction in which the investigation is leading."[4] There was not enough time to explore the dynamics of this case because a considerable chunk of special time was being used to investigate the first case. However, it seems clear that psychoanalytic psychotherapy should have been the treatment of choice in the second case, rather than a medication review of her minor tranquilizer every four weeks and supportive therapy with a community mental health worker who, unfortunately, was not trained in recognizing psychodynamic resistances. This of course raises another issue in the use of psychiatric time in clinical community psychiatry—specifically, staff training and the need for time to follow up on cases that "get lost in the cracks." Fortunately, the clinic director recognized the need for training and set aside time for that purpose. However, patient follow-up was not as easy to handle because of the tremendous flow of patients; thus, it becomes necessary for the patient's worker or therapist to make sure the patient does not get lost.

Case 3 brings up two points in the mismanagement of clinical community psychiatric patients who have neurotic illness. The therapist had known of the existence of another side of the patient for about one year prior to the investigation; however, she assumed that it was a conscious attempt to find an excuse for the patient's "bad, unacceptable behavior." As a result, she employed the Gestalt technique of having the patient talk to her "other self" by switching back and forth on two chairs (each chair corresponding to the role played by Ms. A or Ms. B). While this shows intuitive awareness of the problem, it does not acknowledge the existence of an unconscious and does not acknowledge that the recovery of a repressed memory might alleviate hysterical symptoms. As Freud and Breuer stated: "Thus, a little girl suffered for years from attacks of general convulsions which could well be, and indeed were, regarded as epileptic. She was hypnotized with a view to a differential diagnosis, and promptly had one of her attacks. She was asked what she was seeing and replied, 'The dog! The dog's coming!'; and in fact it turned out that she had had the first of her attacks after being chased by a savage dog. The success of the treatment confirmed the choice of diagnosis."[4]

The second point Case 3 brings up is that it was assumed that this patient's difficulties certainly could not have been psychoneurotic. It was assumed that she was likely experiencing a major psychotic illness; thus, she was given antipsychotic medication and a return appointment in three months. To quote James Comer: "Psychiatric treatment has always been costly, and minorities that experienced legislative discrimination and denial of opportunity in this country have always been poor. Thus, most of those who have manifested signs of severe psychological problems have received custodial care or been treated as criminals, while many middle-class white persons with similar symptoms have received psychiatric treatment."[8] Furthermore, "among patients treated in mental health facilities whites are more likely to be diagnosed with depressive disorders while blacks or nonwhites are more likely to be diagnosed as schizophrenic."[9] One wonders how many cases of hysterical psychosis are diagnosed as schizophrenic, not to mention the hysterics who simply present with a confusing diagnostic picture.

CONCLUSIONS

First, while there is a need for supportive therapy and management of psychiatric patients in clinical community psychiatry, there is also a need for "the practical aim of treatment...to remove all possible symptoms and to replace them with conscious thoughts..."[4] possibly through symptom etiology tracking rather than classical psychoanalytic psychotherapy. As Fenichel points out:

On one hand the therapist may give rest, reassurance, the satisfaction of wishes for passivity and dependence—'take-it-easy' suggestions. On the other hand, he may give catharsis, the opportunity for stormy discharges and for the repeated re-experiencing of the trauma, and a verbalization and clarification of the conflicts involved. The second method is, when applicable, a more direct help; the first one becomes necessary when the ego is too frightened, when a working through of the traumatic event is still unbearable and would still be too much of a repetition of the traumatic character of the experience.[1]

Secondly, clinical community psychiatry more often than not overlooks the needs of the lower socioeconomic neurotic patient, partially because of a myth that such patients do not exist and partly because of economic factors involved in the appropriate treatment of such patients.

Finally, since community psychiatry does rely on the services of nonpsychiatric professionals (who hopefully are as mature as the therapist in Case 3, who upon realizing she did not grasp the patient's dynamics, sought out and accepted consultation), clinical community psychiatric time must also allow for staff development. Therapists tend to seek to ignore their patient's experiences of anxiety to avoid being reminded of their own. Hopefully, this will not prevent us from giving patients the proper treatment.

COMMENTARY

This article could have easily been placed in Section Four, "States of Consciousness," because the three case histories presented illustrate the states of consciousness "dreaming," "repressed memory," "states of fragmentation," and "states of frenzy." However, because the article also addresses intervention and advocacy, it was placed here. Its line of inquiry remains very useful to me in my current work. In many ways, it was my first real experience in trying to relieve traumatic stress and various stress-related disorders in African Americans (see Chapter 3). Since writing it, I've been identified as one of the few African-American psychiatrists who advocates using the psychoanalytic theory in helping African-American patients cope with stress. As a result, fifteen years after I wrote this article, I was invited to write two other papers on the usefulness of psychoanalytic theory in public mental health programs.

The first was "Is Psychoanalytic Therapy Relevant for Public Mental Health Programs?" (In: Kirk SA, Einbinder SD, eds. *Controversial Issues in Mental Health*. New York: Allen and Bacon; 1994:118–130). It presented two new cases of African Americans helped by understanding and applying psychoanalytic theory during their treatment. The first case involved a woman who'd been robbed once and threatened once, but who hadn't been physically harmed in any way. Because of her stress, she developed acute anxiety symptoms. In her fifth session, I came upon an apparent gap in her memory and consciousness. As I pressed her to remember what she was thinking during her second attack, she told me she could not say because her mind was blank. Finally, she told me she was thinking she was glad her young daughter was not with her. The only sense I could make of it was that she was afraid her daughter would see something that was horrible. I asked the patient if she'd ever been raped. The patient fell on the floor and told me she couldn't remember. When I asked why, she told me it was as if there was a wall between her and her memory. When I pressed her to try remembering, she recalled having been raped as a teenager. After she recounted the event in detail to me, she sat back in her chair. With a great sigh of relief, she looked at me and told me she had not thought of that in years. She went on to say she felt as though a great weight had been lifted from her. I never had a clearer case of "symptom removal" by "making the unconscious conscious." The second case I presented involved the same. There, I used dream interpretation to get at the repressed unconscious memory that was causing the symptom.

The second article I was asked to write, "Is Psychoanalytic Therapy Relevant for Public Health Programs?" (*Psychiatr Times*. 1994;11:31–34), was co-written with K. Davis. In this article, I presented the case of the 13-year-old black female with traumatic stress resulting in a Learning Disorder Not Otherwise Specified. I had earlier written about the same patient in "Stress-Related Disorders in African-American Children" (see Chapter 3).

There is concern that Freud's observations don't apply to 21st-century African Americans. He was, after all, middle-class and Jewish, and made his observations in Europe during the late 19th and early 20th century. Until I had the opportunity to attend to these three patients, I too doubted if Freud's theories applied to the poor, African-American population I was treating. In fact, I had doubts that his theories had any validity at all. However, these initial reservations didn't stop me from throwing around terms like unconscious, repression, dissociation, and hysteria during my residency. I was learning this jargon because it was important in the psychiatric culture I was joining. Looking back, I realize very few of us knew what those terms really meant, because only a few of us had directly observed their manifestation. At the time, I wasn't one of the privileged few. Fortunately, though, I had good teachers like Dr. Merton Gill, who taught me to be patient and simply observe human behavior while trying to be helpful. The insights contained in this article came because of that patience and observation. I'll be eternally grateful for the instruction that exposed this universal facet of human behavior to me.

Now at the CMHC, most of my time spent with patients is with both adults and children who are seriously and persistently mentally ill. I haven't been able to apply the psychoanalytic theory to such patients because they most likely suffer from a major imbalance in their brain chemistry, which responds to medication and psychosocial rehabilitation. On the other hand, I've found psychoanalytic theory very helpful in understanding anxiety symptoms that result from children being exposed to traumatic stress. The thread of psychoanalytic theory can also be found in the first case presented in Chapter 3 of this book. By presenting these cases, I hope that other African-American mental health professionals will realize that while the psychoanalytic theory wasn't developed with us in mind, it still holds some useful insights and tools that can help African Americans cope with stress constructively.

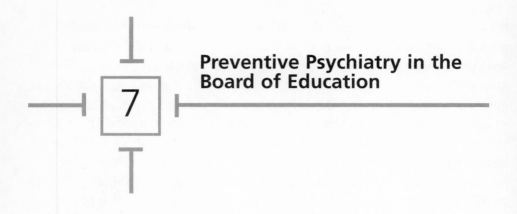

Preventive Psychiatry in the Board of Education

The Board of Education has a significant role in the psychiatric prevention of criminal and psychiatric disorders. Two hundred and seventy-four children were seen over a two-year period, and their diagnostic groupings are presented. Follow-up was possible on 150 of the children, and it was found that 70% of them were better. The findings and conclusions from this sample are presented.

INTRODUCTION

Questions are constantly being raised about what needs to be done about the high incidence of rape, murder, crime, drug abuse, alcoholism, child abuse, child molestation, mental illness, and suicide. It seems clear that in order to decrease these forms of social maladjustment, the children who will become rapists, murderers, criminals, drug abusers, child molesters, psychiatric patients, and suicide victims need to be raised differently right now, rather than waiting to begin corrective measures until after their psychopathological patterns are solidly formed. It is certainly easier to treat an explosive child before he has grown several feet, put on 100 pounds, and becomes legally responsible for himself.

Originally printed as Bell Carl C. Preventive psychiatry in the Board of Education. *J Natl Med Assoc.* 1979;71:881–886.

The Board of Education is the political administrative group responsible for providing the public school environment, the primary social contact (other than family) for children. The school can thus provide programs that counteract "the stressful or potentially harmful social conditions that produce mental illness by promptly intervening when such conditions exist."[1] Children are present in school during the day, five days a week with other children and adults; this social milieu is perfect for direct observation of interpersonal relatedness of children.[2] One can thus observe and identify children with problems that, given time, could develop into full-blown criminal or psychiatric disorders. The school can be a tremendous aid in early identification and treatment (secondary prevention).[1] The Board of Education also has a role in providing tertiary prevention[1] because after treatment has occurred, the Board must aid in the patient's rehabilitation by placing him in the regular school milieu.

This paper primarily focuses on the secondary prevention that the Board of Education is obligated to provide under Public Law 94-142 (outlined later in this chapter), concerning the education of handicapped children.

PROCEDURES

In an attempt to take advantage of the secondary prevention potential of the public school social milieu, the Chicago Board of Education set up a network of Pupil Service Centers (PSC) that were to identify children with learning and behavior problems and provide referral for correction of the problem or the problem's etiology. Children with difficulties were identified on the local school level and referred to the adjustment teacher, who tried to deal with the problem on a local level with the help of local school personnel. If the problem was above the adjustment teacher's head, the student was referred (via the principal) to the PSC serving the school's district. Once at the PSC, the referral was examined, along with other pertinent accompanying information, and the child and parents were screened to identify problems and services needed. On the basis of this initial intake, the children and parents were scheduled to see various members of the team, which included a psychiatrist, pediatrician, public health nurse, vision tester, dentist, hearing tester, laboratory technician, social worker, psychologist, school nurse, adjustment teacher, special education teachers, speech pathologist, and educational diagnosticians specializing in learning disabilities, social maladjustment, behavioral disorders, and mental retardation. Transient classroom settings were provided for the children in order to obtain first-hand observation of classroom behavior. Finally, all of the information was gathered and a staffing was held with parents present to discuss findings and recommendations. These recommendations were then turned over to either the local school, the appropriate central office bureau, or the area's Board of Education task force for implementation.

Psychiatric evaluations were requested if the child had clear indications of being seriously emotionally disturbed or if, after a complete evaluation by the other team members, no reason could be found for the child's inability to learn. Parents and children were seen for an hour. If a clear diagnostic picture could not be obtained in this brief session, the family was scheduled for another hour. First, the parents were asked about their understanding of the difficulties their child was having in school. They were then asked about any problems at home. The referral and school record were reviewed with the parents and child present so that the parents could either be informed or further questioned about the child's behavior, and so the child could be aware of what was documented. Usually, there was information from the social worker (home environment and family relationships), the psychologist (IQ, perceptual-motor difficulties, reading and math scores, behavioral observations, and on occasion, projective tests), the school nurse (medical history, and visual and auditory competence), and other appropriate team members. Occasionally, there was information concerning previous diagnostic evaluations or treatment.

The parents were then excused, and the child was asked to tell his side of the story concerning his difficulties at school or at home. The child was questioned about his feelings of anger, sadness, excitement, happiness, apathy, and fearfulness. Depending on the child's affect and history, he was approached with an affect best suited to enlist his cooperation (e.g., fearful children were approached in a warm, friendly manner; angry children were approached in a realistic, firm but fair manner, etc.). Children were told exactly what was going on from the examiner's viewpoint, and what the child's options were. In all cases, there was an attempt to get a treatment contract (verbalization of the problems and willingness to get help for it) from the child. Finally, the ability of the child to relate inter-personally with the examiner was considered a major factor in the evaluation because it was felt that children who could relate could be better influenced by therapists and teachers than those who could not. Children who did not choose to cooperate with the interviewer (usually due to anger and surliness) were immediately returned to their parents, who were usually able to convince the child to cooperate.

Finally, the parents and child were seen together and told of the findings and recommendations, providing an opportunity for input or additional information. Usually, a clear picture was presented to the parents, which encouraged them to have a bit more confidence in the examiner. Oftentimes, at this point in the interview, they shared information that confirmed the examiner's impressions. The family was asked for a treatment contract, consisting of their recognition of the problem and their cooperation in following through on the treatment recommendations. The report was typed, with one copy sent to one of three locations for implementation: the area's Board of Education task force (if either a therapeutic school milieu outside of the Board, hospitalization, or special alternative school placement was needed); the appropriate bureau—Trainable Mentally Handicapped (TMH), Educable Mentally Handicapped (EMH), or Learning Disability (LD); the local school. If no treatment contract was given, the family was told that the Board would in all probability handle the child's problem in an administrative fashion (suspension for acute acting up, social maladjustment school for chronic acting up, truancy investigation for nonattendance, etc.), rather than using a therapeutic approach.

Children were categorized as "seriously emotionally disturbed" according to the following guidelines in Public Law 94-142:

1. The term means a condition exhibiting one or more of the following characteristics over a long period of time and to a marked degree, which adversely affects educational performance:
   a. An inability to learn which cannot be explained by intellectual, sensory, or health factors;
   b. An inability to build or maintain satisfactory interpersonal relationships with peers or teachers;
   c. Inappropriate types of behavior or feelings under normal circumstances;

     d. A general pervasive mood of unhappiness or depression or a tendency to develop physical symptoms or fears associated with personal or social problems.

2. The term includes children who are schizophrenic or autistic. The term does not include children who are socially maladjusted, unless it is determined that they are seriously emotionally disturbed.[3]

RESULTS OF PSYCHIATRIC EXAMINATIONS

The patients' psychiatric examinations were reviewed over a two-year period, and it was found that 274 children fell into 10 tentative categories of emotional illness (see Table 1). There were 54 females and 220 males (19.7% and 80.3% of the total population, respectively). The average age of both males and females was about 11.5 years.

TABLE 7.1. Diagnostic Categories of Children Studied, with Consideration of Sex as a Variable

Diagnostic Categories	No. of Females (% Total)	No. of Males (% Total)	Total No. Males & Females (% Total)
Organic Brain Syndrome (OBS)/ Trainable Mentally Handicapped (TMH) with explosive behavior	5 (9.3)	17 (7.7)	22 (8.0)
Educable Mentally Handicapped (EMH) with explosive behavior	5 (9.3)	17 (7.7)	22 (8.0)
EMH with neurotic symptoms	2 (3.7)	9 (4.1)	11 (4.0)
Psychotic (autistic, childhood schizophrenia, adolescent schizophrenia, other)	3 (5.6)	23 (10.5)	26 (9.5)
Borderline syndrome	3 (5.6)	15 (6.8)	18 (6.6)
Socially maladjusted behavior (personality disorder)	1 (1.8)	—	1 (0.4)
Minimal Brain Dysfunction (MBD)/ Learning Disability (LD) with explosive and/or neurotic symptoms	14 (25.9)	55 25	69 (25.2)
Explosive behavior	4 (7.4)	23 (10.5)	27 (9.9)
Neurotic (anger/depression) symptoms	17 (31.5)	60 (27.3)	77 (28.1)
Psychophysiologic disorders	—	1 (0.5)	1 (0.4)
Total	54 (100)	220 (100)	274 (100)

The first category of patients was those who had a clear history of organic brain syndrome (OBS) and who according to psychological tests were trainable mentally handicapped (TMH). These children were seen primarily because of poor frustration tolerance, which led to poor impulse or affect control and often ended in violent or hostile behavior. Since not all OBS/TMH children are explosive, these children were also classed as seriously emotionally disturbed. Disturbances in memory, judgment, intellect, orientation, and stability of affect were apparent in this group. In addition, they showed marked global visual, auditory, and tactile agnosias; expressive (speaking), receptive (listening), receptive (seeing), and expressive (writing) aphasias; ideomotor and constructional apraxias; spatial orientation difficulties; and poor right-left body discrimination.[4] They tended to be highly excitable, hyperactive, and highly distractible, with poor attention span. Their average age was 12.5 years old. These children were recommended to TMH occupational schools or to a therapeutic school milieu in order to give them a sense of worth and to provide greater controls. Most of them had been in programs beyond their grasp, thus the reason for their frustration.

The second category was children who were educable mentally handicapped (EMH) who had poor frustration tolerance, leading to poor impulse and/or affect control (explosive), and usually resulting in hostility or violence. Disturbances in memory, judgment, intellect, orientation, and stability of affect were not as severe as in the OBS/TMH group. They did show global difficulty with the agnosias, aphasias, apraxias, spatial orientation, and right-left body discrimination, but again not as severely as the first group. These children were also excitable, hyperactive, distractible, etc. Their average age was 12.9 years old. They were referred to EMH occupational schools (if old enough), therapeutic classrooms, or a therapeutic school milieu in order to be taught better emotional control.

EMH children with neurotic features was the third category. These children had neurological shortcomings similar to the EMH children with explosive behavior; however, these children's behavior was of a different nature. They tended to be sad, because they knew they were "slow" and wanted to be "regular." Occasionally this transformed into anger, though these children tended not to demonstrate their anger by hostility or violence, as did the second category. Their average age was 13.8 years old.

These children were recommended for outpatient psychotherapy, EMH classrooms with sensitive, psychologically oriented teachers, therapeutic classrooms, and occasionally, therapeutic school settings.

The fourth category consisted of psychotic children, who were for the most part schizophrenic in one form or another: autistic children demonstrating mutism, echolalia, no interpersonal relatedness, whirling, and affect storms; childhood schizophrenics with responsive speech, bizarre habits, islands of intelligence, poor interpersonal relatedness, a thought disorder, mechanical speech, and a peculiar affect; adolescent schizophrenics with auditory hallucinations, anhedonia, thought broadcasting, thought blockage, a thought disorder, and a lack of interpersonal relatedness. Their average age was 11.2 years old. There tended to be a greater percentage of males in this group. These children were referred to therapeutic school milieus, therapeutic classrooms, or hospitalized as the case indicated.

Children with borderline syndrome were troubled by chronic impulsive and violent behavior, pan-anxiety, pan-anger, and fair interpersonal relatedness with a strong hostile/dependent component. They were in touch with reality and showed no psychotic symptoms or signs. Their average age was 10.8 years old. These children were referred to therapeutic school settings or, if their behavior was severe enough, to residential treatment milieus or psychiatric hospitals.[5]

There was only one female with a personality disorder of an antisocial type. She related well; denied feelings of anxiety, depression, anger, apathy, or fearfulness; and knew what she had done and why. Neither she nor her parents thought she had a problem; nor did they want any help. She was returned to her local school.

The minimal brain dysfunction/learning disability (MBD/LD) group with explosive or neurotic behavior accounted for more than one quarter of the patients. These children showed focal signs in one or more of the following areas: visual, auditory, or tactile agnosia; expressive (speaking), receptive (listening), receptive (seeing), or expressive (writing) aphasia; ideomotor or constructional apraxia; spatial orientation difficulties; poor auditory or visual memory; poor auditory or visual closure.[6,7] They did not show global difficulties as did the TMH or EMH children. Furthermore, they were of average intelligence and related quite well inter-personally. These children tended to have low self-esteem, which had a great part of its etiology in their inability to achieve educationally. They often reported they did not like being "bad," but always found themselves in trouble. They knew that what they had done was wrong after the fact and understood why they had been punished; yet, this did not prevent them from repeating the same behavior. Oftentimes, these children were seen as incorrigible. However, it is suspected that they lacked the neurological competence to either control their impulses or to be able to connect their behavior with its possible consequences, except during hindsight. They tended to be always fighting, impulsive, unable to sit and watch their favorite television show, hyperactive, excitable, with poor attention span, accident prone, distractible, prone to temper tantrums, and enuretic. They also tended to have poor speech, poor Bender-Gestalt tests,[8] poor conceptual thinking, soft neurological signs, histories of an abnormal EEG, and a tendency to reverse letters.[6,7] They showed a mixture of neurotic and explosive symptoms and were therefore not divided into separate categories on the basis of these features. Their average age was 11.6 years old. While there were more males (55) than females (14), the percentage of males and females in the total male and female populations was about the same (25.9% and 25%, respectively). These children were referred for learning disability classes,[9] or if their behavior was serious enough, to a therapeutic classroom or a therapeutic milieu with facilities for learning disabilities.

The children in the explosive behavior group tended to be chair-throwers who were quite hostile, impulsive, and violent. They showed no signs of neurologic dysfunction, perceptual motor dysfunction, anxiety, depression, fearfulness, apathy, or anger. They had good interpersonal relationships, and their behavior, while best described as explosive, was not as severe as exhibited by the children in the borderline group. Their average age was 12.0 years old. These children were referred to therapeutic settings that could provide firm but fair controls and limits. Private schools were very useful in providing this setting. If the child and parents refused a treatment contract, they were left to face the consequences of the child's behavior, which would be invoked from the Board of Education (e.g., referral to a correctional facility) if the acting up continued.

Children with neurotic disorders were found to be of average intelligence and quite interpersonal, as was the previous group. There was an absence of perceptual-motor problems or MBD/LD. Some were quite candid with their reports and others tended to show defensive structures in an attempt to deal with their problems. Their difficulties mainly involved feelings of anxiety, unhappiness, and anger due to conflicts between various factors in their life. Their average age was 11.1 years old, and they accounted for more than one quarter of the diagnoses. Outpatient therapy, therapeutic school settings, therapeutic classrooms, and family counseling were suggested for these children. There was only one psychophysiologic reaction patient, who was a male with gastrointestinal symptoms with anxiety.

A few of these children were seen to determine if the treatment they had already received made it possible for them to return to a public school, since they had been tuitioned out to private treatment milieus. Differential diagnosis was clearly very important in determining what disorder underlay the overt behaviors that were often similar between groups. Children with MBD/LD and explosive and/or neurotic behavior needed a quite different educational and treatment approach than did the children with similar behavior, but not the MBD/LD. Autistic children had to be differentiated from children who were deaf, aphasic, mentally handicapped, brain damaged, or severely neurotic. Fortunately, a diagnostic team screening usually provided enough information to make a good differential.

Because children are not as set in their ways as are adults, their diagnoses were not written in their evaluations. Such a "label," it was felt, would tend to be seen as a permanent disorder, as opposed to a possibly transient state (especially if treated before the behavior could become a fixed trait). Thus, the disorder was described rather than diagnosed (this was also due to the non-medical nature of the Board of Education). The only exception was in cases where a diagnosis was necessary for placement.

RESULTS OF FOLLOW-UP

Telephone follow-up was done on the 274 patients, with the average time of 13 months between initial contact and telephone follow-up. Of the total 274 children, 150 (54.7%) were contacted, and their average time between initial contact and telephone contact was 12 months. The percentage of patients able to be contacted three to seven months after the initial contact was 82.7%, whereas the percentage of patients able to be contacted 8–13 months after initial contact dropped to 53.9%. The percentage of patients able to be contacted 14–19 months and 20–25 months after initial contact was 49.2% and 50%, respectively. Patients who were not contacted either did not have a phone or had their number changed.

The percentage of the total male and female population able to be contacted was 53.2% and 61.1%, respectively. There was a lower phone follow-up rate for patients classed as borderline (38.9%), while those children classed as psychotic, explosive, and neurotic had the highest percentage of successful follow-up, approximately 60% (see Table 2). The 150 follow-up patients had a percentage of diagnostic categories similar to that of the diagnostic categories in the total 274 patients. The percentage of males and females in each diagnostic category in the follow-up group was similar to that of the total 274 males and females in each diagnostic category. The patients in the TMH and both EMH groups were older than the patients who were not able to be contacted by an average of one year. The psychotic patients available for follow-up were on the average two years younger than those not available for follow-up. The children in the remain-

TABLE 7.2. Diagnostic Categories of Children Studied, with Consideration of Availability for Follow-Up as a Variable

Diagnostic Categories	Follow-up		No Follow-up			Total
	Total	%	Female	Male	Total	
OBS/TMH with explosive behavior	11	50*	2	9	11	22
EMH with explosive behavior	12	54.5*	1	9	10	22
EMH with neurotic symptoms	5	45.5*	2	4	6	11
Psychotic	16	61.5*	2	8	10	26
Borderline syndrome	7	38.9*	2	9	11	18
Socially maladjusted behavior	—	—	1	—	1	1
MBD/LD with explosive and/or neurotic symptoms	35	50.7*	6	28	34	69
Explosive behavior	16	59.3*	1	10	11	27
Neurotic symptoms	47	61.0*	4	26	30	77
Psychophysiologic disorders	1	100*	—	—	—	1
Total	150	54.7	21**	103+	124	274

*The percent of this diagnostic category that was available for follow-up.
**This number was 38.9% of the total female population of 54.
+This number was 46.8% of the total male population of 220.

ing categories available for follow-up were on the average less than a year older than those not available for follow-up.

Children contacted on follow-up were divided into two basic groups: (1) better—those who had shown improvement in their symptoms, had been placed in appropriate facilities, had demonstrated improvement, and had shown improvement in their academic performance; (2) same— those who had not been properly placed and had shown no symptom improvement, or those who had shown no improvement although in appropriate placements (see Table 3).

TABLE 7.3. Diagnostic Categories of Children Available for Follow-up, with Regards to Outcome

Diagnostic Categories	BETTER			SAME			No. Total Pop. (%)
	No. Female (% Tot.)	No. Male (% Tot.)	Total (%)	No. Female (% Tot.)	No. Male (%Tot.)	Total (%)	
OBS/TMH with explosive behavior	2 (66.6)	6 (75)	8 (72.7)	1 (33.3)	2 (25)	3 (27.3)	11 (7.3)
EMH with explosive behavior	2 (50)	5 (62.5)	7 (58.3)	2 (50)	3 (37.5)	5 (41.7)	12 (8)
EMH with neurotic behavior	— —	4 (80)	4 (80)	— —	1 (20)	1 (20)	5 (3.3)
Psychotic	1 (100)	14 (93.3)	15 (93.8)	— —	1 (6.7)	1 (6.2)	16 (10.7)
Borderline syndrome	1 (100)	4 (66.6)	5 (71.4)	— —	2 (33.3)	2 (28.6)	7 (4.7)
MBD/LD with explosive and/or neurotic symptoms	4 (50)	19 (70.4)	23 (65.7)	4 (50)	8 (29.6)	12 (34.3)	35 (23.3)
Explosive behavior	1 (33.3)	10 (76.9)	11 (68.8)	2 (66.6)	3 (23.1)	5 (31.2)	16 (10.7)
Neurotic symptoms	9 (69.2)	23 (67.6)	32 (68.1)	4 (30.7)	11 (32.4)	15 (31.9)	47 (31.3)
Psychophysiologic disorders	— —	— —	— —	— —	1 (100)	1 (100)	1 (0.7)
Total	20 (60.6)	85 (72.6)	105 (70)	13 (39.4)	32 (27.4)	45 (30)	150

The outcome of the children who were followed up was not related to the amount of time between initial and follow-up contact. This was true whether the outcome groups were considered in totality or broken down into male and female subgroups. Follow-up revealed that in most cases, males who were followed up had a better outcome than females in most of the diagnostic categories and in the total follow-up populations as well.

DISCUSSION

The children who were diagnosed as OBS/TMH and EMH with additional emotional problems were on average older than children in the other categories. This is likely due to the fact that children with compromised intellectual functioning have a difficult time dealing with the stresses of adolescence and therefore tend to develop emotional problems during this period of life, reflected in an average referral age of 13 years. There tends to be a greater percentage of males who develop schizophrenia prior to adulthood than females.

Children with a diagnosis of OBS/TMH, EMH, or MBD/LD can be identified by a neurologic examination with careful attention given to cerebral functions.

While the number of males with MBD/LD and emotional problems was greater than that of females, when a total population of children with emotional problems was considered, the percentage of males and females was equal.

Children with emotional problems who are referred for psychiatric evaluation must be evaluated from a standpoint of determining whether some neurologic dysfunctioning is present. This is especially true if the majority of the population is black, as MBD/LD is associated with prematurity, and as black children have a higher percentage of prematurity than do white children.

Children with neurotic problems account for more than one fourth of all children referred for a psychiatric evaluation for difficulty in school secondary to emotional problems. Children with MBD/LD account for more than one fourth of all these children as well. Children with psychophysiologic disorders and personality disorders are rare. Female children were slightly more likely to be able to be contacted for follow-up than males.

Children categorized as borderline syndrome have the least likelihood of being available for follow-up, and children categorized as psychotic, explosive, and neurotic have the greatest likelihood.

Males tend to have a better treatment outcome than females.

Children who have emotional problems in school do not tend to "outgrow" their problems; those showing improvement had psychiatric treatment. As a result, the Board of Education plays a significant role in all areas of prevention of later psychiatric or criminal disorders. The earlier the age of the child when intervention takes place, the better.

The majority of children (70%) of minority status and low socioeconomic status who have behavioral or emotional problems in school can be helped if they are appropriately diagnosed rather than assigning them to the category of disciplinary problems. Over 95% of the children seen were poor and black, and none of them were "bad kids."

It is clear that 27% of black families are on an income below the poverty level.[10] Secondly, "a black baby is twice as likely to die in the first year of life as a white baby,"[11] and black children in families below the poverty level are more likely to be premature and nutritionally deficient.[12] As a result of deficient income, black children are more likely to get medical services through public agencies supported by tax dollars. It is imperative that black people become politically sophisticated in order to direct those dollars to the patients who clearly need the care.

Appropriate identification of a problem is an exercise in futility unless appropriate linkage to a proper treatment facility is obtained. There is a shortage of proper treatment facilities in minority, low socioeconomic areas, and there needs to be a mean for developing such facilities in impoverished areas.

Finally, it will be interesting to try to locate these children to determine their outcome in five and ten years.

COMMENTARY

This article has much of the same relevance as it did in 1979. It appropriately suggests that the Board of Education has a role in prevention of later psychiatric disability. In addition, it outlines all of the necessary components for a complete childhood multidisciplinary assessment. Most importantly, it presents a classification system based on empirical observations of African-American children who were given a thorough evaluation. The APA has developed a new diagnostic system for children and adults, but I still find the broad diagnostic categories found in this article applicable to the children I see. The article also illustrates the need for outcome evaluation regarding the intervention attempted.

Since writing this, I have continued my interest in working with African-American children (see Chapters 3, 17, and 36). A few years ago, I was evaluating about four African-American children per week, which I'd been doing for more than ten years. My focus on prevention for this population has sharpened over the years. My experience has taught me that of all the broad diagnostic categories I developed, the ones that would most respond to prevention work were "explosive behavior" and "neurotic symptoms." My seasoning as a community psychiatrist has revealed to me that these problems are frequently generated when children are in situations that cause traumatic stress. By early identification and by helping the children cope with their traumatic ordeals, many children's "explosive behavior" and "neurotic symptoms" can be improved. It's a lot of work, but if we pay a little on the front end, we'll avoid paying a great deal on the back.

This path has lead me to an invite to present at Surgeon General Dr. Satcher's *Report of the Surgeon General's Conference on Children's Mental Health: A National Action Agenda*, held in September 2000 (see www.surgeongeneral.gov). This report was a critical piece of a public health plan to develop a children's mental health and wellness infrastructure. It was also a very helpful template for my work with the former First Lady of Illinois Lura Lynn Ryan on her "Futures for Kids" initiative.

The children's mental health infrastructure in the US is inadequate. Given the advances in mental health, I predict that in the next several decades, most psychiatrists will be geriatric psychiatrists or child psychiatrists, as we will be able to diagnose and treat children earlier and prevent them from having morbidity and mortality due to psychiatric disorders. If we don't construct the foundation now, when we find out what mental disorders can be treated early, we won't be in a position to deliver prevention treatment to the children who need it the most.

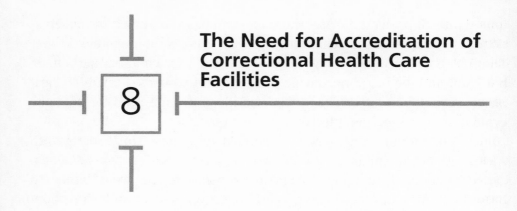

The Need for Accreditation of Correctional Health Care Facilities

8

Approximately 600,000 people are housed in this nation's 5,054 correctional institutions (568 state prisons, 3,493 county and municipal jails, and 993 public juvenile detention and correctional facilities). This year, approximately 7,000,000 people will spend time in these institutions. Most of them will be poor and more than one half will be minorities, who because of their living conditions are at greatest risk for developing communicable diseases and who paradoxically are most likely to be medically underserved. Upon being incarcerated, these people will find themselves in old, poorly ventilated, overcrowded facilities that increase the risk of spreading communicable diseases and likely worsen a non-communicable illness.

These realities should force concerned National Medical Association members to ask about the status of health care facilities in the nation's correctional institutions. The answer is that prisons in 39 states, along with more than one third of the nation's jails, are facing class-action lawsuits alleging inadequate medical care and health services. Often, the courts find the availability and quality of health care in correctional institutions to be inadequate. This nation's correctional institution population

Originally printed as Bell Carl C. Guest editorial on "The Need for Accreditation of Correctional Health Care Facilities." *J Natl Med Assoc*. 1984;76:571–572.

consists of a medically underserved group that by virtue of being in a municipal, county, or state facility, runs a greater risk of becoming ill and being inadequately treated than it would in the community at large. This is a backward state of affairs. The logical next question is what is being done to correct the problem.

This answer is found in a new organization called the National Commission on Correctional Health Care (NCCHC), formed by representatives of 22 nationwide service and professional associations and societies, the NMA among them. It is their goal to offer voluntary accreditation to correctional facilities meeting the health care standards developed by the Commission. The standards require a correctional facility to screen individuals on admission to identify current health care needs and to have a procedure to attend to these needs. There should also be periodic health appraisals, a secure method for handling medical emergencies, and an ongoing system for adequate handling of inmates' physical, mental, and dental problems. The health care providers should not be inmates but rather should be adequately trained and licensed personnel, and the health care delivery system should provide medication in a professional manner and maintain good records. Finally, the correctional facility should allow for good hygiene and regular exercise. The Commission offers technical assistance to help correctional health care facilities improve their delivery system to meet accreditation standards. Research, training, development of publications, and conferences and seminars on correctional health care issues are also provided by the Commission.

The formation of this Commission raises another question, though: how successful can a voluntary accreditation program be at alleviating the inadequate health care facilities in this country's correctional institutions? The fourfold increase in the detection of illness (including communicable diseases) in correctional facilities that have instituted the Commission's standards indicates the answer to this question. If all correctional institutions met these standards, adequate health care for inmates would be ensured. Despite the enormity of the nation's correctional health care deficiencies and the youth of the Commission, the voluntary accreditation program has had a significant impact on the nation's greatest health care problem. The initial focus of the Commission has been on jails. More than 400 have since upgraded their medical services, and 168 have become accredited.

Since it is apparent that the program is effective and that voluntary accreditation does work, the next question is what can be done to maintain the survival of this new national Commission and ensure that all of the correctional institutions in the nation meet the health care standards it has outlined. One way of improving correctional health care is to have the courts order correctional institutions to improve their system of health care delivery. This often resolves the class-action lawsuits. Another way is for municipal, county, and state officials responsible for the operation of correctional institutions under their jurisdiction to realize the extent of the problem, mandate that their facilities be accredited, and allocate the funds necessary to improve the facilities to meet Commission standards.

As a member of the board of directors of the NCCHC, and representing the NMA, I urge NMA physicians to become more aware of these issues and support the need for the accreditation process being set in gear by the Commission. The establishment of minimal correctional health care standards and the institution of on-site visits to validate the process and quality of health care services will ensure that a vast number of poor and minority people will receive screening to detect medical problems and subsequent treatment of the problems identified. As NMA physicians, we must ascertain whether the correctional facilities in our communities have been accredited, providing the minimal requirements for good health care to their inmates. If we find they are not accredited, we should bring this deficiency to the attention of our elected officials and insist that they correct all shortcomings.

Whether the NCCHC and the accreditation of the health care systems in this nation's correctional institutions will be dismissed as a great idea that no one supported, or whether it will emerge as a major institutional force safeguarding the health care of this nation's correctional population, will be determined by this country's citizens' support of the Commission's admirable mission. I would hope the NMA will be in the vanguard to support the NCCHC. After all, the state of this nation's public health is determined by the quality of health of its least fortunate citizens.

COMMENTARY

My work with the NCCHC began 21 years ago in 1983. During my tenure with the Commission's board of directors, I've served as Chairperson of the Accreditation Committee (1985–90; 1997–present), Chairperson of the Board (1991–92), Immediate Past-Chairperson of the Board (1992), and Chairperson of the Policy and Standard Committee (1993–96). I'm still a member of the board, and I still go out on surveys to accredit the health care of jails, prisons, and juvenile detention centers. I frequently ask myself why I'm still involved with this effort, but as I reread this guest editorial, I received my answer: it's good work. While the number of African-American inmates in prisons, jails, and juvenile detention centers has increased greatly since this article was first written, the basic truths in the article remain constant. The editorial speaks for itself.

Currently, the need for this editorial to be heeded is greater than ever, considering the large number of "rats" of diseases in jails, prisons, and juvenile detention centers. Consider the "rat" of tuberculosis—we need to be able to identify and treat this terrible disease within our inmate population. When this underserved population isn't treated, the risk of the disease spreading within the facility and outside the facility is very high. We shouldn't be waiting for tuberculosis to present in the indigent hospitals. We should be actively identifying it in high-risk populations and treating it before it spreads, i.e., "getting rid of the rat." I visited one jail seeking accreditation; it identified one fourth of all of the syphilis cases found within its county. Fortunately, the inmates were treated for the STD on the spot, preventing the infection from spreading further. This is an excellent example of "getting rid of the rat" of STDs. Imagine the disastrous health consequences for that area if the jail hadn't taken on that public health responsibility.

Because the "war on drugs" allowed for the incarceration of people who used and abused drugs from 1980 to now, the prison and jail populations have more than doubled. This population explosion outstripped the correctional health care infrastructure designed to ensure inmates' health and wellbeing. This is a public health crisis. Unfortunately, the NCCHC accredits only about ten percent of all the jails and prisons. Luckily, the Commission's standards are the industry standard. Although 90% of the jails and prisons aren't seeking accreditation from the NCCHC, I suspect they're attempting to follow our standards of health care within their facilities. Naturally, I would feel better if they all sought accreditation, because this way I'd know for sure that the nation's inmates were getting a minimal level of necessary health care.

My work on the NCCHC has been most rewarding to me. It's given me the opportunity to "get rid of rats" within the walls of prisons, jails, and juvenile detention facilities, where some of our least advantaged citizens dwell. Further, it has given me experience as a board director and has allowed me to practice my leadership/organizational skills. I strongly advise individuals interested in health and public health to get involved with a social service organization at the board of directors level. It's an outstanding opportunity to have a role in safeguarding the public's health—no matter how small, and gives great meaning to your life.

JAMA Book Review Editor Dr. Harriet Meyer, who has sent me books to review for the JAMA, gave me the opportunity to review the sixth and seventh editions of the *Comprehensive Textbook of Psychiatry*. While the book struck me as being an outstanding encyclopedia of psychiatric knowledge, my major criticism of the text was its lack of attention to psychiatric care in correctional facilities. The editor did what all good leaders do when someone points out a problem—ask the critic to share their criticism. Thus, my chapter, "Correctional Psychiatry," was added and should be out in late 2004.

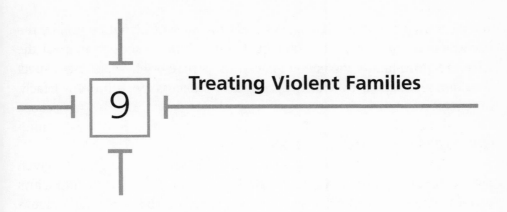

Treating Violent Families

Family violence is responsible for a significant proportion of homicides and is a major cause of premature deaths in African Americans. This article reviews the prevalence of family violence and explores associated risk factors. Treatment principles and tips, as well as a cognitive framework to guide the actual therapy, are outlined. Finally, prevention of family violence is discussed.

INTRODUCTION

Homicide is a significant cause of premature deaths in African Americans,[1] and homicide from family violence has been shown to be disproportionately higher in African Americans than other ethnic groups.[2] Any homicide prevention activities in black communities will therefore have to include the prevention of family violence to have an impact on the rates of homicide for the group.[3]

The purpose of this article is to familiarize the reader with the prevalence of family violence and to explore associated risk factors. Treatment principles and tips are presented to increase understanding of

Originally printed as Bell Carl C, Hill-Chance Gerri. Treatment of violent families. *J Natl Med Assoc*. 1991;83:203–208. Presented at the Annual Meeting of the American Family Therapy Association, Montreal, Canada, June 24, 1988.

treating violent families. The stages and strategies of actual treatment are also presented to increase the skill level of the clinician seeking to make an intervention in family violence. Finally, the article briefly discusses needs of families disrupted by violence and factors necessary to prevent family violence.

PREVALENCE OF FAMILY VIOLENCE

At some point, all intimate relationships must deal with conflict or aggression. Yet, how often does family violence (i.e., behavior that outside the family would call for police intervention) occur? The answer to this question comes from divorce, clinical, emergency room, and general community surveys, as well as family homicide statistics.

Okun's[4] work on the abuse of women noted that the prevalence of spouse abuse in divorce applicants varied but was significant. Levinger[5] reported that 36.8% of women seeking divorce reported family violence, while Fields[6] found that 50% of wives who were applying for divorce reported family violence. O'Brien[7] found that a smaller percentage, 16.7%, of divorce applicants complained of spouse abuse. Parker and Schumacher[8] quantified the assault of wives seeking divorce and noted that 40% reported being assaulted three or more times and that 66% reported being assaulted at least once.

Clinical surveys also show a wide range in the prevalence of family violence. For example, Mowrer and Mowrer[9] found conjugal abuse in 41% of couples seeking treatment, while Sanders[10] found that 15.6% of couples in treatment reported violence between them. Similarly, emergency room surveys reveal a wide range in the prevalence of reported family violence. Rounsaville and Weismann[11] reported that 3.4% of the women presenting to an emergency service were battered by their mates. Stark and Filtcraft[12] reported that 21% of all women who used the emergency surgical service were battered and that half of all injuries occurred from abuse. They noted that one fourth of all women who attempt suicide are battered women, and that for black women, one half who attempt suicide are battered.

In a general community survey by Straus et al.,[13] 16% of marital partners were violent within the past year and 28% have been violent at some time during marriage. Goodwin[14] noted that 25% of all homicides occur between family members, 6% of children are abused each year, 3% of adults have kicked, punched, or bitten a child, 4% of wives are beaten severely each year, and 10% of wives are raped at least once during marriage. She notes that 80% of spouse abuse, intrafamilial sexual abuse, and elder abuse victims are women. In another community survey in Kentucky, it was found that one out of 10 women had been physically assaulted by their partners the year of the survey.[15] Finally, a Texas survey revealed that 8.5% of the women surveyed were assaulted by their mates.[16]

Family homicide statistics are another indicator of the prevalence of family violence. Boudouris[17] found that 50% to 60% of murderous couples living together had not filed for divorce. Gelles[18] noted that in Atlanta in 1972, 31% of the 255 homicides were domestic. More recently, Straus reported that in 1984, 4,408 intrafamilial homicides occurred and that at least 2000 were spouse murders. Of the spouses killed, about two thirds were wives.[19] Block[20] notes that when looking at domestic homicide in blacks, more black wives kill their husbands than black husbands kill their wives. It is important to note that husbands are six to seven times more likely than wives to have initiated abuse and violence that resulted in the husband's murder.

Since the beginning of the 20th century, the annual age-adjusted homicide rate of non-whites has been five to ten times higher than that of any other group,[21] and a significant proportion of these homicides have resulted from domestic violence. This strongly indicates that health professionals treating African Americans should look for risk factors in families to prevent possible domestic violence.

RISK FACTORS

It should be noted that there is a difference between irrational and impulsive behaviors. Family violence is not a sporadic, irrational act; usually, a reason and pattern leads to the violence, although it is often impulsive. Risk factors that increase the likelihood of these impulsive acts of family violence are classified as physiologic, psychologic, current interpersonal/family relationships, cultural/family background factors, and situational risk factors.[22,23]

Physiologic/medical factors that increase the risk of family violence are mental retardation (for child abuse), dementia in adults (for elder abuse), and current hyper-irritability, hostility, or a "short fuse." Past medical history risk factors are perinatal and early childhood brain insult, brain injury from head trauma, childhood history of serious attention deficit disorder and learning problems, and a childhood history of severe hyperactivity and restlessness. Substance abuse, habitual alcohol abuse and dependence, and poly drug use are also biologic risk factors. Other risk factors are partial complex seizures, intense paroxysmal affects, and sudden mood swings.

The psychological risk factors are low self-concept, failure to achieve, low frustration tolerance, inability to delay gratification, inability to tolerate criticism, and inability to examine one's own behavior. Personality problems that lead to interpersonal conflict are also associated with role distortions, dominance and control issues, and distorted dependency feelings. Additional risk factors are recent personal history of assaultive behavior (as well as a past history of recurrent violent and assaultive behavior), a history of child abuse or neglect, and a history of juvenile delinquency with under-socialized features. Impulsivity is a risk factor that may manifest as a history of repeated traffic violations, repeated suicide attempts, hypersexuality, emotional lability with excitability and intense interpersonal emotions, and a propensity for acting out dysphoric feelings. Other psychological risk factors are approval of violence, egocentricity (i.e., self-centeredness, social unconcern, entitlement), cathectic lability (i.e., labile object relationships and non-sustained pursuits), and severe or pervasive psychopathology with persecutory delusions.

The next group of risk factors is the current interpersonal or family relationship factor. There may be a symbiotic relationship between the victim and offender, which results in hostile dependency that often encourages the isolation as well as confused and distorted interpersonal attachments, and an unequal distribution of power and status, commonly found in family violence. A good rule of thumb is that an "out-of-control" adolescent may come from a family with violence amongst family relationships. Another dynamic may be that one or more members of the family may lack interpersonal skills or may become incompetent in the face of stress, which results in interpersonal frustrations that may culminate in violence. There may be jealousy, interpersonal "paranoia" (i.e., blaming oneself for feeling incompleteness), and distorted cognition and attribution (i.e., always expecting an attack). Other factors are pregnancy, previous threats to leave, and child abuse.

The family origin may contribute risk factors such as violence in the early home environment and severe psychopathology (i.e., alcoholism and sociopathy) in parents. The culture of origin may also contribute to or decrease the risk of violence in the family. For example, intrafamilial homicide is much less common in Hispanics than in African Americans or whites.[20,24,25] It is important to obtain a family history of violence to learn who in the family was violent with whom, when, and how often. It is also important to differentiate whether the violence was expressive or instrumental.[26] Such questions help to identify the multifaceted causes of family violence and to identify dynamic family risk factors.

Situational factors may be social or cultural. These two should be conceptually differentiated because it is easier to change situational sociologic factors that contribute to violence than it is to change situational cultural factors. Violence is commonly associated with the situational sociologic variable of poverty. When the variable of poverty is held constant, the disparity between the homicide rates of blacks and whites vanishes.[27] It appears that "the subculture violence"[28] explanations of homicide may be much less important in explaining the higher rates of black homicide, while subcultural factors may explain the lower rates of Hispanic intrafamilial homicide. Other situational factors that increase the risk of violence are the presence of firearms, social isolation, social and structural stress, the perceived level of violence in the immediate community and the need to protect oneself from being victimized, and unstable resources.

PRINCIPLES AND TIPS

Once a violent family has been identified, intervention should be immediate. Unfortunately, the ability of the social service and medical communities to meet the need for intervention is not optimal. There are not enough services or professionals skilled in the intervention of family violence. It is important, then, to clarify essential principles and tips that strengthen a conceptual framework from which to actually intervene.

The therapist must interrupt the escalating cycles of violence and reduce stress in the family. Violence may have begun with one person or sometimes two, but the pattern may now be a functional part of the family's dynamics. The family will need an opportunity to ventilate. They will also need help verifying they are not "crazy" and will need help putting their thoughts, behaviors, and childhood experiences in perspective. The family will need help with referral to other services and agencies, along with specific guidance in personal and non-personal matters. Violent families need help in gaining control over an out-of-control life and help in setting consistent limits.

Although the treatment of family violence should be approached from a systems perspective, clinicians should not overlook an individual cause for family violence in an effort to understand family dynamics. We must look for individual psychiatric diagnoses such as organic brain syndromes, psychosis, affective disorders, and personality disorders. We should be aware of behavior patterns that may be at the root of violence, like habitual delinquency with or without under-socialized or socialized features (i.e., a conduct disorder), ego dystonic destructiveness (i.e., a disorder of impulse), or sudden alterations in consciousness (i.e., a dissociative disorder). Violence in a family can also be generated by an individual who is re-experiencing a trauma (e.g., a post-traumatic stress disorder) or having a maladaptive reaction to a stressor (i.e., an adjustment disorder).[23]

The clinician should be aware that the primary target is not the psyche but the behavior. Intervention must be immediate with no opportunity to rationalize or deny behavior or consequences. Insight does not help, nor does coercion, rescuing, rumination, or emotive directives. One must be very problem-oriented, with the focus on stopping the violence by using supportive confrontation, enhancement of self-esteem, improving problem-solving, structured exercises and practice of skills to control violence, development of affective awareness, and honesty. The therapist must slow down escalation, allow ventilation, clarify stress, develop alternatives, mediate negotiations, encourage perseverance, and remain optimistic. Isolation of the family must be prevented, and the family's resources must be developed and stabilized. The secondary target for intervention is the environment or misinformation that support the violence. The tertiary target is the psyche; the use of insight or traditional therapy is useful in this regard.

There is a therapeutic dilemma involving men who batter due to their feelings of low self-esteem and powerlessness. How does one increase a batterer's self-esteem while rejecting their behavior? The solution is to reject the behavior, not the person, but this distinction is difficult to get across to patients and requires exceedingly clear verbal and affective communications. In this regard, it is good to be aware of the weakness and brittleness of the violent person. Another dilemma is the batterer's motivation for treatment. Is it just to impress the court, or is the motivation for change internally based? Does it make a difference whether the motivation is external or internal? The best predictor of a positive therapy outcome is a batterer motivated enough to accurately report the extent of his violence.[24] Other important principles to keep in mind in the treating of violent families are transference and counter-transference issues, safety of the therapist, and the duty to warn of impending violence, but these are beyond the scope of this article.[29]

There are some controversies about how to approach intervention in family violence. One concern is whether a family therapy approach excuses violent family members for their individual behavior. A traditional family therapy approach may cause the victim to support the perpetrator and to accept too personal a role in their victimization. Different advocates in different geographic regions vary in their philosophy toward intervention and treatment. Some child abuse and elder abuse prevention advocates support decriminalization, while some spouse and intrafamily sexual abuse prevention advocates support recriminalization of their issues. There is also controversy over the ability to predict violence.[30] It is enough to say that the certainty demanded in a legal circumstance is far greater than that needed in a clinical situation. In a family with documented violence, the clinician should always err in favor of the potential victim.

The most rapid impact can be seen by using traditional crisis intervention techniques, with intervention aimed at risk factors in the physiologic/medical category (using medication in a violent bipolar or demented patient) and in the life stress/resource category, i.e., the situational factors. Lasting changes require intervention through the psychological and current interpersonal/family relationship factors. It is important to remember that there is no one answer to every family's problem with violence; however, the preceding principles and tips should be used as guidelines while doing the actual interventions and therapy.

ACTUAL THERAPY

The actual therapy consists of crisis intervention, initial assessment, a complete evaluation, brief therapy, and long-term treatment.[31]

Crisis intervention is most often done by the police but sometimes by the clinician. To prevent intervention in an episode of family violence during a family session, a clinician should be proactive and not allow interpersonal arguments to escalate into physical altercations. Volatile couples should be separated (at least outside of striking distance, possibly with a large table separating them), and it is important that the therapist not take sides, because this can risk antagonizing the aggressor or incurring the wrath upon the victim. Two therapists can be neutral or supportive of each side. Should violence occur, it is important to remain in control and stay calm, but insist that the violence stop. Training in disrupting fights is useful.

The initial assessment and treatment have four steps. The first is to gather basic information about the family but also to pay attention to each individual's story and part. Assess past and present stress, along with the capacity and techniques used to cope. Screen for the quality and quantity of violence and determine what weapons are available. If the information gathering threatens to get provocative and dangerous, separate the family during this phase. Despite the risk of scapegoating or singling out the primary assailant, the therapist must focus on the violent behavior to get it under control. The next step is to assess the family's real needs for reducing stress and dealing with supplying those needs.

The third step is making a contract to stop violence that should be simple and manageable to build short-term control and self-esteem. To accomplish this, the clinician must understand the sequence of events of violence and identify the critical points. Behavior must be specific and structured to stop the violence. Examples include mandating the use of crisis numbers and removing readily available loaded guns. Other ways to structure behavior are mandating the use of time-out behavior by identifying warning signs of impending violence and cues to facilitate de-escalation of arguments, coaching the family to anticipate stress, identifying conflicts, and avoiding disruptions by negotiating instead of dictating. The family should communicate about anger, fears, hopelessness, conflicts, feelings, and worries without verbal or physical abuse. Let the family know the contact is for them and not the therapist. The family should be challenged to avoid self-sabotage by being asked how the contract to stop violence might fail.

The therapist should get an idea about the family's resistance to the contract, as well as get information about flaws, loopholes, or lack of clarity. Cooperation of violent family members can be increased by support and by reducing their sense of hopelessness. The therapist should discuss the worst-case scenario (e.g., legal separation or increase in violence) and should outline specific steps of action in case of possible separation. This preparation may often reduce the stress of anticipating the actual worst-case scenario. The final step teaches the family ways to deal with the most dangerous situations: separation, medicating, hospitalization, and intense family and friend involvement.

The complete evaluation consists of medical histories, identification of more community resources, and histories from other sources. This should be done in the second session. It is important to realize that the second session is usually very different from the first, as the family's defenses will be up, giving a more realistic prognosis.

The brief therapy component should focus on short-term goals, with every session being treated like it is the last. Predisposing factors such as helplessness, intolerance to life's stress, and using the therapist to combat isolation should be tolerated by the therapist and should be met with crisis intervention. The therapist should use firm but gentle confrontation of denial and rationalization. Stabilization of resources during this stage is essential. The family should be guided with tasks that restore normal functioning and increase flexibility, and should be guided with more realistic expectations. Skills training should be used to improve competence of the abuser and the victim in order to increase social skills and assertiveness and to increase social control over behavior. Actual dependency must be replaced by mutual respect. Hostile dependent members must be encouraged to separate and allow each other to develop healthy differentiation. Individuation needs to be encouraged by advocacy of a family member's right to emotional comfort, self-fulfillment, and adequate role performance. The family should learn to identify maladaptive thoughts and self-statements prior to, during, and after an event; in other words, cognitive restructuring may be useful.

New techniques for the expression of anger and the resolution of conflict must be developed. Techniques to consider are relaxation-training, development of a signal to break off communications, nonviolent conflict resolution skills to build negotiation skills, "fair fight" training (practiced in session), and "blaming without response" exercises performed by both parties equally (designed to extinguish the mutual blaming that prevents identification and modification of behavior).

When to start the final phase of treatment, e.g., long-term, varies. Some families drop out before the assessment and contract phase. Most drop out with symptom remission following brief treatment. A few, however, stay for the long term. Because the completeness of treatment varies, relapse is very common; therefore, treatment may occur in stages. Couples' groups, multifamily groups, and long-term family therapy are the treatments of choice aimed at changing psychological and interpersonal/family interaction dynamics. Such group modalities reduce isolation and give support. A good prognosis is indicated by the number of sessions attended, the perception that the violence was severe, and an accurate report of the violence from all involved. Unfortunately, some families come for help after the violence has disrupted the family, and clinicians need information about what these families need. For example, disrupted families with victims in a shelter need help with assertiveness, anger, and self-esteem. They will also need life-planning options such as help with child support, child care, welfare, property issues, public housing, and unemployment, as well as help with sex roles, separation, divorce, independence, and problem-solving.

CONCLUSIONS

Family violence results in significant damage to the public's health. Health care and social service professionals should try to intervene as early as possible to prevent having to get involved after the loss of life, during postmortem activities. This article was written to try to fill a perceived gap in the knowledge and skills necessary to make secondary homicide prevention efforts possible.[26]

It is hoped that public health initiatives can be effective in primary prevention of homicide by preventing attitudes and values that promote initiation of family violence. Such efforts include reducing readily available loaded guns, eliminating violent norms, reducing stress (e.g., providing full employment, eliminating poverty, guaranteeing health care, preventing unwanted children), ceasing sexism, changing child-rearing habits, and changing a legal system that does not intervene.

COMMENTARY

When I presented this paper at the American Family Therapy Association in Montreal, Canada, I hadn't done a great deal of family therapy. As a result, I was anxious about lecturing to a group of family therapists about how to treat violent families. My fantasy was that everyone in the room would already know what I was spouting about. After I gave the lecture, though, it became apparent to me that only about 10% of the members were conversant with my topic. One family therapist, who congratulated me on my address and told me I was absolutely on target, asked me for help with a case of his. He said he was treating a couple in which the husband had gotten so angry with his wife that he'd attempted to run her over with their car. It seemed to me that with such "out and about" anger, there was considerable danger of an interpersonal altercation homicide. I strongly suggested that the therapist discover if the family kept a gun in the house. He sheepishly agreed. At the time, I was confused why this professional group was not more sophisticated in the area of family violence.

While I was consulting with the APA's Task Force on Clinician Safety, the reason many family therapists were uncomfortable with treating violent families occurred to me. I had asked the task force about their recommendations if a patient got angry with and attacked their psychiatrist in his office. They misunderstood the question and assured me that they never recommended that a psychiatrist get directly involved with restraining a patient on an inpatient unit. I clarified the question by reframing it: what if the patient was seeing their psychiatrist in his private office late at night? Essentially, I was asking them what their self-defense policy was. The question caused them to come up short. They hadn't even considered it! This experience taught me that most clinicians are uncomfortable about managing violence because they aren't trained to respond to "potential," "urgent," or "emergent" violence (see Chapter 5). As a result, many therapists avoid exposure to anyone they presume to be violent. I've always recommended that people who work in this field figure out ways to manage violence should it befall them. Since writing this article, I've also come to understand that unless clinicians can assure their own safety, they tend to be in denial about the prevalence of violence in our society. Thus, clinician safety has been a major focus of my work and is the reason why I edited a small book, *Psychiatric Aspects on Violence: Understanding Causes and Issues in Prevention and Treatment* (San Francisco: Jossey-Bass; 2000). One of my major messages these days is that before we do anything about the problem of violence within our community, we must first assure our own safety.

Though there's been a greater commitment to addressing violence in families in the years since writing this article over a decade ago, not much has changed. However, in 1999, I learned that the work of others and myself who were trying to reduce domestic violence had an impact on intimate murders between people aged 20–44. I was appointed to the Violence Against Women Advisory Council in 1995. When I first became interested in 1976 in doing something about black-on-black homicides— the bulk of which were intimate murders between African-American husbands and wives or lovers—the intimate homicide rate in black folk was 14.5/100,000. By 1996, the rate had dropped to 3.5/100,000. I believe this effect was due to the proliferation of spousal abuse shelters as a result of work that myself and others had begun to do in 1984 (see Chapters 1 and 2).

Several years ago, Attorney General Reno and Secretary Shalala asked the advisory council to "think out of the box" in figuring out how to prevent violence against women. Since I'd been working on violence prevention strategies within the Chicago Public Schools, I took my ideas to the council during our Fall 1998 meeting. That evening at a reception, Attorney General Reno came up to me and asked me to look at her violence prevention strategies and let her know what I thought by the next morning. The alignment between the strategies she had outlined and the strategies contained in the Chicago Public School was remarkable. The same principles of re-establishing the village and the adult protective shield; bonding and attachment work between mothers and children; increasing self-esteem, social skills, and access to health care; and identifying children traumatized by violence were all contained in her document, although they were conceived probably under the rubric of "creating social capital," rather than under the federal government's usual rubric.

Section Three

VIOLENCE

AND

VICTIMIZATION

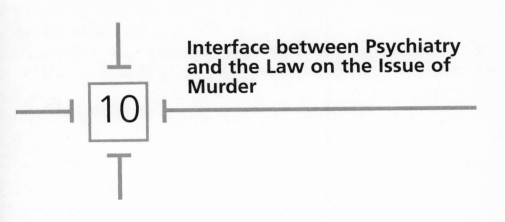

Interface between Psychiatry and the Law on the Issue of Murder

"Not guilty by reason of insanity" is a legal defense for murder. The acquittal of such an act is based on the court finding that the crime was due to the defendant's mental illness and not to criminal intent. The author presents characteristic case histories, as seen by him in the role of expert witness, that may serve as paradigms when the doctrine "not guilty by reason of insanity" is an appropriate defense.

INTRODUCTION

In Illinois, as in most other states, "not guilty by reason of insanity" is a legal defense for the crime of murder. The court, basing its opinion on expert psychiatric testimony, acquits the defendant of murder if the crime was caused by the defendant's mental illness rather than criminal intent. Recently, with such cases as the John Wayne Gacy trial, the defense of "not guilty by reason of insanity" has been brought into question. Those opposing use of this defense have pointed to the often contradictory opinions of different psychiatrists about the defendant's state of mind at the time of the crime and about what constitutes mental illness and criminal intent.

Originally printed as Bell Carl C. Interface between psychiatry and the law on the issue of murder. *J Natl Med Assoc*. 1980;72:1093–1097.

This article seeks to present several characteristic case histories of murderers, as seen from the standpoint of the expert witness, which hopefully will serve as paradigms for when "not guilty by reason of insanity" is an appropriate defense.

CASE REPORTS

Case 1

Case 1 is that of a 29-year-old black male who allegedly murdered his ex-wife. A review of police reports indicates that the defendant turned himself in to the police two days after the stabbing (with blood still on his clothes) and confessed to having stabbed his ex-wife. A statement was properly taken and charges of murder were brought against the defendant.

The defendant's past history revealed psychiatric problems for three years before the incident. His first symptoms occurred while in military service, when he began to have numerous somatic complaints and felt as if he had lost control of his body. A year later, he was discharged from military service with total disability stemming from mental illness (schizophrenia). Shortly after discharge, he experienced a recurrence of somatic pains, delusions of being controlled by some outside force, and bizarre behavior such as eating out of the toilet. There were several other hospitalizations at a veteran's hospital, but as time progressed, he began to get turned away from the veteran's hospital. When his request for admission was denied, he was quite upset (he had thought there was a plot to kill him and that the only safe place was the hospital). He never complied with requests that he attend an outpatient clinic and take medication. One month prior to the murder, the defendant had been denied admission to a hospital despite his reporting that there were electronic devices controlling his body, that he felt himself losing control, and that he was increasingly convinced of a plot against him.

The defendant reported that on the day of the murder, he went to his ex-wife's house to ask for some food. He took some rope, tape, and handcuffs in order to tie her up so he could find the electronics responsible for his mental discomfort. He reported that he felt very confused and heard voices telling him to kill her. He stated that he told her to call the police, as he was dangerous and needed to be taken away. He reported taking a kitchen knife with the intent to hurt her, but that he then gave it to the victim. He took the knife back and began cutting the victim, not with the intent of killing her but to give proof to the authorities of his dangerousness. He did not remember stabbing her, just cutting her. This part of his report was quite fragmented and confused. He reported leaving her alive and being chased by her relatives (who had heard the commotion from upstairs and had come down to investigate), but he got away. He remembered turning himself in later and being shocked when he was informed that his ex-wife was dead. He stated that in some ways, he felt that she was not really dead—that this was part of a plot, and she was really still alive.

During the interview, the defendant had an extremely small range of emotional expressiveness, which caused his affect to be flat and bland. He had delusions of being controlled by outside forces and of there being a plot to kill him; at the same time, he experienced auditory hallucinations that supplied a running commentary of his behavior and thought blockage. He reported that he still felt dangerous and that if he were not placed in an institution, he might harm someone else.

Case 2

Case 2 is that of a 43-year-old black male who was accused of murder of a five-month-old child, attempted murder, and aggravated battery. A review of the police report shows that the defendant turned himself in 36 hours after emptying a 38 caliber revolver into a crowd of people consisting of his estranged wife, their five-year-old daughter, his wife's five-month-old child (the victim), and his wife's sister. A statement was taken in which the defendant admitted to and gave details of the incident.

The defendant's past history revealed no previous psychiatric problems and showed that he had worked two jobs—one as a police officer—in an attempt to support his family to keep a good lifestyle. He reported having mild diabetes and that he had not had any insulin in three months; however, he had been able to continue his two jobs with no decline in performance.

The defendant reported that he had seen his wife (whom he had been legally separated from for three years) and other members of her family walking down the street on their way from church. He remembered parking his car and getting out to talk to his wife. He reported that he took his gun case with him, since the windows of his car were rolled down (as a police officer, he frequently carried his gun in this fashion). He reports that he was deeply in love with his wife, but that she did not want to be with him. He stated that despite the fact that he had worked two jobs for sixteen years, had a five-year-old daughter by his wife, and had bought her a house and car, she had felt he was "too easy" and had needed a challenge. She had left him three years prior to the incident and obtained a legal separation. She had filed for a divorce and even had a baby by another man, but between the time she filed and the shooting, she and the defendant had had an "on again, off again" relationship. This was characterized by her sometimes being cooperative in letting him see his daughter and accepting money for her support and other times being uncooperative and sending his checks back. Sometimes she told him she was coming back to him, but other times told him she never wanted to see him again. He wanted to talk to her about their problems, as they were in the "off" stage of their relationship, but when he met her on the street, she refused to speak to him. The next thing he remembered was driving in his car and hearing all the details on the radio. He reported being extremely upset, but figured he must have committed the crime, since he had a blank memory concerning the incident. He reported being confused and frightened, but after he pulled himself together, he turned himself over to the police. He reported that his "confession" was actually a composite of what he had heard on the radio and what the police interrogating him had "fed" him.

During the interview, the defendant was extremely remorseful about what he felt he had done but did not remember. This was evidenced by his frequent outbursts of tears. His history was relevant and coherent, and he showed no signs of psychosis. He further denied any history of having temper problems or dissociative phenomena (with the exception of the incident). He was interpersonal and had insight into his present difficulties. Finally, there were no signs of organic brain damage.

Case 3

Case 3 is that of a 37-year-old white male who was charged with the murder of a young adolescent male. The police report revealed that the defendant had been picked up several times previously for charges of sexually abusing adolescent males, with accompanying charges of assault and battery. None of the charges were successfully prosecuted, and the defendant was released with a recommendation to seek psychiatric treatment. The report stated that a maid had found the victim dead in a motel room, with his hands tied. In addition, there was evidence that the victim had recently experienced an episode of anal intercourse. The police were able to identify the defendant as a prime suspect due to various reports from witnesses and from clues left in the room. The cause of the victim's death was strangulation. The defendant was picked up. While he did not admit to the murder, the bulk of evidence was so substantial that his lawyer suggested he plead "not guilty," his crime being the product of a mental illness.

The defendant's past history revealed that he had made an attempt to obtain psychiatric treatment for his homosexuality, accompanied by a need to induce suffering in order to achieve sexual arousal. However, he only stayed in treatment a short time since his behavior excited him (though he felt tremendous guilt afterwards). During the psychiatric interview, the patient denied remembering exactly what had happened in the room that night, but he plead "not guilty" to the charges as his lawyer suggested. He had vague memories of inducing the victim to being tied up so the defendant could be sufficiently stimulated to have sex, but that in the heat of passion, things went blank. The next thing he remembered was waking up at home the following morning.

While the defendant was giving this vague historical sketch of what he remembered, he demonstrated no behavioral abnormalities other than an effeminate manner of expressing himself. He denied having any symptoms of psychotic illness nor any form of daily anxiety. He did express guilt about his sexual behavior and was remorseful over the death of the victim. His history revealed numerous sexual and physical traumas at the hands of an older brother, who later in life had to be institutionalized due to psychosis. The defendant was interpersonal and showed no signs of organic brain disease. There had been several episodes of suicidal gestures (aspirin overdoses) in response to his being left by a lover who could no longer tolerate the defendant's sexual/physical abuse.

DISCUSSION OF CASES

These three histories are characteristic of cases that call for an interface between psychiatry and the law. There is a problem of establishing the defendant's probable state of mind during the murder, which involves an exploration of not only the behavior but of, more importantly, the intent of the behavior.

In Case 1, the defendant clearly has paranoid schizophrenia with homicidal impulses. It was felt that he had not lost the total capacity to differentiate right from wrong, although this ability was impaired. More significantly, it was concluded that he was unable to adhere to what is right and was compelled by his auditory hallucinations and delusional need to protect himself. The murder was a product of the defendant's mental illness rather than criminal intent. Because the defendant's homicidal intent stemmed from a mental illness, it was felt that he should be committed to a mental institution for long-term treatment. Since the defendant's illness seemed chronic in nature, it was further suggested that if he should be released from the psychiatric hospital, he should be ordered to attend outpatient therapy and should comply with treatment until cured.

Case 2 is a bit more difficult to formulate, as the defendant did not evidence psychiatric problems prior to the murder. In fact, he could have been characterized as a model husband in light of his efforts to provide for his family. Cases of this type have to be defended with a diagnosis of "transient situational disturbance," which can occasionally reach proportions of acute psychotic illness. However, there must be sufficient evidence to show that the defendant suffered an altered state of consciousness[1] prior to the murder, rather than after the incident in an attempt to repress the abhorrent behavior. There was insufficient evidence of this in Case 2, and as a result, no opinion could be given about the defendant's state of mind at the time of the crime. In another very similar case, the defendant was observed as being asleep, lethargic, in a daze, and unable to adequately perform a job he was quite good at the day he murdered his girlfriend; he was noted as "not being himself." The defendant himself reported experiencing visual hallucinations as well as feeling stuporous, in a trance, and fragmented prior to the stabbing of his girlfriend 64 times (such a high number further indicated a state of frenzy). Thus, with this evidence, in addition to his not having remembered the act and a history of drug ingestion on the day of the murder, it was judged that the crime had been the product of a mental illness.

An interesting point about Case 2 is that the defendant gave a statement to the police in which he described and admitted to the murder but later reported not remembering what had happened and having to piece together information from the radio and the police. This may be a valid explanation, although it it sounds rather suspicious (the defendant could have conferred with his lawyer to come up with the explanation for his incriminating confession in order to get acquitted). In another case, a defendant confessed to the stabbing murder of a man in a YMCA lobby, explaining that the man had followed him there after harassing the defendant just a few moments before they reached the entrance door. However, witnesses reported that the defendant entered the hotel brandishing a knife and announced he was going to "kill every nigger in the house." After the stabbing, the defendant was reported to have walked up to a witness and said, "I did my job didn't I?" The defendant had a long history of alcoholism, having been committed several times for dangerousness to others, schizophrenic-like symptoms, and organic brain disease. He had confabulated the incident that had been lost from his deficient memory. Similarly, defendants who lose memory of their behavior may fill in the missing details from outside sources.

Case 3 poses a different problem—it raises the issue of what to do with the mental illness of characterologic proportions, but that does not manifest itself by causing the defendant to lose touch with reality. This defendant had a clear history of sexual deviation consisting of homosexuality and sadism, which, in this case, represented a mental illness. While he did not remember actually killing the victim, he did remember some sadistic behavior on his part before "things went blank." As in the second case, there was insufficient evidence to warrant a diagnosis of "transient situational disturbance with psychotic proportions," but the act was felt to be the product of a mental illness. It may have also been the result of an impulse that the defendant was unable to resist, due to the nature of his characterologic psychiatric disorder.

Cases like the above bring into question the liberal Durham rule[2]: "an accused is not criminally responsible if his unlawful act was the product of mental disease or mental defect."[3] The Durham rule was issued in 1954 because it was believed that the existing rules were inadequate. For example, the M'Naughten rule held that "a man is not guilty by reason of insanity if he labored under a mental disease such that he was unaware of the nature, quality, and consequences of his act, or if he was incapable of realizing that his act was wrong."[3] This rule relied on only the ability to distinguish right from wrong. The "irresistible impulse" concept held that a person is "irresponsible for his act when the act is committed under an impulse which the prisoner was by mental disease in substance deprived of any power to resist."[3] The "irresistible impulse" concept did not cover mental illnesses, which cause people to commit a crime on the basis of a well thought out delusion, not on the basis of an impulse.

Fortunately, the American Law Institute proposed rules that "provide that responsibility for an act can be negated if, as a result of mental disease or defect, substantial capacity was lacking to appreciate the criminality of conduct or to conform conduct to the requirements of the law."[4] With regard to Case 3, it was held that the defendant was not disturbed enough to have begun the act (which likely led to the murder of the adolescent) if a policeman had been present; his behavior was therefore not the product of an "irresistible impulse." In another case, a defendant who had a long history of an explosive personality went into a rage and attempted to kill his supervisor with a bar he had pulled out of the wall. A security guard pulled his gun and threatened to shoot the defendant in the head if he did not stop beating the victim. The defendant told the guard that he did not care, that he should go ahead and shoot. He continued to beat the supervisor until several other workers pulled him off. While this defendant clearly had an "irresistible impulse"—he was unable to resist due to the nature of his characterologic psychiatric disorder—the problem remains of what to do in this type of case. Fortunately, this is not a psychiatric decision, but one that is left up to the courts.

DISCUSSION

It is reported that violence is more common among minorities and the poor than among persons of affluence.[5-7] "The most common type of murder—the young black man who lives in a central city and kills an acquaintance, also young, black, and urban—has been characterized as the subculture-of-violence murder..."[6] It has been reported that "of the urban murders in this country, sixty-six percent are between blacks, twenty-four percent between whites, six percent entail blacks killing whites, and four percent whites killing blacks. The black murder rate is sixteen to seventeen times that of the white rate, and black females murder three times as frequently as white males."[6] Finally, it was reported that "the homicide rate has risen dramatically and over 20,000 persons are homicide victims each year; homicide is the seventh leading cause of death among nonwhite males of all ages, ranking second only to accidents in the deaths of both black and white males ages fifteen to twenty-four."[8]

Despite these statistics, it is important to note that a high crime rate is not characteristic of all black groups, since criminality is not an inherited black characteristic. Economically secure blacks have a far lower crime rate than poor blacks, and a similar differentiation occurs between well-educated and poorly educated black groups. The murder rate is also several times lower in certain black African tribes than among black or even white Americans.[9] There is evidence that cultural factors are responsible for the high homicide rate among American blacks. Furthermore, though blacks are heavily involved in raising homicide statistics, there has never been (to the author's knowledge) a black person who has committed heinous crimes like Richard Speck, John Wayne Gacy, and others have done. One also finds that:

> ...the mentally ill are perhaps less dangerous than so-called normal people. When one reflects on the rise in violence in this and many other countries during the past two decades, it becomes apparent that the great majority of capital crimes, serious assaults, and crimes against property are committed by persons who are not thought to be mentally ill.[5,10]

While the most dangerous patients are paranoid schizophrenics[11,12] (such as in Case 1), murder by acutely psychotic patients is rare.[13]

CONCLUSIONS

It is very apparent that blacks are involved in more homicides than are whites, and that a black is nine times as likely as a white to be placed in a correctional facility as an adult, and four times as likely to be sent there as an adolescent.[14] Thus, it is very important that black psychiatrists get involved with issues of forensic psychiatry. This involvement is recommended not so that a black psychiatrist can give more "breaks" to a black defendant who may not be guilty by reason of insanity. A fairer assessment might be obtained by a black psychiatrist than by a white psychiatrist with no knowledge of black culture, an inability to establish rapport with a black defendant, and no interest in broadening the knowledge and skills necessary for assessing and treating black populations.

In the case briefly mentioned about the patient who tried to kill his supervisor with a bar he pulled out of the wall, for example, the author made a diagnosis of explosive personality and indicated that the defendant had in fact suffered an "irresistible impulse." A white psychiatrist, on the other hand, gave the same defendant a diagnosis of antisocial personality. The white psychiatrist had spent only a very brief time with the defendant and had not elicited the history of temper outbursts, intense remorse after his crime, and his strong sense of loyalty. It was further ignored that though the defendant's life was threatened if he did not cease his outburst and the defendant did not desist, it was felt there was sufficient information gathered to chalk up this black male's behavior as antisocial. It is the author's opinion that such a diagnosis was a misrepresentation of the situation. The author also feels that regardless if the true diagnosis of explosive personality with an "irresistible impulse" altered the legal outcome, it is the expert's responsibility to give the court as accurate an assessment of the behavior and the intent of behavior as possible. The court can then make a determination as to the guilt and disposition of the defendant. The aim of expert psychiatric testimony, then, is to consider only the facts of the case and report them as the expert sees them, regardless of the issue of race or criminal responsibility.

COMMENTARY

This paper reflects several beginnings in my career and illustrates my initial grappling with violence in the African-American community. It was my first effort at presenting the fact that there are many varying motivations for violence. This paper documents the first time I used altered states of consciousness as a way to understand psychiatric issues in African Americans (see Chapter 18). I advocated here for the first time that black psychiatrists get involved with forensic psychiatry (see Chapter 8) as well. While I was doing this work, I hadn't yet left my office to "get rid of the murder rat" in the black community; I was dealing with the problem after the fact, not taking efforts to prevent it (see Chapter 2). Despite this, this early paper is still relevant, as it clearly presents some basic dynamics of varying motivations for murder.

I got involved with work on violence in a very unusual way. When I went to work at Jackson Park Hospital after getting out of the Navy, there was a psychiatric technician who worked in Jackson Park's Psychiatric Emergency Service and who helped in restraining patients. His case was described in this article. Although the employee had been doing an outstanding job, I noticed that his work had been deteriorating drastically and that he'd been falling asleep at work. I asked him about his recent poor performance and if he was having any problems, but he told me he was doing all right. A few days later, while his girlfriend was visiting him in the clinic under construction next door to our service, they apparently got into an argument. He stabbed her 64 times until she died.

When he went to trial, I was asked to testify about his mental status at the time of the murder. Although I'd been involved with some aspects of forensic psychiatry during my psychiatric residency, this was my first real forensic case. When I interviewed the defendant, he was in the psychiatric section of Cook County Jail because of his jail suicide attempt. At the time of the interview, he was extremely depressed. Because of my testimony, he was found not guilty by reason of insanity. During my testimony, though, I made it clear that I was functioning as an impartial expert witness.

It's been my experience that frequently, expert psychiatric witnesses don't act impartially. Some of them always determine that a defendant's murderous behavior was a product of antisocial personality, regardless of tons of evidence that the person was insane long before the crime. "Insanity" is a not a psychiatric term, but a legal term, rather, indicating that an individual was suffering from a mental disorder that prevented him from differentiating between right and wrong and/or conforming his conduct to the letter of the law. On the other hand, some expert psychiatric witnesses find the defendant "not guilty by reason of insanity" regardless of the absence of any evidence of insanity before the murder. Because I firmly believe in the ethics required to be a good physician, I've always found such bias reprehensible. As a result, when I do forensic psychiatry work, I make it a point to make it clear to whichever side that hires me that I'm functioning as a truly impartial expert. As a consequence, some of my opinions might hurt or help the defense. Similarly, some of my opinions might hurt or help the prosecution. I believe it's because of this approach of mine that I was asked to be a consultant for the Murder Task Force of the Cook County Public Defender's Office. Another reason was expressed to me while I was involved in a murder trial as a resident. After my testimony about the psychiatric status of a patient who had witnessed a murder, Cook County Judge Eugene Pincham told me I was the first psychiatrist he'd ever had in his courtroom who could explain something in a way he understood!

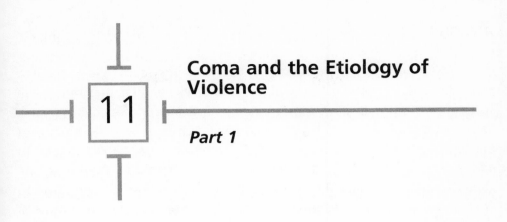

Coma and the Etiology of Violence

Part 1

Coma and the etiology of violence are explored by the author through a review of the literature. Animal studies, post-traumatic psychic disorder studies, post-traumatic anger and violence studies, tumor and lesion of the limbic system studies, temporal lobe epilepsy studies, and episodic dysfunction syndrome studies, minimal brain studies are reviewed here. Part 2 (see Chapter 12) will conclude the review with clinical surveys on violent individuals and studies on clinical treatment of violence.

These studies reveal the etiologic significance of central nervous system dysfunction in the production of violent behavior. Because central nervous system factors are involved in some instances of violent behavior, physicians clearly have a role in the early identification of potentially violent subjects and in the intervention or treatment of individuals who have been violent toward others. Studies have consistently found that lower socioeconomic groups are more predisposed to brain injury from trauma, and several studies have indicated that this is true for segments of the black community. Therefore, investigation of the relationship between central nervous system injury and violence should be a major goal of the black community. Black physicians should assume a lead role in these inquiries and in the prevention and treatment of violence, specifically black-on-black murder.

Originally printed as Bell Carl C. Coma and the etiology of violence, part 1. *J Natl Med Assoc.* 1986;78:1167–1176. Presented at the 91st Annual Convention and Scientific Assembly of the NMA, New York, NY, July 19–24, 1986.

INTRODUCTION

Nationally, the homicide rate is ten times higher for black men than for white men, and five times higher for black women than for white women.[1] Black men have a 1:21 chance of becoming homicide victims; white men have a 1:131 chance. Black women have a 1:104 chance of becoming homicide victims, and white women have a 1:369 chance. In 1983, black people accounted for 43% of the homicide victims in the United States, although they represented only 11.5% of the population. One black in forty will be murdered, and 90% of blacks who are murdered will be murdered by other blacks. Two thirds to three fourths of black homicides occur in families or among friends and acquaintances. Black-on-black homicide is the leading cause of death in black men aged 15–44 years. One in three black men who die between the ages of 20 and 24 are murdered.[1] More blacks lost their lives from black-on-black murder in 1981 than were killed in the twelve years of war in Vietnam.[2]

The National Institute of Alcohol Abuse and Alcoholism has estimated that about one half of all homicides in the United States are related to the use of alcohol.[3] Seventy percent of individuals convicted for manslaughter had been drinking.[3]

Considering these facts, it becomes apparent that black-on-black homicide is a major threat to the wellbeing of black Americans. The situation is even more grave when one considers that for every homicide, there are 100 assaults.[4] Furthermore, car accidents, rapes, and muggings cause fewer injuries requiring medical treatment than husbands cause their wives. Without doubt, the prevention and alleviation of violence among blacks should be a major goal of the National Medical Association.

To take a public health approach to black-on-black homicide, the epidemiology of homicide will need to be more thoroughly studied to learn where best to focus primary, secondary, and tertiary prevention efforts. It seems reasonable to slate the prevention of interpersonal violence as a primary prevention effort. A secondary prevention or intervention effort should be the early identification and treatment of individuals who have been violent toward others but who have not yet murdered. Assisting relatives and friends of victims of violence and murder should be a tertiary prevention effort[5] or post-intervention.[6]

Currently, homicides are divided into two basic types, primary and secondary. Primary homicides, which account for two thirds to three fourths of all murders, are "crimes of rage" that occur between family or friends and acquaintances. Secondary homicides are murders committed during a felony, such as robbery (usually involving strangers).[7]

An additional effort to develop a conceptual framework from which to intervene has been the classification of murderers. Because of the high number of black-on-black homicides, one of the most prominent descriptions of murderers in general has been the "subculture-of-violence" murderer classification. This classification proposes that blacks have a subculture (developed from the violence of slavery, racism, and the effects of discrimination, unemployment, and poverty) that not only tolerates violence but expects and promotes it.[8] The theoretical basis for this type of murderer partly arises from the finding that the urban ghetto environment produces a murderer who is characteristically young, black, and of lower socioeconomic class and who is quick to respond to narcissistic injury with lethal aggressive intent. This environment is thought to predispose individuals to using lethal aggression as a means to an end and using criminal violence to obtain material goods ordinarily out of their reach. The descriptive nature of this type of murderer is an accurate portrayal; however, the etiology, focused in subcultural dynamics, is questionable and leads to inappropriate rationalizations for murder. This thereby discourages further research and hinders the development of intervention strategies short of major subcultural change.

The other categories of murderers are suggestive of some clear and logical intervention strategies. For example, the "family-of-violence" murderer characteristically has witnessed and been the target of impulsive behavior and attacks of rage because of parental lack of control. The intervention strategy for this etiology of black-on-black murder involves early identification of violent families (e.g., gynecologists could detect such families by doing routine assault histories on all of their patients) and enactment of child and spouse abuse laws and interventions (e.g., strengthening black families).[9]

Problems associated with classifying what constitutes a psychiatric disorder and the legal ramifications of being judged mentally ill during a homicide make the "psychiatric-disordered murderer" category a controversial one. The question whether mentally ill patients are more predisposed to violence is hotly debated, with one camp asserting that acutely psychotic murderers are rare[10] and another camp asserting that there is a substantially higher prevalence of schizophrenic illness among men convicted of homicide (11%) than one would expect in the general population (0.1-0.4%).[11] It should be noted, however, that the conclusions that the researchers make are directly related to the population surveyed. Most surveys of psychiatric populations reveal a lower prevalence of violence than in the general population, but most surveys of correctional populations reveal a higher prevalence of psychiatric illness among prisoners convicted of violent crimes than in the general population. For this reason, it remains unclear if there is predisposition to and causality of violence in psychiatric patients. If, however, some psychiatric patients are more predisposed to murder than in the general population, the intervention strategy is clear: there must be tighter control of the mentally ill who show a history of violence. It is apparent that the rate of homicidal death among psychiatric emergency room patients is twice as high as that of the general population,[12] and steps need to be taken to prevent victimization of the victimized population.

Finally, the incidence of "biologically induced" murderers also is debated strongly; however, this type of murderer would be most clearly in the purview of physicians to identify and treat before they commit the endpoint of interpersonal violence—murder. Some estimate that 30% of all murderers fall into this category. These murderers have a subclinical brain dysfunction that produces an "epileptoid" mechanism responsible for impulsive rage.

In a previous study, Bell et al.[13] found that 45.4% of 108 black subjects (36 normal, 36 anxious, and 36 psychotic) had experienced a coma at least once in their lives. Of the 49 subjects reporting at least one episode of coma, 18 (36.7%) reported having had a coma of moderate severity (lasting more than 30 minutes but less than 24 hours) and seven (14.3%) reported having a severe coma (lasting more than 24 hours). As there is some evidence that cerebral insult resulting in unconsciousness or neuropsychological impairment may be partly responsible for interpersonal violence, a thorough literature review was made to substantiate further investigation into whether the large number of comas seen in a black population are causally related to the high rate of black-on-black homicide. The purpose of this article is to present a review of the literature on the central nervous system components of violence.

ANIMAL STUDIES

In 1937, Papez[14] proposed that the hypothalamus, anterior thalamic nuclei, gyrus cingulus, hippocampus, and their interconnections constitute a harmonious mechanism that may elaborate the functions of central emotion. Kluver and Bucy[15] in 1937 noted that bilateral temporal lobectomy could cause a profound change in emotional behavior. Specifically, bodily expressions of emotions associated with aggressive tendencies could be observed in some monkeys a few months after the surgery. Bard and Mountcastle[16] found that animals with hypothalamic lesions are predisposed to ferocious behavior after bilateral removal of the neocortex. There was a time latency of several weeks in this response. In 1974, Glusman[17] found that bilateral localized destruction of the ventromedial nuclei of the hypothalamus in cats results in the development of permanent "savage" behavior (develops two weeks after surgery). Other animal studies indicating the limbic system's role in the production of aggression show that septal forebrain lesions in the rat produce continuous fighting in experimental rats placed in the same cage.[18,19]

Looking at neurochemical animal studies, particularly stimulation and ablation studies in cats, it has been found that norepinephrine plays a significant role in affective aggressive behavior,[20,21] and the same holds true for central cholinergic mechanisms. Further, shock-induced aggression is correlated with catecholamine metabolism, and especially with norepinephrine. Thus, there is increased shock-induced fighting during morphine withdrawal as dopamine, serotonin, and norepinephrine turnover is increased; lithium lowers shock-induced aggression by decreasing functional availability of norepinephrine.[21] A connection between anatomical and neurochemical studies is found in the fact that septal lesions, which facilitate shock-induced and spontaneous fighting, are related to catecholamine systems and to some extent, cholinergic systems. Anatomical and neurochemical studies are connected by the fact that there is a relationship between septal lesions (which facilitate shock-induced and spontaneous fighting), catecholamine systems, and to some extent, cholinergic systems. Isolation-induced aggression and predatory aggression in rats seem regulated by catecholamines, specifically serotonin. Various medications are also able to raise or lower aggression in animal studies, depending on how the aggression is induced.[21]

Other animal studies relevant for a review of the relationship between head injury and violence are those examining experimental concussions. These studies tell us that the amount of damage to nerve cells is proportional to the number and strength of the blows inflicted.[22,23] Mild cases of trauma affect the rough surfaces of the brain (with the temporal lobes, frontal poles, and orbital cortex suffering the most).[24] There is evidence of decreased cerebral dopaminergic and serotonergic activity in frontotemporal lobe contusion, presumably from dysfunction of subcortical pathways involving mesolimbic areas (septal nuclei and hippocampus); it has been demonstrated in the animal studies cited above how these areas relate to aggression.[25]

POST-TRAUMATIC PSYCHIC DISORDERS

Several studies have documented that delirium, delayed psychotic states, personality disorders, and mental deterioration can occur following head injury (open and closed types).[26,27] There is some disagreement about how late a clinical problem may present. Some researchers report that post-traumatic encephalopathy is progressive,[28] while others note that changes occur within a few years and do not progress beyond that time.[26-29] Some investigators have found degeneration of cerebral matter with severe dementia.[30] Others have found that cerebral atrophy is secondary to head trauma.[26] Various degrees and types of head injury have been examined, and both the strength and number of blows are important variables in closed head injuries.[22,31] Mild, closed head injuries tend to lead to post-concussion syndrome[32-35]; however, some have speculated that this syndrome is due to neck and head injury as opposed to brain injury.[36] Others have found depression occurring after mild head injury.[37] Other clinical studies on moderate[38] and severe[39] head injury document the occurrence of headaches, memory loss, and a prevalence of lower socioeconomic patients at risk for these types of injury.

In a recent review of psychiatric complications of head injury, Kwentus et al.[40] noted that abnormal sleep patterns have been documented for up to five years after head injury. These authors maintain that in addition to the development of post-concussion syndrome, depressive and schizophrenic-like symptoms follow head injury. In their reviews, Lishman[41] and Davidson and Bagley[42] also quoted several studies that noted schizophrenic-like and affective symptoms after head injury. Since the 1930s, articles have reported the connection of head injury and schizophrenia, paranoia, or manic-depressive psychoses.[43-45] Shapiro[46] reported that the cases he collected with schizophrenic-like symptoms after head injury also had confusion, dizziness, memory defects, defects in orientation, and persistent headaches. These symptoms imply an organic etiologic factor. This author has also noted a delay in the appearance of psychic symptoms following head injury, as have others.[28,47,48] Other authors have reported that some patients, immediately following a head injury, recover from post-traumatic organic psychosis with hallucinations and delusions in a clouded or confused state and regain their premorbid intellectual state, but retain hallucinations and delusions.[49] Hillborn[50] noted that dementia, Korsakoff's psychosis, characterological changes, depressive psychoses, Manic-Depressive psychoses, reactive psychoses, paranoid psychoses, and schizophrenic-like psychoses can occur after head injury.

These studies are relevant because they point to the possibility of a head injury resulting in the delayed appearance of a schizophrenic-like syndrome. As it is apparent that the prevalence of "schizophrenic" symptoms is higher in the incarcerated population of murderers than in the general population.[11,12] Since it seems that the clinical manifestations of "schizophrenic" symptoms may not appear until some years after the murder,[51] one must wonder how much of the "schizophrenia" noted in murderers in correctional facilities is actually a delayed onset schizophreniform illness resulting from head injury. The murder may also be a result of head injury, as the next group of studies suggest.

POST-TRAUMATIC ANGER AND VIOLENCE

Several studies have documented that following head injury (open and closed types), anger and violence sometimes results.[44-45] Patients presenting to emergency settings exhibiting violent behavior have been found to be suffering from neurologic disorders resulting from head trauma, central nervous system infections, epilepsy in ictal and posttctal psychotic forms, degenerative dementia, and cerebrovascular disease.[51-53] Levin and Grossman[54] have reported agitated behavior during the transition from a coma of moderate severity (comatose for more than a half hour but less than 24 hours) to alertness manifested by hallucinations, delusions, and aggressively explicit behavior.

An early report by Strecker and Ebaugh[55] indicated that children who experienced cerebral concussion with loss of consciousness later developed explosive outbreaks in school or at home that were characterized by threats to kill, destructive behavior, and temper tantrums. Blau[56] found evidence of post-traumatic psychopathic personality in such children characterized by hyperkinesis, irritability, violent tempers, unrestrained aggressiveness, lying, stealing, destructiveness, quarrelsomeness, and cruelty to animals and younger children.

In a study of head-injured patients from World War II, Lishman[57] noted that in 144 patients, ten had signs of overt aggression. In a later review,[41] he noted that psychiatric sequelae of head injury may result in reduced control of aggression in episodic dyscontrol syndrome. Goethe and Lewin[58] reported that head trauma is the most common etiologic factor in organic personality syndrome, which is characterized by emotional lability, poor impulse control, apathy, or suspiciousness. Others[59-60] have noted that families of closed head injury patients have reported that the patients after the head injury were irritable, "hot tempered," restless, labile, and stubborn. Others have reported that this change in behavior occurs in a delayed fashion and may take a year to manifest.[61] Kwentus et al.[40] have noted that both frontal[62] and temporal lobe damage may lead to reduced control of aggressive impulses, with patients becoming subject to sudden violent outbursts with minimal provocation.

An interesting special perspective on post-traumatic anger and violence can be obtained from studies on boxers, which report on cases of boxers showing signs of cerebral atrophy, cavum septum pellucidum, and episodes of violence.[63-68] Casson et al.[65] suggest that even less powerful subconcussive blows cause microscopic damage to deep medial structures of the brain. Patients with these injuries may become extremely intolerant to small amounts of alcohol and become hostile and aggressive when ine-briated.[65,68–69] Corsellis et al.[70] suggest that the unprofessional outbursts of rage or aggression they found in fifteen boxers who had abnormalities of the septum pellucidum, scarring of the cerebellum and other areas, degeneration of the substantia nigra, and neurofibrillary tangles are due to post-traumatic lesions in the limbic structures, and especially in the septal area. This clinical hypothesis has gained support from animal studies men-tioned previously.[18,20] Others have noted that encephalopathy of boxers seems to progress through stages, one of which is characterized by psychic phenomena like increased arrogance, irritability, suspiciousness, and pos-sibly aggression[71] or uninhibited violent behavior. Encephalopathy may be a progressive condition resulting in neuropsychiatric impairment long after the trauma has occurred.[72] This observation is supportive of animal stud-ies[15–17] and studies[26,28,47–48] on brain injury that show a delayed onset of psychic disorders.

TUMORS AND LESIONS OF THE LIMBIC SYSTEM

Pilleri and Poeck[73] noted that pathological rage might appear after lesions in the limbic system. They point out that mild cases of this prob-lem occur in patients with temporal lobe epilepsy, which is manifested by irritability. More severe cases occur because of tumors of the temporal lobe or diencephalon or because of viral encephalitis (rabies and herpes encephalitis). Rage in these instances appears as an integrated pattern of angry behavior directed at surrounding people or objects and may be in response to delusions or misinterpretations. Finally, Pilleri and Poek note that in neoplastic or inflammatory lesions of the anterior midline and par-ticularly diencephalic structures, a maximal outbreak of rage may occur. It is often not related to the situation but is triggered by trifling nonspecific stimuli. Malamud[74] reported on eighteen cases with tumors of the limbic system that presented with psychiatric symptoms. Zeman and King[75] reported on four cases with midline tumors, which produced temper flare-ups and outbursts of anger and violence. Charles Whitman, who in 1969 killed his wife and mother then climbed to the top of a tower at the University of Texas to shoot 38 people (killing 14), was found to have had a large malignant tumor in his amygdala. Although rare, these occurrences support the notion that central nervous system factors are important for understanding violence[76] and that limbic dysfunction may be an important area of study.

TEMPORAL LOBE EPILEPSY

Mark and Sweet[77] note that young men after craniocerebral injuries often go through a phase of hyperactivity and belligerence. While the injury is often too diffuse to correlate a specific brain area with the symptom of violence, there are reports of restlessness and combativeness in patients with contusions of the temporal lobe. It has been estimated that post-traumatic epilepsy develops in 5% of closed head injuries, and most of this epilepsy is temporal lobe.[41] Animal studies[24-25] on the general nature of concussion note that the temporal lobe is at risk. Finally, Gastaut[78] in his study of temporal lobe epileptics reports that trauma may be responsible in a majority of cases.

The relationship between trauma and temporal lobe epilepsy (TLE) is significant to this review because of the number of head injuries found in blacks in general and that because TLE is associated with violence. Several authors[77-80] have noted the following occurring in an otherwise adjusted individual with TLE: irritability, explosiveness of affect, outbursts of aggressiveness, rage, personality disorders (characterized by episodic impulsiveness, irritability, destructiveness, and combativeness), hostility, anger, paranoid trends, psychopathic syndromes, ictal clinical manifestations characterized by violent impulses, rage in patients with 14 and 6/sec temporal spikes on their electroencephalograms (EEGs), ictal and interictal violence and assaultive behavior, paraoxysmal rages, and pathological aggressiveness. Nuffield[81] studied children with epilepsy and found that children with TLE were significantly more aggressive. Ounsted[82] studied children with TLE and found that although disorderly homes and rage outbursts were statistically linked, they may be found independent of each other in kids with TLE. In this study, 36 of 100 children with TLE had outbursts of catastrophic rage. Davis[83] proposed that children with explosive or episodic behavior disorders were probably suffering from a disorder of organic origin and reported on a number of studies indicating abnormal EEGs present in the posterior temporal lobe in this population. Treffert[84] found that aggressiveness and ictal-aggressive symptoms in the form of rage episodes and assault were more characteristic of patients with temporal lobe EEG focus (with and without clinical epilepsy) than psychiatric patients without temporal lobe EEG foci. Liddell[85] noted that psychiatric patients with TLE showed more aggressiveness and hostility, along with a tendency for violent, short-lived, and unprovoked outbursts before a seizure.

Serafetinides[86] and Taylor[87] found a significant amount of overt aggressiveness and character disorders associated with aggression in temporal lobe epileptics, but attributed these findings to deficient learning and stresses of epilepsy. These authors thought that epilepsy produced intolerance to frustration rather than an interference of neurologic mechanisms that control aggressive behavior.

Goldstein[21] notes that TLE as a cause of aggression is hotly debated. Studies done by Stevens[88] and Rodin[89] found TLE does not predispose patients to aggressive behavior or to character disorders associated with aggression. These authors speculate that the misconception that TLE predisposes patients to aggressive behavior is the result of previous studies using patients from psychiatric populations. There is similar controversy about whether TLE predisposes patients to paranoid schizophrenic symptomatology[90-91] or not.[92] Despite these controversies, the fact remains that Jack Ruby was defended with a diagnosis of psychomotor epilepsy,[89] and epilepsy is several times more common in prisoners than in noncriminals.[93] Current consensus on the relationship between violence and seizures is that violence and ictal phenomena are rare; however, subjects who demonstrate violent behavior have had seizures, which implies a role seizures have in subjects with poor impulse control.

EPISODIC DYSCONTROL SYNDROME

In 1971, a group of researchers[94] described 130 patients who presented to psychiatric emergency rooms with fears of losing control and harming someone. The patients had had homicidal ideation, repetitive aggressive behavior under the influence of alcohol, impulsivity, rage outbursts, dangerous misuse of an automobile, or repeated arrests for violent acts. Patients often had past histories of birth injuries, mental retardation, coma-producing illness such as meningitis, febrile convulsions in infancy, or head injury with prolonged unconsciousness. In the study, violence was viewed as a symptom of psychodynamics, social disorganization, and brain dysfunction. These researchers noted five groups that had episodic dyscontrol syndrome: temporal lobe epileptics (7 patients), those with seizure-like outbursts (30 patients), those with diffuse violence (57 patients), those with pathological intoxication (25 patients), and those with repetitive violence (11 patients). Seventy-two patients reported having been unconscious due to injury or illness, and 25 of 130 had had childhood febrile seizures or adult seizures. Finally, of the 79 that had EEGs, 37 were abnormal (20 with spikes in the temporal region). Twenty-nine of 50 questioned had a history of hyperactivity.

Maletzky[95] reported on 22 subjects who demonstrated episodes of violence upon minimal or no provocation and whose outbursts occasionally were preceded by an aura and followed by headaches and drowsiness. Sixteen subjects had a history of hyperactivity, twelve reported a history of febrile convulsions, and seven had a history of head trauma severe enough to cause loss of consciousness. About one half of the subjects had seizure-like symptoms of auras of hyperacusis, visual illusions, numbness of extremities, nausea, headaches, drowsiness, and altered states of consciousness. Eleven had soft neurological signs (left-right ambivalence, dysdiadochokinesis, mild ataxia, astereognosis, dysgraphia, and perceptual reversals). Fourteen of 22 had abnormal EEGs, six with spiking in the temporal region and eight with nonspecific rhythm abnormalities in the temporal lobe, including some theta activity. Since 19 of the 22 responded to anticonvulsant treatment, Maletzky suggests that the episodic dyscontrol syndrome may be the manifestation of a subclinical epileptogenic foci of the temporal and limbic regions.

Elliott[96–99] has written extensively on the neurology of explosive rage. He has collected 286 cases in which episodic dyscontrol had developed in 102 formerly stable individuals after a specific brain insult. In the remainder of the cases, the explosive rage began as temper tantrums, which had developed prior to puberty. Fifty-one subjects had the explosive rage develop after head injury, 119 had minimal brain dysfunction, 40 had TLE, and 7 had generalized epilepsy. For the remainder, the explosive rage developed from other assorted neurologic disorders. In 148 cases in which computerized axial tomography was done, structural abnormalities were uncovered in 41%. Elliott noted that explosive rage might occur many months after a head injury, or as a result of repeated minor head injuries. He reviewed several articles that support the argument that head injury may lead to explosive rage, and remarks that the percentage of cases may have been larger had the follow-up been longer, because explosive rage may develop one to two years after the initial trauma. He notes that severe and mild head injuries can produce subtle changes in the personality that may occasionally lead to aggression; further, an acquired liability to small quantities of alcohol, which can trigger off attacks of uncontrollable rage, may develop.

An interesting aspect of Elliott's work is that the subjects of his study were mostly all middle- or upper-socioeconomic-class private patients, 96% of whom were white. This raises a question of how serious the problem must be for lower socioeconomic groups, which have been shown to be at greater risk of head injury.[100] Further, considering Clark's[101] observation that far more children and young adults are killed by cars in Harlem than in the rest of New York City (6.9:100,000 in blacks compared with 4.2:100,000 in whites), one must wonder at the number of children hit by cars who are not killed but get head injuries. Similarly, a recent report of free falls from heights notes a disproportionately high incidence of falls among minority group children (45% of the falls being accidental).[102]

Currently in the DSM-III,[103] episodic dyscontrol syndrome is classified as "intermittent explosive disorder." Because of the nature of this disorder, it is apparent that there would be a higher prevalence of this disorder in correctional populations. Thus, it would be reasonable for correctional health care standards[104] to highlight the identification and treatment of this disorder in an effort to reduce this public health problem.

MINIMAL BRAIN DYSFUNCTION

Morrison and Minkoff[105] reported on three cases of hyperactivity in which a decreased ability to concentrate was outgrown, leaving behind incapacitating aggressiveness with a hair-trigger temper. Hertzig and Birch[106] examined 100 psychiatrically disturbed male adolescents (75% of their presenting symptoms were antisocial, i.e., running away from home, aggressiveness at home or school, assaultiveness, theft, and attempted homicide). Compared with a normal population, these male adolescent psychiatric patients were found to have indications of neurologic dysfunction six times more often, adventitious movements twelve times more often, auditory-visual integrative deficiency fifty times more often, and subnormality in intelligence eight times more often. Similarly, other authors[107] have studied emotionally unstable character disorders in antisocial, impulsive patients with short, nonreactive, bipolar mood swings and found that these patients have soft neurologic signs, indicating that central nervous system damage may be involved in their etiology. Andrulonis et al.,[108-109] in studying the relationship between the borderline personality syndrome (patients with hyperactive, impulsive, and aggressive behavior) and organic brain dysfunction, have found that individuals with minimal brain dysfunction (attention-deficit disorder and learning disabilities) and trauma or encephalitis or epilepsy are often lumped in the borderline syndrome category as adults. Further, patients with these subcategories of the borderline personality also have "spectrum" disorders on an organic brain dysfunction continuum, and frequently display symptoms of the episodic dyscontrol syndrome. These authors suggest episodic dyscontrol syndrome is a subcortical temporal lobe-limbic system dysfunction that is best treated with anticonvulsants, while patients with minimal brain dysfunction subcategories are best treated with stimulant medication.

COMMENTARY

This article continues the effort I'd made in classifying the various motivations for murder outlined in Chapter 10 and also focused on coma, a state of consciousness we'd found to be quite prevalent within African-American communities (see Chapter 24). This article was published in JNMA along with the editorial Doctors Prothrow-Stith and Smallwood-Murchison and I did on the NMA's responsibilities in eliminating black-on-black homicide (see Chapter 1). This work was so long, I had to break it into two parts. Part 1 reviews the central nervous system's components of violence, while Part 2 (see Chapter 12) is more clinically based and covers clinical surveys of violent individuals and studies on clinical treatment of violence.

Currently in the African-American community, there is controversy about biologic causes of violence. Much of the concern regarding this issue is based on the fear that white scientists are looking for a genetic cause of violence. If they find one, there's the additional fear they will use it as an excuse to put black children on various medications or engage in some form of genocide. Much of this fear is being fueled by various fringe anti-psychiatry groups that go around saying that psychiatry kills and is a destructive force when the reality is that doctors don't go to medical school to harm people. A close examination of the actual research on the biology of violence reveals that currently no one puts much stock in genetic causes of violence, though there's some proof that some individuals are genetically predisposed to developing antisocial personality disorder and alcoholism. However, so far, genetic predisposition for these disorders has been found only in European-American and European populations. It's clear that the most prevalent type of violence isn't genetically based.

In addition to genetics, other types of biologic problems can contribute to an individual's becoming violent. An example is the "acquired" biology of a head injury or lead poisoning that produces an explosive behavioral problem. It seems to me that this could be prevented, which would reduce violence in society. African Americans must always be concerned about sundry ways that "science" might try to denigrate us. However, we should also be careful not to become too anti-scientific, lest we throw the baby out with the bath water.

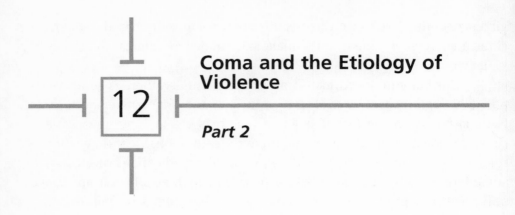

Coma and the Etiology of Violence

Part 2

Coma and the etiology of violence are explored by the author through a review of the literature. Animal studies, post-traumatic psychic disorder studies, post-traumatic anger and violence studies, tumor and lesion of the limbic system studies, temporal lobe epilepsy studies, episodic dyscontrol syndrome studies, and minimal brain dysfunction studies were reviewed in Part 1 (see Chapter 11). Part 2 concludes the review highlighting clinical surveys on violent individuals and studies on clinical treatment of violence. These studies reveal the etiologic significance of central nervous system dysfunction in the production of violent behavior. Because central nervous system factors are involved in some instances of violent behavior, physicians clearly have a role in the early identification of potentially violent subjects and in the intervention or treatment of individuals who have been violent toward others. Studies have consistently found that lower socioeconomic groups are more predisposed to brain injury from trauma, and several studies have indicated that this is true for segments of the black community. Therefore, investigations in the relationship between central nervous system injury and violence should be a major goal of the black community. Black physicians should assume a lead role in these inquiries and in the prevention and treatment of violence, specifically black-on-black murder.

Originally printed as Bell Carl C. Coma and the etiology of violence, part 2. *J Natl Med Assoc.* 1987;79:79–85. Presented at the 91st Annual Convention and Scientific Assembly of the NMA, New York, NY, July 19–24, 1986.

INTRODUCTION

There have been several studies on psychopathic or delinquent children and adolescents who have exhibited violent behavior and who have been brought to the attention of psychiatrists.

CLINICAL SURVEYS OF VIOLENT INDIVIDUALS

In 1925, Healy[110] reported on 4,000 cases of delinquency, noting cases in which a change of personality had directly followed a severe concussion. Further, he reported that there was a larger number of head injuries among delinquents than among non-delinquents and that 3.5% of his sample had had a head injury of some severity, each having suffered at least one period of unconsciousness. Kasanin[111] found (in 5,000 cases at the Judge Baker Foundation) that among 120 cases diagnosed as psychopathic personalities, 10% had had a serious brain injury during childhood and adolescence, with conduct disorder following the trauma. Bender,[51] who studied 33 children and adolescents who had killed, found that 16 of 19 subjects who had stabbed, repeatedly struck, or shot their victims had schizophrenia, brain disease, and/or epilepsy. The final diagnostic count of Bender's cases was as follows: 3 with intellectual defects, 12 with schizophrenia (none were diagnosed as such at the time of the incident; 9 had been recognized in childhood and 3 in adulthood), 3 with epilepsy, 7 with chronic brain syndrome with no epilepsy but impulsive disorders, 10 with psychoneurotic depressions reactive to the situation.

Lewis and her colleagues[112–116] have done extensive research on violence in children and have found several interesting trends relevant to this review. In one study[112] where Lewis reported on 285 children referred to juvenile court, she found psychomotor epileptic symptoms in 18 (6%). Psychomotor epileptic symptoms have been found to be frequently associated with aggressive behaviors and offenses. These patients had episodes of loss of full conscious contact with reality and long staring spells or falling; 16 of the 18 also had paranoid symptomatology in the form of delusions. Eleven of the fourteen available electroencephalograms (EEGs) showed an abnormality, but only three had a temporal lobe focus. Lewis notes a striking finding of serious trauma to the central nervous system in 15 of the 18.

In another study,[113] Lewis et al. found that incarcerated adolescents had significantly more accidents and injuries, specifically head or face injuries, than hospitalized adolescents had. In addition, Lewis found that 18% of the violent incarcerated male adolescents she studied had psychomotor seizures.[114]

In a later study Lewis[115] and her colleagues studied 55 children, 21 of which were homicidally aggressive. The most significant behavior distinguishing the homicidally aggressive from the non-homicidally aggressive children was suicidal behavior (57% vs. 23%). Of the 21 homicidal children, 48% definitely had a history of seizures (many had experienced febrile seizures), compared with 7% of 30 non-homicidal children. Furthermore, an additional 10% of the homicidal children probably had seizures. There was a tendency for more of the homicidally aggressive children to have had a history of head injury (57% vs. 30%) and to have averaged a greater number of head injuries as well. In 62% of the households producing the violent children, the fathers had been physically violent toward the mothers, compared with only 13% in the non-homicidal children. Alcoholism was also significantly more common in the fathers of homicidally aggressive children (52% vs. 10%). The most significant factor distinguishing mothers of homicidally aggressive children from non-homicidally aggressive children was a history of psychiatric hospitalization (43% vs. 7%).

In a prospective study of children who murder, Lewis et al.[116] noted five characteristics (history of extreme violence, psychotic illness in a first-degree relative, witness or victim of violence in the family, psychotic symptoms, and major neurologic impairment) that when taken collectively, significantly differentiated nine children (six had severe head injury) who murdered from those 24 who did not. Lewis et al.[116] speculate that the prevalence of head trauma, perinatal problems, or seizures in their samples indicates a problem of central nervous system dysfunction—the kind often associated with lability of mood and impulsivity. The theory is that the central nervous system dysfunction, combined with a vulnerability to psychotic disorganization, contributes to children's self-destructive and homicidally aggressive behaviors.

Malmquist,[117] in a study of 20 adolescents charged with murder, found that suicidal preoccupations may be common the week before the homicide. Inamdar et al.[118] studied violent and suicidal behavior in psychotic adolescents and found that 27.5% had been both violent and suicidal, with male subjects significantly more likely to be violent and suicidal. These findings parallel a study by Whitlock and Broadhurst[119] comparing 50 suicidal patients, 50 non-suicidal psychiatric patients, and 50 healthy persons; they found that suicidal patients had significantly higher violence indices than did either of the controls. The relationship between suicidal and homicidal impulses is also seen in the finding that 12% to 18% of the calls to suicide hotlines are in fact calls related to homicidal impulses.[6] Of interest to this review is the finding that suicidal and homicidal impulses have been correlated in blacks,[120] and that at least one study notes a significant prevalence of head injury (14%) occurring in a black population during the year of a completed suicide.[121]

In clinical studies of prison inmates who have committed violent crimes, neural factors in the generation of this violence have been indicated. Gunn and Bonn[122] found that the prevalence of epilepsy in prison was several times greater than in the general population and noted that other studies found that murderers were more prone to epilepsy than were the general population. A representative sample of epileptic prisoners was no more criminally violent than a matched control group of prisoners without epilepsy. However, this study found epileptics to be more impulsive than controls, which fits with previous observations that individuals with abnormal EEGs are more likely to commit motiveless homicidal violence.

Hill[123] has written on "epileptoid" features in psychopathic personalities that cause abnormal irritability, resulting in attacks of rage with poor reflection, a twilight state, and markedly clouded memory; jealousy and alcohol are the precipitants. He notes that of the aggressive psychopaths (patients whose histories repeatedly show hostile acts against individuals and a tendency to self-injury) he studied, 65% had abnormal EEGs and 33% had had head injuries. However, Hill notes that EEG abnormalities in aggressive persons are independent of previous head injury and that although head injury can produce aggressiveness and dysrhythmia, these results are probably not related; he feels dysrhythmia is more common in naturally aggressive psychopaths than in psychopaths whose aggression results from head injury.[124] Hill[125] studied 110 murderers and found that they had 11% more theta wave excess and 6.2% more post-temporal slow wave focus than did controls. Of these murderers, there were ten with temporal lobe foci, and nine of these were in the posterior regions.

Williams[126] studied 1,250 prisoners in which more than half were incarcerated for a crime of major violence (murder, attempted murder, inflicting bodily harm, rape or attempted rape). The remaining prisoners had committed crimes that involved bodily violence, such as robbery with violence. A random sample of 333 was closely studied. It was found that the EEGs of the habitually aggressive inmates were abnormal in 65% of the cases, compared to 24% of inmates who had committed major violent crimes but who were not habitually aggressive, and to 12% of the inmate population at large. When those who were mentally retarded, epileptic, or had had a major head injury were removed from the tally, it was found that the EEG was abnormal in 57% of the habitual aggressive inmates, but in only 12% of the non-habitually aggressive inmates who had committed a major violent crime (the same as the population at large). The EEG abnormalities in the habitual aggressives were seen bilaterally in 64% of the cases and involved the frontal cortex. In addition, the temporal lobes were affected in all (the anterior part three times as often as the posterior), while rhythms known to be associated with temporal lobe dysfunction (theta wave, four to seven second) were present in 80%.

Another study of legally insane murderers showed that these individuals had EEG abnormalities about four times more often than the control group.[127] Stafford-Clark and Taylor[128] studied 64 murderers and found that the murders could be grouped in the following manner: (1) murder incidental to committing another crime, (2) a clear motive for the murder or intended violence while committing another crime, (3) essentially motiveless murders, (4) murders with a strong sexual element, (5) murders in which the murderer was legally insane. For murderers in groups 1 and 2, there was a preponderance of normal EEGs, but those committing unmotivated murder (group 3) there was a preponderance of abnormal EEGs. There was a marked preponderance of abnormal EEGs in murderers in groups 3 (73%) and 5 (86%), which strongly suggests that the cerebral dysfunction such abnormal records indicate is significantly correlated with a capacity to commit apparently motiveless violent acts. In contrast, less than 10% of murderers in group 1 (accidental murder) had abnormal records, which approximates the proportion in the general prison population.

Other miscellaneous clinical studies on criminal populations include the work by Gibbons, Pond, and Stafford-Clark.[129] They noted that nearly half of the criminal psychopaths studied who had suffered prior head injury were originally convicted for violent offenses, and this proportion was much higher than in psychopaths without complications, or psychopaths with epilepsy.

Frazier[130] studied 23 one-time murderers and 8 multiple murderers and found organic brain factors in four one-time murderers (temporal lobe epilepsy in two and mental retardation in two) and in two multiple murderers (organic brain syndrome caused by neoplasm in one and early dementia from central nervous system infection in another). He noted that episodic dyscontrol was present in eight one-time and three multiple murderers, and episodic psychosis without external reality testing was present in 15 murderers (three of whom were multiple murderers).

Finally, Langevin et al.[131] studied sexually aggressive inmates. Though they found no significant difference between sexually aggressive inmates with temporal lobe pathology (30%) and controls with temporal lobe pathology (11%), they did find that the sadistic sexually aggressive inmates had significantly more temporal lobe pathology (56%) than did non-sadistic sexual aggressive inmates (0%). One third of the sadists had indices over the cutoff point for significant brain damage, compared with 8% of the non-sadistic sexually aggressive inmates and 18% of the controls.

Clinical studies of patients who come to emergency rooms for treatment because of violent tendencies have already been discussed in the section on episodic dyscontrol syndrome (see Chapter 11). A study by Climent and Ervin,[132] however, has particular relevance to this review. These authors compared 40 violent emergency room patients with 40 controls and found that violent subjects were more likely to have been beaten as children and more likely to have owned and used knives. Alcoholism in the father and mother was more common in the parents of the violent group. Of the 19 violent subjects who reported head injuries before 15 years of age, 9 reported unconsciousness along with the injury; in contrast, unconsciousness was reported by only three of twelve controls who had had head injury before the age of 15. Significantly more violent subjects reported head injury with unconsciousness (the severity of injury being judged by coma). Five of the violent subjects reported convulsions before the age of ten, compared with none in the control group. After ten years of age, 15 of the violent subjects had suffered from convulsions, as opposed to none in the non-violent group. The violent subjects suffered significantly more headaches. The authors hypothesize that these findings point to the likelihood of violent behavior being influenced by organic brain disease. Violent subjects also had more suicidal thoughts.

STUDIES ON CLINICAL TREATMENT OF VIOLENCE

Lion, Bach-y-Rita, and Ervin[133,134] raised significant questions to determine which patients exhibit violent behavior that might be caused by a neurologic disorder. These questions included the following: Were there symptoms such as headaches or altered states of consciousness that accompanied the violent act or impulsiveness? Are there subtle personality changes over time (implying neoplasm)? Is there a marked alteration in sexual function or memory (implying temporal lobe process)? Is there a past history of infection such as meningitis or head injury that may have led to brain impairment? Is there an impairment of intellectual ability or a history of learning difficulty? Is there a family history of epilepsy or a history of convulsions in childhood? Do aura or seizure-like states exist? Is there a history of repetitive rage reactions or periodically reoccurring temper tantrums that suggest temporal lobe epilepsy? Similarly, Elliott[97] suggested asking the following: Do you have difficulty in controlling your temper? Have you been charged with traffic violations for dangerous driving? Are you especially sensitive to alcohol? Such questions asked during a standard review of systems would identify patients who are at risk for violent behavior due to central nervous system causes. Physicians who routinely asked for a history of assault could uncover families of violence and could initiate the appropriate intervention—sociologic, interpersonal, intrapsychic, or biologic.

Lion[135] notes that aggression is a symptom that may stem from psychosis—severe character disturbance of the explosive, antisocial, or passive aggressive type. Impulsivity is a common feature in all of these types, and their violence is usually episodic and paroxysmal, indicating that organic factors may or may not underlie such problems as hypersexuality, depression, or mania. Lion further notes that various types of medication may adequately treat the underlying causes of violence.

As previously reported, several authors have noted gross clinical psychopathology (usually schizophrenia) in murderers.[11,21,51,116] Although there is considerable controversy about the dangerousness of mentally ill patients,[136–139] it is important to note that several authors have indicated the efficacy of antipsychotic medication in treating aggression stemming from psychosis.[21,140–142]

Lithium has been noted to reduce aggression in several animal studies.[21,143] In addition, Sheard[144] studied twelve maximum security prison inmates who were selected on the basis of a prehistory of three or more episodes of violent crimes of assault, prison behavior characterized by continuous verbal and physical aggressive behavior, and high scores on aggressive scales. He found a significant reduction in aggressive affect (self-rated) and a reduction in the number of tickets received for physical or verbal aggression secondary to treatment with lithium. Tupin et al.[145] studied 27 male convicts with a pattern of recurrent violent behavior (in and outside of prison) and who reacted rapidly to slight provocation with anger or violence. They found several other common characteristics in the patients' medical profiles, such as a history of brain injury, nonspecific abnormal EEGs, and mixed psychiatric diagnoses (eight schizophrenics, four possible schizophrenics, twelve explosive personalities, and three others). These authors found a significant decrease in the mean number of disciplinary actions for violence for identical time periods before and after lithium. Prisoners reported a decrease in aggressive feelings, an increased capacity to reflect on consequences of action, an increased capacity to control angry feelings when provoked, diminished intensity of angry affect, and a more generally reflective mood. Staff consistently reported a decrease in aggressive behavior in the inmates studied as well. Sixteen of the 21 deemed to have improved had an abnormal EEG or a history suggestive of brain damage (including head trauma with unconsciousness) or known central nervous system disease (e.g., meningitis or epilepsy). Morrison et al.[146] studied 20 inpatients (11 with frequent seizures, abnormal EEGs, and hyperaggressiveness; 2 with hyperaggressive behavior but normal EEGs; 7 with EEGs showing 14/6 per second positive spiking but without clinical seizures). They found that 15 of the 20 inpatients treated with lithium showed a reduced frequency of hyperaggressiveness and assaultive behavior, a decreased tendency to quarrel, and greater self-control when provoked. Finally, Rifkin et al.[147] reported that lithium aids overaggressive patients with character disorders.

As a result of the findings that associate EEG abnormalities with violence, several authors have investigated the use of anticonvulsants in the treatment of violent subjects. Several authors[148,149] have discussed the efficacy of carbamazepine in violent patients with abnormal limbic system discharges and temporal lobe pathology with sham rage attacks. Monroe[150] and his colleagues[151,152] have noted that a significant number of violent acts are committed by individuals in whom central nervous system instability can be demonstrated by special EEG activation procedures using alpha-chloralose as the activating agent. This instability is suggested by the circumscribed ictal phenomenon in the limbic system, demonstrated on subcortical EEGs. These authors note that chlordiazepoxide or primidone led to dramatic improvement in 23 of 55 acutely disturbed patients with episodic, impulsive, aggressive behavior. Maletzky[95] reported on 19 of 22 subjects with episodic dyscontrol syndrome who responded favorably to phenytoin.

Elliott[153] reported on seven patients whose belligerence (secondary to acute brain damage) was successfully controlled with propranolol. Yudofsky and his colleagues[154-156] have made several reports on the usefulness of propranolol in treating rage that occurs secondary to organic brain damage. One study[154] indicated that propranolol controlled the rage and violent outbursts in four patients with irreversible chronic organic brain syndromes. A second more extensive study[155] examined 30 children and adolescents with uncontrolled rage outbursts and organic brain dysfunction (9 with minimal brain dysfunction, 11 with uncontrolled seizures and 3 others with history of definite neurogenic seizure, and 4 with anticonvulsant medication for suspected seizures) and found that over 75% of the patients showed either moderate or marked improvement in response to propranolol treatment, although propranolol did not do much for the seizures. These authors[156] presented a case of rage and violent behavior in a patient with Korsakoff's psychosis, in which propranolol controlled the rage and violent behavior. Elliott[153] suggested that catecholamine access to the brain stimulates alpha- and beta-adrenergic receptors to induce dyscontrol of anger and violence. Animal studies reported on earlier[20,21] support this hypothesis.

Other authors have reported that psychostimulants[157] are useful in treating children and adolescents with hyperactivity problems (resulting in fighting, defiance, and impulsiveness) by reducing violent behaviors, and suggest that some adults with residual minimal brain dysfunction resulting in hyperaggressiveness may be aided by similar medication. Although there is some controversy about whether minor tranquilizers cause a reduction in aggressive behavior or cause "paradoxical" rage reactions, one author[158] reports that in his experience, this type of medication has helped anxious, aggression-prone individuals, and suggests further research in this area.

Lastly, it must be noted that most authors who advocate a chemotherapeutic approach to managing violent individuals underscore the additional need for psychotherapy in these persons. Lion[159] notes that patients who have aggressive personality disorders are unable to handle depression-arousing stimuli and that a major goal of therapy is to establish an ability to feel and appreciate depression stemming from frustration. He also notes that these patients need practice fantasizing and imagining possible consequences of their behavior. He suggests that the therapist needs to be supportive, empathic, and firm and available in times of need. Lion and Bach-y-Rita[160] reported on their experiences with group psychotherapy and violent outpatients. They noted that two therapists in the group helped to create an atmosphere of control. This was accomplished by seating the group around a large table and constantly emphasizing the need for verbal rather than physical expression of emotions, which helped ease the group's tensions. This group was viewed as an ongoing therapeutic modality available to members in time of stress, so intermittent member attendance was acceptable. It was also felt that insight was less a factor in helping than was the social experience of a group.

CONCLUSIONS

From this review of the literature on the central nervous system and the causes and treatment of violence, it should be clear that physicians have a role in the early identification of potentially violent subjects and the intervention or treatment of individuals who have been violent toward others. It is only through this active role taken by physicians that there will be a substantial reduction of black-on-black homicide.

This paper's review of the animal studies, post-traumatic anger and violence studies, tumor and lesion of the limbic system studies, temporal lobe epilepsy studies, episodic dyscontrol syndrome studies, minimal brain dysfunction studies, clinical surveys on violent individuals, and studies on clinical treatment of violence all point to central nervous system factors being involved in some instances of violent behavior. Considering the consistent finding that lower socioeconomic groups are more predisposed to brain injury from trauma and considering that several studies[13,101,102] have indicated this is indeed true for segments of the black community, investigations of the relationship between central nervous system injury and violence are a must for the black community. Black physicians should assume the lead role in these inquiries.

COMMENTARY

Most of the confusion about what should be done about violence comes from a lack of understanding of the various types of violence. Much of my current work tries to inform people of the various types of violence I've identified. In Chapter 10, I described violence that occurs because of severe mental illness resulting in insanity (a legal term indicating that an individual was suffering from a mental disorder that prevented him/her from differentiating between right and wrong and/or being unable to conform his/her conduct to the letter of the law). Violence that occurs as a result of one having a psychopathic personality was also identified. I also discussed violence that occurs because of an acute rage reaction stemming from a personal relationship with the victim. In Parts 1 and 2 of "Coma and the Etiology of Violence," I would go on to differentiate between primary and secondary homicides. Primary homicides encompass violence resulting from an acute rage reaction between two people who know one another and get into an interpersonal altercation. In secondary homicides, violence occurs during a felony like a robbery and usually occurs between two strangers. More recently, I've begun to describe primary homicides as "interpersonal altercation violence" and secondary homicides as "predatory violence." These two terms are more descriptive of the relationship between the victim and offender. The "Coma and the Etiology of Violence" articles would also identify biologic violence such as a head injury as another type of violence.

In addition, physical violence can also be described as group violence, as in the case of mob violence, or can be perpetrated by an individual. Systemic violence such as racism can be less direct in its manifestation and yet can be just as damaging as direct physical violence. Hate-crime violence is another type that calls for its own particular response. Gang-related violence also requires a tailor-made reaction. Drug-related violence falls into four subcategories, all requiring different answers. Systemic drug-related violence occurs when one drug dealer kills another to sell drugs to his competitor's customers. Pharmacological drug-related violence occurs when a drug user is violent because of the drugs in his system. Economic drug-related violence happens when a drug user engages in violence to get money to buy drugs. Negligent drug-related violence transpires when a person high on drugs harms someone accidentally. I thank Dr. Paul Goldstein for making these differences between the various types of drug-related violence clear to me.

Violence can be described as legitimate verses illegitimate or non-lethal verses lethal. Terrorism, mass murder, murder sprees, and serial killing are also other more rare forms of violence. Although there may be some overlap in these classifications, they can be separate and distinct in many ways. The most important thing to recognize is that we must consider the type of violence targeted in order to form prevention strategies appropriate for each type. Once we are well informed about the different types of violence, we can all develop strategies to prevent each of them.

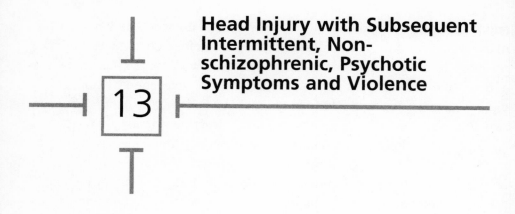

Head Injury with Subsequent Intermittent, Non-schizophrenic, Psychotic Symptoms and Violence

13

A black, young adult, female presented to an outpatient clinic for treatment with a history of intermittent, non-schizophrenic, psychotic symptoms. Because of their situational sociology, blacks may be more predisposed to severe head injuries, and this acquired biologic factor may be, in part, responsible for the high rate of black-on-black murder. The use of beta-blockers is discussed as an adjunct in the treatment of violence occurring in patients with a past history of severe head injury.

INTRODUCTION

A black, young adult, female presented to an outpatient clinic for treatment with a history of intermittent, non-schizophrenic, psychotic symptoms. Her post-psychotic, psychosocial functioning lacked the significant deterioration found in post-psychotic adjustment of schizophrenics. It was, however, characterized by irritability, an inability to get along with significant others, and a tendency to have intermittent episodes of explosive violence. The patient's past history revealed that her intermittent, non-schizophrenic, psychotic symptoms and violent behavior began after a severe head injury.

Originally printed as Bell Carl C, Kelly Ruby P. Head injury with subsequent, intermittent, non-schizophrenic, psychotic symptoms and violence. *J Natl Med Assoc.* 1987;79:1139–1144.

CASE HISTORY

The patient was born in the early 1960s following an essentially normal gestation and delivery. She was considered an average baby who had achieved all developmental milestones within the normal range. Her relationship with family members during her early development was described as affectionate, outgoing, and playful. Her biological parents separated when the patient was three years old, but the patient was not reported to have manifested any separation issues as a result. Overall, the patient's early developmental years showed no significance for poor frustration tolerance, temper outbursts, or violent tendencies. Her mother remarried while the patient was in kindergarten, and she and her stepfather developed a close relationship. It was reported that because the patient was the youngest of three girls, her stepfather tended to be a bit indulgent with her. Her relationship with her mother and eldest sister was close, with elements of respect and identification, but her relationship with her next older sister was competitive for the mother's attention. However, their sibling rivalry was not considered as unusual.

The patient's academic standing throughout elementary school was slightly below average. Socially, however, she was very outgoing and had lots of friends and good relations with her teachers. She was active in sports, cheerleading, dancing, and other activities. There were no reports of truancy, fights, temper outbursts, or impaired relationships with others throughout her elementary school years. She graduated on time and went on to attend a local neighborhood high school, but continued to achieve slightly below average. Popularity among peers and teachers continued, and she participated in various organizations, sports, cheerleading, and dancing activities. Her family relations continued as they had through childhood, and the patient began heterosexual relationships by dating a high school sweetheart off and on for four years.

During her late adolescence, the patient experienced a traumatic event that resulted in a significant change. When the patient was a senior in high school, she and her best friend went on a double date with their boyfriends. All of them had been drinking and subsequently were involved in a tragic auto accident in which everyone was killed except the patient. She sustained a head injury and was comatose for ten days. After recuperating from the accident, she returned to high school, but this proved to be difficult, since she encountered too many associations that reminded her of her deceased friends. She began to withdraw and imagined seeing her deceased friends on the school grounds. Her mother transferred her to another area high school, where the patient completed her high school requirements, although she continued to withdraw and failed to make any new friends.

During the six months after the accident, the family noticed several behavioral changes. The patient was abrasive toward others, had paranoid thoughts that others were "out to get her," evidenced difficulty in concentrating, and had crying spells. This made a sharp contrast to her behavior before the accident, which was described as cheerful, playful, active, competitive, affectionate, easy to get along with, outgoing, and charismatic. Despite these behavioral changes, the family was not overly alarmed, feeling the patient was going through a normal grieving process. After her high school graduation in 1980, the patient was employed as a waitress in a fast-food restaurant but was terminated after a three-week period because of her inability to get along with others.

The patient next attended a beauty culture school for six months, but again, her success was curtailed because of her inability to get along with the teacher. She was terminated from her next employment in a clothing store because she generated interpersonal friction. During this year after graduation, the family noticed additional behavioral changes: rages, temper outbursts, slamming doors, physical and verbal confrontations with others, and suicidal ideation.

During the patient's young adult years, her level of functioning became increasingly worse. Although motivated to seek gainful employment, she seldom could stick with a vocation because of her poor frustration tolerance and equally poor impulse control. In 1982, she successfully completed a four-month program at a local vocational training center and received a certificate in medical technology. During this same year, she worked in two blue-collar jobs that ended in termination because of her inability to get along with supervisors and coworkers. Her sporadic temper outbursts and impaired relations with others continued until the early months of 1984. At this point, the family became more concerned over the patient's constant complaint of boredom, increased withdrawn behavior, excessive sleeping pattern, destruction of property, frustrations regarding her lack of employment, and inability to move out on her own. As a result, in June 1984, the family sought help from a local city mental health clinic. It was seven years after the accident, and the patient was 23 years old.

The family's main motivation for seeking help at this time was that the patient had become "unmanageable." The patient was diagnosed as being schizophrenic, paranoid type and was placed on oral fluphenazine. She was later switched to fluphenazine decanoate injections. Her mother stated that her daughter's behavior improved with this treatment; however, the patient became noncompliant, complaining that the medication slowed her down and made her feel "like a mummy." In September 1984, the mother had the patient admitted to a private university psychiatric hospital because the patient had spent one week in bed, was irritable, and exhibited poor concentration.

Upon admission to the hospital, the patient underwent a thorough physical examination, laboratory tests, and psychiatric evaluation. The physical examination was within normal limits. The neurologic examination showed the patient to be alert and oriented to person and place but not to time. Her cranial nerves were intact; her motor functions were appropriately strong and symmetrical bilaterally; and her sensory functions were intact regarding touch, temperature, and pain. She revealed a normal capacity for cerebellar coordination on the right, as she was able to successfully complete the finger-to-nose and heel-to-shin tests on that side; however, there was some awkwardness on the left side. Her gait was normal, but the presence of Romberg's sign was questionable, because the patient fell asleep when she closed her eyes. Routine laboratory results were all within normal limits. The electroencephalogram results showed a normal tracing while the patient was in the awake and drowsy state, and there were no focal paroxysmal or epileptiform patterns seen. However, nasal leads were not recorded.

The psychiatric evaluation revealed anxious behavior, restlessness, incoherent speech, flight of ideas, and loosening of associations. Her mood was sad and constricted. She reported a ringing sound of bells and other noises in her ears and paranoid ideation. She also evidenced impaired memory. Initially, the diagnosis was questionable: post-traumatic stress disorder, schizophrenia, major depressive episode with psychotic features, and possibly an organic affective disorder were all considered. She was hospitalized for six weeks and was placed in a structured day program, which included occupational therapy, music therapy, dance therapy, multiple family meetings, small verbal groups, and individual therapy. During her hospitalization, the patient continued to exhibit psychotic symptoms and later admitted to infrequent auditory hallucinations.

As a result of the diagnostic uncertainty, she was given psychological tests (Holtzman Ink Blot, Sentence Completion) that indicated slightly abnormal thought processes. The Minnesota Multiphasic Personality Inventory (MMPI) was also administered, and the patient was found to have characteristics compatible with a schizophrenic disorder. At discharge, she was diagnosed as schizophrenic, disorganized type. Her aftercare plans included medication management (trifluoperazine, 20 mg at bedtime, and benzotropine, 2 mg, if needed) and follow-up at an outpatient day-treatment program. She failed to comply with the aftercare plan.

After discharge, the patient was able to function without psychotic symptoms for over a year, although she was not on medication. During this period, however, she continued to evidence sporadic temper outbursts and impaired relations with others. In the fall of 1985 (approximately around the anniversary of her accident), her family noted an exacerbation of depressive symptoms. These symptoms persisted for several months, after which the patient began to develop signs of agitation that progressively worsened. In the summer of 1986, she was re-hospitalized at a state psychiatric hospital for disrupting the household, becoming easily enraged, being always angry because of feelings that everyone was plotting against her, getting into a fight with her next older sister in which the patient pushed her sister down a flight of stairs, and throwing firecrackers at children playing downstairs. She was hospitalized for two weeks and was managed on haloperidol, 5 mg three times a day, and benzotropine, 2 mg twice a day. She was discharged earlier than anticipated because she did not return to the hospital after she had been issued a pass. Her discharge plan was to participate in a structured day-treatment program and vocational training.

The patient followed the recommendation for aftercare treatment at the Community Mental Health Council. The psychiatric evaluations completed in August 1986 revealed most of the previously reported history. The patient's current mental status was evaluated as follows: the patient was appropriately and neatly dressed and behaved in an uncooperative and hyperactive fashion. Her speech was characterized by confusion, circumstantiality, and pressure. Her affect was constricted in range and representative of a dysphoric mood. She denied current homicidal or suicidal ideation and auditory or visual hallucinations. She was oriented to person and place but marginally oriented to time. Her recent memory was fair for events of the day, and her ability to differentiate the current mayor of Chicago from the current president of the country was initially poor. She was able to correct herself with prompting and more labored concentration. Her mathematics skills were below what one would have expected from a high school graduate, which seemed to indicate poor concentration. The patient demonstrated an instability of affect because of a tendency to switch from a sullen, dysphoric affect to unreasonable anger, and this instability decreased the patient's ability to maintain age-appropriate social judgment.

Diagnostic formulation described the patient as a 25-year-old, single, black woman who had a history of crying spells, fluctuating sleep patterns, violent outbursts, destruction of property, verbal and physical confrontation with others, suspiciousness, paranoid ideation, poor sensorium and cognition skills, and two episodes of psychiatric hospitalizations due to intermittent, non-schizophrenic, psychotic symptoms. These behaviors became manifest six months following an accident in which the patient sustained a head injury and was comatose for ten days. Before the accident, she was functioning at a perceptually higher level of psychosocial functioning. Based upon this formulation, the diagnoses of organic affective disorder and intermittent explosive disorder were assigned. Initially, the patient was placed on loxapine, 25 mg, and benzotropine, 2 mg twice a day, but because the patient complained of excessive fatigue, her medication was gradually reduced to the current level of loxapine, 10 mg at bedtime. She was also placed on propranolol, the dose of which was gradually being increased while her loxapine dose was being decreased, until a final dose of propranolol of 40 mg twice a day was reached.

The patient is currently compliant with treatment, and her affective disorder with psychotic symptoms (presumably due to an organic cause) and her intermittent explosive behaviors have ceased. While her relationships with significant others have improved markedly, she continues to show subtle sensorium and cognitive deficiencies that hamper her adjustment, and she maintains a tendency to deny her difficulties, although she is much more satisfied with her current outpatient treatment.

DISCUSSION

This case illustrates how a head injury causing a coma may later result in an organic affective disorder with psychotic symptoms and an organic personality disorder, explosive type (referred to in DSM-III[1] as "intermittent explosive disorder"). Organic affective disorder with psychotic symptoms[2–4] has been discussed elsewhere and thus will not be extensively discussed here, except as the problem relates to blacks. Bell et al.[5] demonstrated that a substantial proportion of blacks with prior psychotic episodes reported a history of having had an episode of coma. Over half the patients studied reported having had a coma, with 15% of the aftercare sample reporting that their unconsciousness had lasted longer than 24 hours. These findings imply that a significant proportion of psychotic illness in blacks may be related to a prior head injury. Another point of interest is that the patient discussed here was diagnosed as schizophrenic based on psychiatric evaluation and psychological testing (MMPI). There are records of misdiagnosis of blacks with affective disorders[6–9] and of the excessive diagnosis of schizophrenia in blacks based on psychological testing,[10,11] but the question of how a substantial prevalence of head injury in blacks obscures diagnostic assessments has yet to be investigated.

Organic personality disorder, explosive type, is characterized by a persistent behavior pattern of recurrent outbursts of aggression or rage often resulting in serious assault or destruction of property. According to revised DSM-III criteria, the explosive behavior is grossly out of proportion to any precipitating psychosocial stressor and is not due to psychotic symptoms, major affective disorders, or clouding of consciousness. Unfortunately, this revision does not clearly consider that head injury may also cause intermittent, psychotic, non-schizophrenic symptoms. The exclusion criteria (in the authors' opinion) should refer only to clearly "functional" psychotic or affective symptoms and not to psychotic or affective symptoms that seem to be related to an organic cause. Patients such as the reported case, who have intermittent, psychotic, non-schizophrenic symptoms secondary to head trauma may need treatment with low doses of antipsychotic medication, but this should not preclude the recognition of their explosive disorders. The revised DSM-III criteria also require a history of unconsciousness for at least fifteen minutes following a head injury, seizures, drug or alcohol use, infection, or physical illness; or evidence of the patient exhibiting an abnormal brain function or structure (e.g., history of seizure disorder, neurologic "soft signs," or history of an abnormal electroencephalogram).

A recent review of the literature[12,13] documents some research that led to establishing the understanding that head injury may have some significance in the origin of violent behavior and recommends this for further study. Lewis et al.[14] have recently furthered this understanding through their work on the neuropsychiatric impairment of death row inmates who had murdered. All of the individuals studied had a history of significant head injury, one third had evidence of major neurologic impairment, and an additional one half had less serious neurologic problems that were identifiable by neurologic examination.

The understanding that head injury may have some causative significance for violent behavior has particular relevance for blacks. Several studies have shown that blacks are more at risk for such head injury. Whitman et al.[15] found that the head trauma rate for blacks living in the suburbs was 394 per 100,000 and 403 per 100,000 for inner-city blacks. The head injury rate for suburban whites was 296 per 100,000. In their study, falls were the most common cause of head injury for inner-city black children aged under sixteen years. Rivara and Mueller[16] found that for "...all races, injury death rates [from head trauma] are inversely related to income level, and much of the difference seen in death rates between racial groups may be the result of existing discrepancies in income." Further, the incidence of head injury in nonwhites has been shown to be nearly 50% higher than in whites. The male-to-female ratio is slightly higher among nonwhites as well.

Blacks have a greater incidence of head injury, and head injury has been associated with causing a predisposition to violence. This casts significant doubts on the "subculture of violence" explanation that has been expounded concerning the high rate of black-on-black murder. This high rate may be due more to the high incidence of head injury in poor black neighborhoods than to a supposed "subculture" existing in those neighborhoods.

It has been proposed that physicians pay attention to the situational sociologic conditions that predispose blacks to head injury (e.g., inadequate housing leading to a disproportionate number of free falls from heights among black and Hispanic children).[17] This will help reduce situational sociologic conditions rather than addressing the "red herring" of subcultural shortcomings of black people.[18,19] In addition to reducing the acquired biologic factors contributing to violence, it has been suggested that physicians and health professionals address the situational sociologic conditions that cause psychological factors (e.g., self-hatred that predisposes blacks to violence).[20,21] Physicians and health professionals can also directly repair those psychological factors that predispose blacks to violence.[22]

It has been suggested that physicians directly treat acquired biologic conditions leading to violence by thoroughly studying medications that seem to have promise in reducing violence partly stemming from acquired biologic factors like head injury. Propranolol, which has shown significant promise in this regard, was used in this study's patient and saw good results. This medication has been shown to be useful in reducing violence in several studies,[13] but the bulk of these studies' subjects were white. Propranolol has been reported to be less effective in the treatment of black hypertensives. Schorer[23] has also noted, "too few black patients have been included in studies [on explosiveness] to reach any conclusions about the efficacy of propranolol, or whether race is a differentiating factor." Propanol's lack of effectiveness in hypertensive blacks taking propranolol may be unrelated to the effect the medication might have on reducing violent behavior. Should propranolol be useful in treating intermittent explosive disorders in blacks (as has been the experience of the author), however, its anti-hypertensive ineffectiveness in blacks may be a boon in disguise, since a physician treating a black patient for intermittent explosive disorders would not need to be concerned about cardiovascular side effects of the medication. More studies are urgently needed to elucidate these important questions, as it is clear that the answers would greatly benefit blacks.

It is hoped that discussing this case history will give physicians some motivation for presenting their own case studies. It is also hoped they embark upon more controlled clinical research to test the hypothesis that propranolol may be useful in reducing intermittent explosive violence resulting from head injury, and the hypothesis that head injury may attribute significantly to the high rate of black-on-black murder.

COMMENTARY

After more than a year of successful treatment, the patient discussed in this paper stopped coming to the clinic and was lost to follow-up. Years later, after this paper was published, I learned that Dr. E. Evelina Powers, the CMHC's medical director, had been treating her at the clinic. The patient had started using crack cocaine. Because of her drug use, she hadn't been compliant with treatment and had deteriorated. A couple of years ago, a public defender called me and told me she'd committed a homicide. These developments surprised me, but it only shows that one can never be too sure when and how unexpectedly an ex-patient might appear into a psychiatrist's life. I sent the public defender a copy of this paper, but I haven't heard anything about the outcome.

One of my biggest frustrations in treating patients is that though I know I can help most of them live more satisfying lives with less difficulty, many of them, unfortunately, refuse the help and would rather go through life plagued by treatable problems. The patient discussed here is a perfect example. The biggest tragedy is that despite a careful assessment and an individualized treatment plan, when a patient doesn't fully agree with the assessment or doesn't fully comply with the treatment, they rarely get better. They halfway go along, only to show up in my office years later telling me, "If only I'd listened to you five years ago, I wouldn't be in the mess I'm in today." I try never to tell them, "I told you so." I just try to help them where they are. Deep down, though, it's quite painful for physicians to see lives hurt and productive years lost because of hard heads. But you know what your grandmother told you about hard heads making for soft behinds.

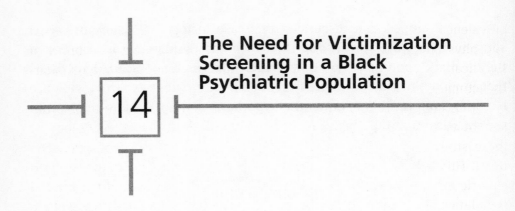

The Need for Victimization Screening in a Black Psychiatric Population

14

Recent reports indicate that violence toward others is a major public health problem in the black community; however, there are very few empirical studies that delineate the severity of the problem. In an effort to add to the meager data on violence in the black community, the authors compiled the results of a victimization screening form obtained from a black outpatient psychiatric population. Recommendations are made that black psychiatric populations be screened for histories of victimization, as victimization is common in this population group and will have a significant impact on treatment.

INTRODUCTION

In 1983, black-on-black homicide was the leading cause of death in blacks aged 15–34 years.[1] Furthermore, it has been estimated that for every one homicide there are one hundred assaults.[2] These indications of the prevalence of violence in the black community lead one to wonder about the prevalence of violence (sexual and physical) that might affect black psychiatric patients. The purpose of this study is to delineate the

Originally printed as Bell Carl C, Taylor-Crawford Karen, Jenkins Esther J, Chalmers Deborah. Need for victimization screening in a black psychiatric population. *J Natl Med Assoc.* 1988;80:41–48.

prevalence of black psychiatric outpatients who report a history of sexual and physical assault and to determine the number of them who know of significant others (relatives, friends, or neighbors) who have been similarly victimized.

A review of the literature reveals that few studies address the problem of violence in a psychiatric population. Since the methodology of these studies varies greatly, it is difficult to make comparisons between them. Hillard et al.[3] reported that the rate of homicidal death among psychiatric emergency room patients was twice as high as that of the general population. Rounsaville and Weissman[4] reported that 3.4% of the women presenting to a psychiatric emergency service had been battered by men they knew intimately. Stark and Flitcraft[5] noted that battered women were five times more likely to use psychiatric facilities than were non-battered women, and that battering accounted for one in four suicide attempts in all women and for one in two suicide attempts in black women. Hilberman and Munson[6] reported that half of the women referred for psychiatric consultation in a rural medical clinic were in battering relationships. Only a handful of studies exist on the prevalence of a positive victimization history among inpatients. Post et al.[7] reported that 48% of the inpatients they interviewed had a history of battering relationships. Fifty percent of the women (compared to 14% of the men) reported having been battered, and 21% (compared to 27% of the man) had abused their partners. Carmen et al.[8] reviewed psychiatric records of 188 adolescent and adult inpatients and found that 43% had a history of physical or sexual abuse, or both. Thirty-two percent had been physically abused, 8% had been sexually abused, and 12% had been both sexually and physically abused. 53% of the women and 23% of the men had been abused. These authors noted that blacks were slightly more likely than whites to have been victims of abuse, but attributed this finding to the high percentage of women (85%) in the black sample. Jacobson et al.[9] obtained complete histories from 100 psychiatric inpatients and found that 81% had experienced major physical and/or sexual assault. Barnhill et al.[10] reported on the prevalence of physical violence in a community mental health center setting and found that 49.4% of the inpatients and 38.6% of the outpatients reported present or past concerns about violence (either as victims or assailants).

METHODS

A total of 427 patients were screened for this study. This number represents all the open cases at the Community Mental Health Council, Inc. (CMHC), in May 1986. At the time of the screening, the clients were in one of the agency's four programs: Screening and Medical Assessment (SMA), Family Systems, Outpatient, and Community Day Treatment (CDT). With the exception of SMA, the programs reflect the severity of the clients' emotional disturbance. If they can function independently, they go into the outpatient program, but if they need more direction to get through life, they go to the day treatment program. The SMA program, which performs entrance assessment, is designed to evaluate patients who request treatment so they can be referred to an appropriate treatment program. Family Systems takes a family therapy approach to its patient population, which consists of children and adolescents under 18 years of age and adults with no history of psychotic illness but who need psychotherapy. The Outpatient Program population consists of patients who have had a psychotic illness and need ongoing chemotherapy to prevent a relapse, but who have sufficient psychosocial living skills to live fairly independently. The CDT program population consists of patients who have had a psychotic illness and need ongoing chemotherapy to prevent a relapse, in addition to intensive psychosocial rehabilitation. Ninety-nine percent of the total patient population is black, 68.3% live on $7,400 or less annually, and 61% live alone. A breakdown by age, sex, and program of the 427 patients screened is displayed in Table 1. Over 58% of the patients were women, and approximately 20% were under the age of 18. Most patients were in the Outpatient Program.

TABLE 14.1. Sex, Age, and Program of Clients

	SMA Prog. No. (%)	Family Sys. Prog. No. (%)	Outpatient Prog. No. (%)	CDT Prog. No. (%)	Total No. (%)
18 Years and Older					
Men	14 (3.0)	12 (2.8)	74 (17.3)	28 (5.3)	123 (28.8)
Women	14 (3.0)	50 (11.7)	138 (32.3)	18 (4.2)	220 (51.5)
Under Age 18					
Men		54 (12.6)			54 (12.6)
Women		30 (7.0)			30 (7.0)
Total	28 (6.0)	146 (34.1)	212 (49.6)	41 (9.5)	427 (99.9)

The CMHC's Victimization Screening Form (see Figure 1) was administered to the patients by their therapists or by an intake worker if a therapist had not been assigned. The staff had previously received in-service training on the problem of victimization in the black community and

FIGURE 14.1. Victimization Screening Form

Name: _____ Age: _____ Sex: _____

YES   NO

               I. **Child/Adolescent** (*Note: must be at least 6 years of age*)
                    A. Has anyone ever:

_____   _____ 1. Forced or threatened you into letting him/her touch any part of your body, e.g., breast/chest, vagina, penis, anus, buttocks (molested)?

_____   _____ 2. Forced or threatened you into letting him/her sexually assault/rape you, i.e., put penis or any other object in either your mouth, vagina, or anus (raped)?

          If yes, specify when and by whom: _____

                    B. Have you ever been:

_____   _____ 1. Robbed? Was a weapon used? Specify: _____

_____   _____ 2. Physically assaulted (beaten up)?

          If yes, specify when and by whom: _____

                    C. Has someone close to you (relative, friend, neighbor) ever been:

_____   _____ 1. Molested?

_____   _____ 2. Raped?

_____   _____ 3. Robbed (stuck up)?

_____   _____ 4. Physically assaulted (beaten up)?

_____   _____ 5. Murdered (killed)?

          If yes, specify when and by whom: _____

              II. **Adult** (*Note: 18 years and older*)
                    A. At any time in your life, have you been:

_____   _____ 1. Molested (forced or threatened into letting someone touch any part of your body)?

_____   _____ 2. Sexually assaulted/raped?

          If yes, specify when and by whom: _____

                    B. At any time in your life have you been:

_____   _____ 1. Robbed? Was a weapon used?

_____   _____ 2. Physically assaulted?

          If yes, specify when and by whom: _____

                    C. Has someone close to you (e.g., relative, friend, neighbor) ever been:

_____   _____ 1. Molested?

_____   _____ 2. Raped?

_____   _____ 3. Robbed?

_____   _____ 4. Physically assaulted?

_____   _____ 5. Murdered?

          If yes, specify when and by whom: _____

Intake Worker: _____ Date: _____

Referral to Victims Assistance Program: Yes _____ No _____

on the use of the form. The Victimization Screening Form, developed in the CMHC's Victims Assistance Program, asks about the patient's incidence of sexual and physical victimization and about the victimization of individuals close to the patient.

RESULTS

Adults

The adult mental health patients (aged 18 years and older) reported considerable victimization of themselves and individuals close to them. Twenty-four percent (N = 82) of the 343 adults had been sexually molested, 23% (N = 78) had been sexually assaulted, and 40% (N = 138) had been physically assaulted. Forty-three percent (N = 147) of the adults had been robbed, and 43% (N = 61) of these robberies involved a weapon.

A clearer indication of the extent of assault experienced by the patients is reflected in the number of patients who have been sexually assaulted only, physically assaulted only, and both sexually and physically assaulted. Almost half (48%, N = 163) of the adult patients at the agency had been sexually or physically assaulted, or both. Sixteen percent (N = 27) had been sexually assaulted only, 53% (N = 87) had been physically assaulted only, and 31% (N = 50) had been both physically and sexually assaulted.

At least one in five of the patients was aware of a relative or friend who had been victimized. Nineteen percent (N = 65) reported that someone close to them had been sexually molested, 24% (N = 81) knew of someone who had been sexually assaulted, and 31% (N = 105) had a relative or friend who had been physically assaulted. Over one third of the adults (35%, N = 121) reported that a relative or friend had been robbed, and one fourth (N = 87) reported that someone close to them had been murdered.

Data for men and women in the four programs are presented in Tables 2 and 3. When the ten items measuring victimization of self and others were analyzed for all adults and separately for men and women, no significant relationship was found between program and victimization. Analysis of the sexual assault only, physical assault only, and physical and sexual assault measure, however, found a significant relationship between type of victimization and program for women ($x^2 = 15.51$ [6], $p < 0.02$). Women in the Family Systems program (the least severely disturbed) were more likely to have suffered physical assault and less likely to have experienced sexual assault than women in the other programs (see Table 4). Of the 25 women in the Family Systems program reporting assault, 56%

TABLE 14.2. Adult Male Patients Sexually and Physically Assaulted

	SMA Prog. No. (%)	Fam. Sys. Prog. No. (%)	Outpatient Prog. No. (%)	CDT Prog. No. (%)	Total No. (%)
Personally:					
Molested	2 (14.3)	3 (25.0)	6 (8.1)	1 (4.3)	12 (9.7)
Sexually assaulted	0 (0)	0 (0)	4 (5.4)	1 (4.3)	5 (4.1)
Robbed	7 (50.0)	4 (33.3)	31 (41.9)	9 (39.1)	51 (41.1)
Robbed with a weapon	4 (28.6)	2 (16.7)	18 (24.3)	3 (13.0)	27 (22.0)
Physically assaulted	7 (50.0)	5 (41.7)	25 (33.8)	13 (56.5)	50 (40.7)
Know of someone:					
Molested	0 (0)	3 (25.0)	12 (16.2)	2 (8.7)	17 (13.8)
Sexually assaulted	1 (7.14)	3 (25.0)	12 (16.2)	1 (4.3)	17 (13.8)
Robbed	6 (42.9)	3 (25.0)	28 (37.8)	5 (21.7)	42 (34.1)
Physically assaulted	2 (14.3)	5 (41.7)	18 (24.3)	7 (30.4)	32 (26.0)
Murdered	2 (14.3)	4 (33.3)	19 (25.7)	7 (30.4)	32 (26.0)
Total No. of patients	14	12	74	23	123

TABLE 14.3. Adult Female Patients Sexually and Physically Assaulted

	SMA Prog. No. (%)	Fam. Sys. Prog. No. (%)	Outpatient Prog. No. (%)	CDT Prog. No. (%)	Total No. (%)
Personally:					
Molested	6 (42.9)	13 (26.0)	42 (30.4)	9 (50.0)	70 (31.8)
Sexually assaulted	5 (35.7)	11 (22.0)	48 (34.8)	9 (50.0)	73 (33.2)
Robbed	4 (28.6)	18 (36.0)	67 (48.6)	7 (38.9)	96 (43.6)
Robbed with a weapon	1 (7.1)	8 (16.0)	23 (16.7)	2 (11.1)	23 (10.5)
Physically assaulted	9 (64.3)	22 (44.0)	51 (37.0)	6 (33.3)	88 (40.0)
Know of someone:					
Molested	4 (28.6)	15 (30.0)	24 (17.4)	5 (27.8)	48 (21.8)
Sexually assaulted	4 (28.6)	14 (28.0)	39 (28.3)	7 (38.9)	64 (29.1)
Robbed	4 (28.6)	21 (42.0)	3 (34.8)	6 (33.3)	79 (35.9)
Physically assaulted	5 (35.7)	19 (38.0)	41 (29.7)	8 (44.4)	73 (33.2)
Murdered	5 (35.7)	14 (28.0)	31 (22.5)	5 (27.8)	55 (25.0)
Total No. of patients	14	50	138	18	220

TABLE 14.4. Sexual and/or Physical Assault in all Adult Patients

	Sexual No. (%)	Physical No. (%)	Both No. (%)	Total (%)
Screening and Medical Assessment Program				
Men (N=14)	0	7 (50.0)	0	7 (50.0)
Women (N=14)	0	4 (28.5)	5 (35.7)	9 (64.2)
Family Systems Program				
Men (N=12)	0	5 (41.6)	0	5 (41.6)
Women (N=50)	3 (6.0)	14 (28.0)	8 (16.0)	25 (50.0)
Outpatient Program				
Men (N=74)	2 (2.6)	22 (30.6)	2 (2.6)	26 (35.8)
Women (N=138)	18 (12.9)	21 (15.1)	28 (20.8)	67 (48.8)
Community Day Treatment Program				
Men (N=23)	0	13 (56.5)	1 (4.34)	14 (60.8)
Women (N=18)	3 (16.6)	1 (5.5)	6 (33.3)	10 (55.4)
Total				
Men (N=123)	2 (1.6)	47 (38.2)	3 (2.4)	52 (42.2)
Women (N=220)	24 (10.9)	40 (18.1)	47 (21.3)	111 (50.)
Total (N=343)	26 (7.5)	87 (25.3)	50 (14.5)	163 (47.6)

reported physical assault only, compared with 44% in SMA, 43% in Outpatient, and 33% in CDT. The majority of the assaulted women in SMA (56%) and CDT (60%) reported both physical and sexual assault. Women in the Outpatient Program were more evenly divided across the three assault categories.

A comparison of men and women indicates a significant relationship between sexual victimization and sex. Women were more likely to report that they had been sexually molested ($x^2 = 19.9$ [1], p < 0.0001), that they had been sexually assaulted ($x^2 = 36.43$ [1], p < 0.0001), and that they knew of a friend or relative who had been sexually assaulted ($x^2 = 9.37$ [1], P < 0.01). Analysis of gender differences within each program indicate that in those programs with the most severely disturbed patients, women were significantly more likely than men to have been sexually victimized. Compared with the men, women in the Outpatient Program were more likely to have been sexually molested ($x^2 = 20.90$ [1], p < 0.0001) and sexually assaulted ($x^2 = 12.46$ [1], p < 0.0001), as was the case with women in CDT for molestation ($x^2 = 9.07$ [1], p < 0.01) and assault ($x^2 = 9.07$ [1], p < 0.01). Women in SMA were more likely than men to have been sexually assaulted ($x^2 = 3.89$ [1], p < 0.05) but were no more likely to have a history of sexual molestation. In the Family Systems program, there was no significant relationship between victimization and sex. Women were no more likely than were men to report that they had been sexually molested or sexually assaulted.

Data on the co-occurrence of sexual and physical assault (Table 4) indicate that one half of the women and 42% of the men had been sexually assaulted, physically assaulted, or both sexually and physically assaulted. Twice as many women had been both sexually and physically assaulted as those had been sexually assaulted only. Women appear to have been at equal risk for physical assault and both physical and sexual assault. Analysis indicated that men and women experienced a different pattern of sexual and physical assault ($x^2 = 46.7$ [2], $p < 0.001$). Women were nine times more likely than men to be sexually and physically assaulted, and men were twice as likely as women to be physically assaulted only. Although it is not clear from the data whether physical assault accompanied the sexual assault, it is interesting to note that of the 73 women reporting sexual assault, 48 (66%) had also been physically assaulted.

Youth

Data on the boys and girls (under 18 years of age) are presented in Tables 5 and 6. As indicated, nine (11%) of the 84 young clients, all of whom were in the Family Systems program, had been sexually molested,

TABLE 14.5. Adolescent Patients under 18 Years Old, Sexually and Physically Assaulted

	No. Male (%)	No. Female (%)	Total (%)
Personally:			
Molested	3 (5.6)	6 (20.0)	9 (10.7)
Sexually assaulted	1 (1.9)	4 (13.3)	5 (6.0)
Robbed	10 (18.5)	1 (3.3)	11 (13.1)
Robbed with a weapon	4 (7.4)	1 (3.3)	5 (6.0)
Physically assaulted	21 (38.9)	10 (33.3)	31 (36.9)
Know of someone:			
Molested	6 (11.1)	6 (20.0)	12 (14.3)
Sexually assaulted	11 (20.4)	8 (26.7)	19 (22.6)
Robbed	4 (7.4)	10 (33.3)	14 (16.7)
Physically assaulted	13 (24.1)	9 (30.0)	22 (26.2)
Murdered	5 (9.3)	7 (23.3)	12 (14.3)
Total No. of patients	54	30	84

and 5 (6%) had been sexually assaulted. Over one third (37%, N = 31) had been physically assaulted, ten (13%) had been robbed, and about half of the robberies involved a weapon.

Data on sexual assault only, physical assault only, and both sexual and physical assault (Table 6) showed that 39% of the boys and girls had been physically or sexually assaulted, or both, with the majority reporting physical assault only. Of the 33 youth reporting physical and/or sexual assault, 81% reported physical assault only.

TABLE 14.6. Sexual and/or Physical Assault in all Patients under 18 Years Old

	No. Sexual (%)	No. Physical (%)	No. Both (%)	Total (%)
Men (N=54)	0	19 (35.2)	1 (1.9)	20 (37.0)
Women (N=30)	2 (6.7)	8 (27.0)	2 (6.7)	12 (40.4)
Total (N=84)	2 (2.4)	27 (32.1)	3 (3.6)	32 (38.1)

The boys and girls did not differ in their reports of victimization. Although more girls than boys reported having been molested and sexually assaulted, the association between sex and victimization was not statistically significant. The boys and girls differed significantly only in their reports of close others who had been robbed ($x^2 = 7.56$ [1], $p < 0.01$). Girls were five times more likely than boys to know of a close other who had been robbed.

Disregarding sex in the Family Systems program, a comparison of adults and youth indicated that in general, the youth were less likely to be personally victimized and were less likely to be aware of relatives who had been victimized. Adults were twice as likely as the youth to report that they have been sexually molested ($x^2 = 4.71$ [1], $p < 0.05$) and sexually assaulted ($x^2 = 3.94$ [1], $p < 0.05$). Adults also were significantly more likely to know of close others who had been sexually molested ($x^2 = 3.89$ [1], $p < 0.05$), robbed ($x^2 = 7.89$ [1], $p < 0.005$), or murdered ($x^2 = 3.89$, $p < 0.05$). There was no significant relationship between age and physical assault. Thirty-one percent of the adults and 26% of the youth reported that they had been physically assaulted.

Separate analysis of females (older vs. younger) and males (older vs. younger) found no significant relationship between age and victimization within these groups. That is, girls were not significantly less victimized than women 18 years and older, except for reports of robbery. The women were three times more likely than were girls to have been robbed ($x^2 = 9.32$ [1], $p < 0.01$). Boys were not significantly less likely to be victimized than were the men, nor were they any less likely to be aware of relatives or friends who had been victimized.

DISCUSSION

In this survey of black psychiatric outpatients, 48% had a history of victimization. These figures are comparable to those of Carmen et al.[8] in their study of psychiatric inpatients; however, they are much higher than the victimization rate for the general population. The Bureau of Justice Statistics for 1985 reports that the incidence of assault in individuals twelve years of age and over is 24.1 per 1,000 and reports that robbery occurs at a rate of 6.0 per 1,000 in the United States. From these statistics, the overall assault rate is reported to be similar among whites and blacks, although the rate of aggravated assault is higher among blacks and the rate of simple assault is higher among whites.[11] These figures are probably an underestimate of the occurrence of such crime, since it is estimated that crime occurs at a rate of four times of that actually reported. In addition, blacks may underreport crime more than whites do because of the different responses accorded to both groups by the criminal justice system. However, even taking into account the estimated underreporting as well as the fact that data were analyzed only for those CMHC patients presenting with a complaint of mental illness, the mental health patients at the CMHC were four to five times more likely than the general population to have experienced assault. Clients who presented with a complaint of only victimization and not mental illness were referred to the agency's victims assistance program and were excluded from the analysis.

Although it has not been differentiated in this screening program whether the assault occurred before the development of clinical illness, it is interesting to note that there was no difference in incidence of victimization by severity of mental disorder, if the results for both sexes are summed. The data indicate, however, an impact of illness severity on women: women in the more severely disturbed treatment groups reported the highest incidence of both sexual and physical assault.

The finding that women are more likely to be victimized than men, owing to their much greater incidence of sexual victimization, is consistent with findings from other studies.[8,9] Indeed, women in this sample were eight times as likely as men to report an incidence of sexual assault, with two thirds of these victims reporting having also been physically assaulted. The findings on the sexual assault of women take on particular importance in light of evidence that victims of sexual victimization suffer from more severe mental health problems than do victims of robbery and physical assault.[12]

The data on the youth indicate that the boys and girls did not differ in their reports of victimization, but girls were five times more likely to have knowledge of others having been victimized. Does this sensitivity to the hostile environment have an impact on girls' sense of self, or is it indeed society's pronouncement of her as the weaker sex that makes her more sensitive to violence around her? A comparison of all female subjects showed no significant relationship between age and sexual or physical assault. This indicates that except for their lower chances of being robbed, girls were equally as likely to be victims of physical and sexual assault as adult women. Again, although the boys and girls were equally likely to be victimized, further study is required to assess what impact girls' awareness of victimization has on the development of clinical symptomatology.

Although it has been well documented that an episode of violent or sexual victimization has an impact on the individual's sense of psychological wellbeing, many questions are yet to be answered. What causal effect, if any, is there between psychiatric disorders and victimization? Does victimization precede psychiatric deterioration, or does the deteriorated individual become a more likely prey to be victimized? If there is an effect on the individual who suffers sexual or physical assault, does the effect differ if the victim is a child as opposed to an adult? What are the long-term effects of victimization?

It would seem incumbent for all mental health care providers to follow the enjoinder of Hillard et al.[3]: "... it is important for psychiatric emergency facilities to try to minimize patient mortality from all causes and not just from suicide. The excess mortality in the emergency room from nonsuicidal violent deaths suggests that homicide prevention and accident prevention are goals worth striving towards." With early preliminary findings such as these presented here, it can only be speculated how a history of violence might impact morbidity, treatment, and the client-therapist relationship. However, exploration to discover a history of violent and sexual victimization early in a patient's treatment is clearly warranted, given these findings.

SUMMARY

This study underscores the need for routine screening for victimization in the black mental health population. Such screening may identify individuals who are at greater risk for being a victim of future violence and possibly, murder. The finding that 48.1% of a community mental health population had been victimized implies that a community mental health center that does not actively identify and address its victims' needs does not serve the needs of the community it is mandated to serve. Although this study answered some questions, it raised many other important ones. These questions will only be answered through basic empirical, applied clinical research. It is hoped that those of us who realize the importance of this line of investigation will be inspired to continue researching violence and victimization in our communities and find some of our own solutions to our problems.

COMMENTARY

Being a psychiatrist, it's impossible to ignore the trauma caused by sexual assault. Too many patients come in with psychiatric symptoms that can be traced back to their sexual victimization. Understanding this dynamic, the CMHC started its Victims' Services Program in 1984. That year, we launched our attack on violence on several fronts. We began to explore the various causes of violence from a psychiatric perspective, as well as formally explore violence from a public health perspective and advocate for this approach. In 1984, the CMHC completed its first survey of children regarding their experiences with violence. We set up a rape victims' identification and referral system at the local hospitals serving our community and began to provide rape counseling. In these ways, we'd begun to actively address identifying and treating victims of violence. As we delved deeper, though, it occurred to us that we didn't know how serious a problem victimization was for our psychiatric patients. This article describes the work we did to answer this question.

Regarding our advocacy activities, the Victims' Services Program provided consultation to public service departments in several states and in more than 30 cities. We displayed models for violence prevention and intervention, screening clients for victimization, and alternate methods of conflict resolution. This advocacy work had some influence. For one, some of the medical staff at Cook County Hospital grew interested in our work. They did a larger study similar to the one here to identify the extent of the problem of violence in their institution. They went on to show an association between comprehensive health functioning/wellbeing and violence victimization.

Another example of the impact of our advocacy efforts occurred in late 1986 after I'd demonstrated our models in Richmond, Virginia. Because the CMHC had already begun screening for victimization, I was able to give our screening form to the nurses in Richmond. I later learned that they began to do victimization screening while doing home visits to check blood pressure and diabetes. They found a surprising level of unreported violence in their community, much of which was domestic. As a result, the Richmond community began to strengthen its domestic violence intervention efforts by increasing its number of domestic violence shelters. Richmond's city council also began supporting Blacks Mobilizing against Crime, a group formed to combat black-on-black murder (see Chapter 1, Letter to the Editor). It's significant to note that such efforts would later have a huge impact on the African-American homicide rate (see Chapter 9).

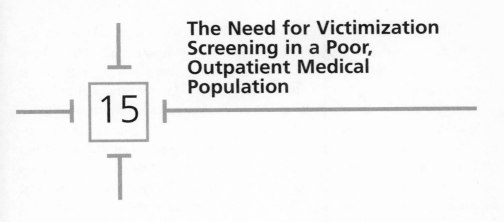

The Need for Victimization Screening in a Poor, Outpatient Medical Population

15

Recent reports indicate that violence toward others is a major public health problem in the black community; however, there are few empirical studies that delineate the severity of the problem. The authors have compiled the results of a victimization screening form obtained from a poor outpatient medical population. These results are compared with those from a similar survey performed on a poor outpatient psychiatric population. The authors recommend that poor medical populations be screened for history of victimization, because early identification of at-risk patients may reduce their chances of victimization in the future.

INTRODUCTION

In 1986, blacks accounted for 44% of the murder victims in the United States, and, as in previous years, 95% of the black victims were slain by black offenders.[1] Partly responsible for this disparity is the fact that blacks are disproportionately represented among perpetrators and victims of spouse killings.[2,3] Thus, domestic murder, which often stems from family violence, is a significant contributor to the high murder rates in blacks.

Originally printed as Bell Carl C, Hildreth Carolyn J, Jenkins Esther J, Levi Deborah, Carter Cynthia. The need for victimization screening in a poor, outpatient medical population. *J Natl Med Assoc.* 1988;80:853–860.

It has been estimated that 30–40% of women murdered in the United States are killed by their husbands or lovers, usually after being beaten by those men for years.[1,4] Unfortunately, wife-beating is the most common but least reported crime in the United States.[4] Straus et al.[5] estimated that each year, 15–30% of US couples experience marital violence and about two million women are beaten by men. This study also estimated that one half of all married women experience physical violence from their husbands at least once during their marriage. More recently, Straus and colleagues[6] have estimated that 1.5 million women receive medical attention because of an assault by a male partner each year. Stark and Flitcraft[7] estimated that three to four million women are beaten each year, with battering accounting for one of every five visits to emergency services by women and accounting for half of injuries reported. They also noted that battered women suffer more frequently from general medical problems, rape, and psychological symptoms of stress (e.g., suicide attempts, alcoholism, drug abuse, depression).

Because non-lethal violence is a frequent antecedent to homicide[6] and because blacks have a disproportionately higher rate of domestic murder than the rate for whites, one would expect that the domestic violence rate for blacks would also be disproportionately higher than that for whites. However, studies on domestic violence and abuse of women reveal contradictions. For example, Straus et al.[5] found that abuse of women occurred three times more often in blacks than in whites. Contrary to that observation, the Department of Justice when examining violent crimes by spouses or ex-spouses, found no difference in the victimization rates for blacks and whites; however, more blacks than whites reported violence by relatives other than spouses.[8] The reason for this disparity is unclear. It may have to do with other variables that are more prevalent in blacks than in whites, such as unemployment status, poorer educational opportunity, lower class status, and lower income.[9,10]

Arguments and altercations between relatives and friends are frequent precursors to homicide.[1,2,5,11-13] Several studies[14,15] have shown that perpetrators and victims of homicide have histories of more frequent fighting than do controls. Since the rate of aggravated assault victimization is higher among blacks when compared to whites, physical injury is more common in blacks and in low-income assault victims.[12]

Although only 1% of gun robberies lead to a death, robbery is a violent crime, and the rate of robbery is higher for men, blacks, and the unemployed. Thus, robbery is still very physically and psychologically damaging to the black community.[12] Unfortunately, very little is known about the effects of the higher robbery rate on blacks' physical and psychological health. For example, post-traumatic stress disorder is known to occur in robbery victims, but how often it occurs is unknown.

Forcible rape is another violent crime that rarely results in death but exacts a heavy toll on society. Several studies note a high prevalence of sexually abused women in psychiatric populations and propose that their sexual abuse may have etiologic significance in their psychiatric disorders.[16–18]

In summary, violent crime is a serious problem in America. It causes high rates of mortality and physical and psychological morbidity. A murder occurs every 25 minutes; a forcible rape occurs every 6 minutes; a robbery occurs every 58 seconds; an aggravated assault occurs every 38 seconds.[1] There is every reason to believe that poor people and blacks are at great risk of these violent crimes. Despite these findings' gravely serious implications for the medical community treating victims of these violent crimes, the medical community seems wholly unaware of the prevalence of victimization in their patients. As a result, the medical community has been negligent in developing strategies and interventions to reduce the problem of violent crime in society. This has been especially true when considering patients from the black community.

Because the early identification of violence allows for interventions that may preclude a future homicide, the investigation of the prevalence and dynamics of violence should be a major priority. Because the homicide rate is higher among blacks and low-income persons, studies of these populations should receive first priority.[11–13] It is extremely important that the medical profession take the lead in such investigations, since physicians and other health professionals are responsible for treating the damage that stems from domestic violence. Taking a public health philosophy toward violence is especially crucial since, according to the FBI, "...the fact that three out of every five murder victims in 1986 were related to (sixteen percent) or acquainted with (forty-two percent) their assailants..." supports the "philosophy that murder is primarily a societal problem over which law enforcement has little or no control"[1]

The purpose of this paper is to present some research findings on the prevalence of victimization in a poor, predominantly black outpatient medical population. These results are compared with those from a similar study of a black outpatient psychiatric population[16] (see Chapter 14). Finally, recommendations are made on how the medical profession can begin to intervene to prevent further victimization of its patients.

METHODS

Sample

A total of 262 patients at a neighborhood outpatient medical center were screened for the study. The sample was 80% black, about 13% Hispanic, and 5% white and other. Their ages ranged from 4–80 years, with 59% of the sample aged 18 years and over. Of the 155 patients over 18, the vast majority was female (N = 141). The clients younger than 18 were more evenly split between boys (N = 42) and girls (N = 65).

All of the respondents were visiting a neighborhood medical clinic on the Near North Side of Chicago in an area that is predominantly black, Hispanic, and poor. The clinic has a total yearly patient population of 16,000, 78% of whom receive either Medicare/Medicaid or pay a minimal fee. Over the two month period when the data was collected (July–August), the agency saw 6,359 patients, 66% of whom were black and 29% of whom were Hispanic. The blacks were somewhat overrepresented in the study's sample, and Hispanics (despite a Spanish-language version of the screening form) were underrepresented. Analysis of the client population indicates that women over the age of 18 years were also somewhat overrepresented (by 20%), and youths younger than 18, who made up over 60% of the agency's caseload, were underrepresented.

Procedure

Adult patients in the waiting room of the clinic were approached by an interviewer (a fourth-year medical student or a nurse), who explained the nature of the study and requested the participation of the individual and his or her children. Consenting patients either completed the Victimization Screening Form alone or had the form administered to them by the interviewer. All children younger than sixteen years were administered the form. Parental consent was obtained for all children younger than 18 years.

Originally developed for use with a mentally ill population, the Victimization Screening Form (see Chapter 14) is a one-page questionnaire that asks about the incidence of sexual and physical victimization of the individual and of the individual's relatives, neighbors, and friends.[16] The form specifically asks if the individual and close others have ever been molested, raped, robbed with or without a weapon, or physically assaulted. In addition, the form asks if a close other has ever been murdered.

RESULTS

Adults

Data for adult female and male patients reporting victimization of self and of close individuals is presented in Table 1. Responses for black, white, and Hispanic patients are combined because analysis indicated no significant difference in numbers between these groups. Analysis is reported by gender.

Women. Approximately one in seven of the adult women indicated that they had been molested (14%), and a similar number had been raped (14%) and physically assaulted (15%). Looking at the number of victimized patients as opposed to the number of isolated incidents reported, 6% (N = 8) of the women had been sexually assaulted, 7% (N = 10) had been physically assaulted, and 8% (N = 11) had been both sexually and physically assaulted. A total of 21%, or roughly one in five, of the women had experienced sexual and/or physical assault. Approximately one in five of the women as well indicated that they had been robbed, and over half of the 29 robbery victims indicated that a weapon had been used.

All of the women knew of a relative, neighbor, or friend who had been victimized. Fifteen percent (N = 21) of the women reported that someone close to them had been molested, and 19% (N = 26) knew of someone

TABLE 15.1. Victimization Reported by Medical Outpatient Victims, Age 18 Years and Older

	Medical Outpatients			Psychiatric Outpatients		
	Female No. (%)	Male No. (%)	Total No. (%)	Female No. (%)	Male No. (%)	Total No. (%)
Personally:	**(N=141)**	**(N=14)**	**(N=155)**	**(N=220)**	**(N=123)**	**(N=343)**
Molested	19 (14)	0 (0)	19 (12)	70 (32)	12 (10)	82 (24)
Raped	19 (14)	0 (0)	19 (12)	73 (33)	5 (4)	78 (23)
Robbed	19 (21)	5 (36)	34 (22)	96 (12)	51 (41)	147 (43)
Robbed with weapon	11 (8)	4 (29)	15 (10)	23 (10)	27 (22)	50 (15)
Physically assaulted	21 (15)	5 (36)	26 (17)	88 (40)	50 (41)	138 (40)
Know of some- one:*	**(N=140)**	**(N=14)**	**(N=154)**	**(N=220)**	**(N=123)**	**(N=343)**
Molested	21 (15)	7 (50)	28 (18)	48 (22)	17 (14)	65 (19)
Raped	26 (19)	5 (36)	31 (20)	64 (29)	17 (14)	81 (24)
Robbed	60 (43)	7 (50)	56 (44)	79 (36)	42 (34)	121 (35)
Physically assaulted	43 (31)	5 (36)	48 (31)	73 (33)	32 (26)	105 (31)
Murdered	39 (28)	6 (46)	44 (29)	55 (25)	32 (26)	87 (25)

*Number of female medical outpatient respondents: 140; male medical outpatient respondents: 14; total medical outpatients: 154.

who had been raped. Sixty (43%) of the women reported that a close other had been robbed, 43 (31%) knew of someone who had been physically assaulted, and 39 (28%) reported that a close other had been murdered.

Men. Only 14 adult men visited the clinic and completed the screening form. Of those 14, none had been sexually victimized (molested or raped), but over one third (36%) indicated that they had been physically assaulted. The same number indicated that they had been robbed, and four of the five robbery victims reported that a weapon had been used.

A relatively high percentage of the men reported that someone close to them had been victimized. One half (N = 7) of the men knew of someone who had been robbed, and six (46%) reported that someone close to them had been murdered. Five (36%) knew of someone who had been raped and physically assaulted.

A comparison of male and female subjects suggests different victimization experiences, although the differences, with one exception, were not statistically significant. Only women reported sexual victimization, whereas men were twice as likely to report that they had been assaulted and were 1.5 times more likely to report that they had been robbed. Men were also more likely to report that a close other had been victimized and were significantly more likely to report that a close other had been sexually molested ($x^2 = 8.25$ [1], p < 0.01).

Youth

Data for male and female medical patients under the age of 18 years are presented in Table 2. Similar to the findings seen for adults, only female patients reported instances of sexual victimization; five (8%) of the girls had been molested and two (3%) had been raped. Four male (10%)

TABLE 15.2. Victimization Reported by Medical Outpatients, Age 17 Years and Younger

	Medical Outpatients			Psychiatric Outpatients		
	Female No. (%)	Male No. (%)	Total No. (%)	Female No. (%)	Male No. (%)	Total No. (%)
Personally:	**(N=65)**	**(N=42)**	**(N=107)**	**(N=30)**	**(N=54)**	**(N=84)**
Molested	5 (8)	0 (0)	5 (5)	6 (20)	3 (6)	9 (11)
Raped	2 (3)	0 (0)	2 (2)	4 (13)	1 (2)	5 (6)
Robbed	4 (6)	4 (10)	8 (7)	1 (3)	10 (19)	11 (13)
Robbed with a weapon	1 (2)	0 (0)	1 (1)	1 (3)	4 (7)	5 (60)
Physically assaulted	12 (18)	7 (17)	19 (18)	10 (33)	21 (39)	31 (37)
Know of some- one:	**(N=50)**	**(N=33)**	**(N=83)**	**(N=30)**	**(N=54)**	**(N=84)**
Molested	7 (14)	1 (3)	8 (10)	6 (20)	6 (11)	12 (14)
Raped	7 (14)	3 (9)	10 (12)	8 (27)	11 (20)	19 (23)
Robbed	19 (38)	9 (27)	28 (34)	10 (33)	4 (7)	14 (17)
Physically assaulted	22 (44)	11 (33)	33 (40)	9 (30)	13 (24)	22 (26)
Murdered	13 (26)	3 (9)	16 (19)	7 (23)	5 (9)	12 (14)

and four female patients (6%) had been robbed, but only one, a 16-year-old girl, reported that a weapon had been used. The boys and girls were almost equally as likely to report having been assaulted (17% and 18%, respectively). It must be noted that in the questionnaire administered to the youths, the word "whipped" was used to clarify the term "physical assault." Therefore, it is unclear how many of these reported "assaults" were reasonable disciplinary actions taken by family members (eight were specified as such) and how many were actual physical assaults.

Data from 83 of the youths on victimization of close others are also included in Table 2. In comparison to boys, girls were more likely to know of the victimization of close others in all five areas and were three times more likely to report that a close other had been murdered.

A comparison by age found that male adults were significantly more likely than were boys to have been robbed ($x^2 = 3.57$ [1], $p < 0.05$) and to know of someone who had been molested ($x^2 = 12.20$ [1], $p < 0.001$) and murdered ($x^2 = 5.95$ [1], $p < 0.01$). Female adults were significantly more likely than were girls to have been raped ($x^2 = 4.18$ [1], $p < 0.05$) and robbed ($x^2 = 5.84$ [1], $p < 0.01$).

COMPARISON OF MEDICAL AND PSYCHIATRIC OUTPATIENTS

In a recent report by Bell et al.[16] performing victimization screening of 427 psychiatric outpatients (see Chapter 14), the data indicated that the mentally impaired experienced considerable victimization, with almost one half of the adult mentally impaired clients reporting sexual and/or physical assault. Data from the current survey of medical (MED) patients was compared with that from the psychiatric (PSY) group to gain a better perspective on both. Analysis was done separately for female and male adults and for females and males younger than 18 years.

The results indicate that in general, the mentally ill were significantly more likely to be victimized. This was particularly so for female adults (see Table 1). The female PSY outpatients, compared with the adult female MED patients, were more than twice as likely to have been sexually molested ($x^2 = 16.49$ [1], $p < 0.001$), raped ($x^2 = 16.41$ [1], $p < 0.001$), and robbed ($x^2 = 18.62$ [1], $p < 0.001$). They were more than 2.5 times as likely to have been physically assaulted ($x^2 = 23.71$ [1], $p < 0.001$). The mentally ill are seen to be more likely to be victimized because of their vulnerability, which makes them less of a threat to their attacker. Consistent with this notion is the finding that the female PSY outpatients were more likely to have been robbed without a weapon, as opposed to the female MED patients, who were significantly more likely to have been robbed with a weapon. Of the 21 female MED patients who had been robbed, 11 (51%) indicated that a weapon had been used, while 23 (24%) PSY female patients had been robbed without a weapon ($x^2 = 23.7[1]$, $p < 0.001$). Although MED and PSY females did not differ significantly in their knowledge of the victimization of close others, PSY women were somewhat more likely to report a close having been sexually victimized, whereas more MED women reported a close other having been robbed. The two groups of women were about equally as likely to know of someone who had been assaulted or murdered.

Although a reliable comparison of male adults is difficult due to the small number of male medical patients, the figures suggest that PSY and MED male adults experience, or at least report, comparable levels of personal victimization. However, male MED patients were more likely than male PSY outpatients to indicate that a close other had been victimized and were significantly more likely to indicate that a close other had been sexually victimized. MED patients were 3.5 times more likely to know of someone who had been sexually molested ($x^2 = 11.41$ [1], $p < 0.001$) and 2.5 times more likely to have had a close other raped ($x^2 = 4.47$ [1], $p < 0.05$).

A comparison of the MED and PSY youth outpatients indicates that in general, the PSY youths were more likely to report personal victimization (see Table 2), although few of the differences were statistically significant.

Girl outpatients at the mental health center were 2.5 times more likely than girl outpatients visiting the medical clinic to have been molested and more than four times as likely to have been raped. Girl outpatients from the mental health facility were more likely to have been assaulted, but the girl medical outpatients were twice as likely to have been robbed.

More of the PSY girls also reported that they knew of someone who had been raped and molested. More MED girls reported that someone close to them had been assaulted. A comparable number in both groups knew of someone who had been murdered. 23% of the PSY girls and 26% of the MED girls reported that a relative, friend, or neighbor had been murdered.

Among boys, the PSY outpatients were more likely to have been victimized and were significantly more likely to have been assaulted ($x^2 = 5.6$ [1], $p < 0.05$), even considering the somewhat inflated numbers for the MED youths mentioned previously.

Similar to the girls, more PSY male patients knew of someone who had been molested and raped, but the boy outpatients from the medical center were significantly more likely to report that a close other had been robbed ($x^2 = 6.39$ [1], $p < 0.05$) and somewhat more likely to have known of someone who had been assaulted. Interestingly, PSY and MED boys were equally likely to report that a close other had been murdered. This percentage (9%), considerably lower than that for girls or for male and female adults from either group, raises some interesting questions about young black males' perception and recall of threatening events.

DISCUSSION

The sample of 262 patients represents approximately 4% of the patient population seen during the two months of the study. Although patients were randomly requested to participate in the screening, the sample is not representative because the patients had the option of refusing to participate, which made the study sample self-selected. Hispanics seemed reluctant to participate despite a Spanish version of the screening form and, as a result, were underrepresented. Children were also underrepresented due to the technical difficulty of getting their parents' consent to allow them to participate in the study. The sampling procedures used in the study were influenced by a number of extraneous variables that could not be controlled, and any discussion of the findings must consider this factor. Despite this shortcoming, the authors feel that the data gathered from this survey have heuristic value.

The adult females who participated in the screening reported a significant amount of sexual and/or physical assault and robbery, and an even greater percentage of them knew of others who had been similarly victimized. In contrast, while over one third of the adult males reported physical assault and robbery, none reported being sexually assaulted; yet, adult males were significantly more likely than females to report knowing of someone who had been sexually molested. Like the adults, the girls screened for victimization reported a significant incidence of sexual assaults while the boys denied experiencing such events.

The finding that females reported experiencing more sexual abuse than males is not surprising, as females are more often the target of such attacks. However, the finding that none of the males reported experiencing a sexual assault contradicts other studies on the subject. Risin and Koss[19] reported that 7.3% of their male sample had experienced an abusive sexual experience before the age of 14. This figure is consistent with Finkelhor's[20] study revealing that 6.4% of boys under 14 had been sexually victimized. The authors suspect that the lack of reporting of sexual victimization in this predominantly black male sample was due to a significantly greater difficulty for the males to admit such an emasculating event and due to the lack of a stable clinical relationship with the screening professional.

The finding that the whole population experienced significant amounts of robbery (with and without a weapon) and physical assault is not surprising, since the victimization rate for these crimes are high for poor people and blacks. Similarly, the finding that men report more robbery with and without a weapon and report more physical assault than women is not unusual because men become robbery and assault victims more frequently; the less vulnerable the robbery victim, the more likely the robber will wield a weapon in the robbery.[12]

Growing up in a predominately poor, minority community, one is fraught with recognizable real dangers, which may be denied or faced at different ages for different sexes. What was unexpected is that more adult males than adult females knew of someone who had been sexually molested. The authors suspect that the males may know more victims of sexual assault because males are usually the perpetrators of such assaults and as a result may have more knowledge of such attacks as either perpetrators or confidants of perpetrators. Males may also have less reason to deny such threatening events, while females, in an effort to deny the danger, may not discuss such issues. The girls knew of significantly more murder victims than did the boys, which may be due to the boys' denial of the risk of murder. Rates of reported robbery and physical assault were low in both the girls and boys (several of the youth included spankings as physical assault, so this category may be exaggerated for them). Finally, in looking at age as a variable, it appears that as males get older, their chances of getting robbed increase and their awareness of sexual molestation and murder in others increases. Older females have a greater chance of being raped and robbed.

In comparing the reports of victimization between the MED and PSY patients, some interesting differences became apparent. First, the economic indicators in both populations revealed that a greater proportion of the MED patients screened were poor when compared with the PSY population. While poverty may be a predisposing factor for some types of victimization,[12] adult PSY female patients (who were economically more well off) were more likely to be victimized (molested, raped, robbed, and physically assaulted) than were adult MED females. However, adult MED females were significantly more likely to be robbed with a weapon, a finding consistent with the literature, which indicates that more "difficult" victims are likely to be robbed with a weapon.[21] These findings suggest two possibilities. One is that being victimized might increase one's risk for developing a mental illness. Thus, when screening for victimization in a mentally ill population, more episodes of past victimization will become apparent. Second, these findings could indicate an additional dynamic suggested by Bell et al.,[16] that perpetrators may perceive mentally ill patients as more vulnerable, which makes these patients more likely to be victimized.

Another interesting finding is that although the PSY females were significantly more likely to be victimized, the MED and PSY female adult populations did not significantly differ in their knowledge of others who had been victimized. Thus, both populations have a similar view of risks of victimization to others. How this influences their self-protection behaviors is not clear and needs further investigation.

Unlike MED males, the PSY males were willing to admit sexual assault at levels similar to those in reported by the literature previously cited. Despite a lack of personal experience with sexual assault, MED males reported significantly more knowledge of others who had been molested than PSY males. The authors speculate again this finding may be related to the MED men having more personal knowledge of such assaults as either perpetrators or confidants of perpetrators. Similar to the adults, PSY youths were more likely to have been victimized.

This initial pilot study on screening for victimization in a medically ill population has some important implications for a public health approach to handling violence toward others, which the Surgeon General has deemed a major[22] public health problem. Although minority populations are at significantly greater risk for a number of violent crimes (due to the inordinately high proportion of minorities who are poor), there is very little empirical epidemiologic research on victimization in a medically ill, minority population. More data needs to be collected, as it is evident there is a considerable area to be explored. Because reporting sexual assaults is a difficult task, the authors suspect that both the adults and youths underreported their experiences. However, histories of physical or sexual assault are not often elicited in routine clinical assessments,[23] and standardized screening offers an opportunity to regularly inquire about an assault history. Therefore, the authors recommend screening, as underreporting is better than receiving no information at all. In addition, it is the authors' experience that as patients start knowing the clinical setting for being seriously concerned about patients' victimization, it becomes more acceptable for patients to discuss such previously taboo subjects.

By instituting routine screening, it becomes possible as well to identify victims who are not identified in routine clinical assessments. Once identified, more in-depth information can be obtained, and various secondary prevention efforts can be started to reduce future morbidity and mortality from a past or future assault. For example, such screening could identify battered women when they seek medical services for their battery-related injuries or distress. A handbook on victimization[4] could then be given to the woman, along with a referral to a victim's service program. Of course, this would entail medical facilities establishing a solid relationship with such services. Such a case finding and referral procedure may help to reduce future domestic violence in blacks,[24] as well as homicides from domestic and peer violence. Similarly, such screening may allow for early intervention in a number of medical and behavioral problems that seem to stem from victimization. The following have all been reported to stem from sexual and physical abuse: suicidal ideation and attempts,[18,25,26] nervous breakdowns,[18,25,26] drug abuse, juvenile delinquency,[27] criminal behavior,[18,27] self-destructive behaviors (biting, cutting, burning, head banging, suicide attempts) in children,[28] assaultive behaviors,[18] psychosomatic symptoms,[7,18] depression,[29] alcoholism,[7] sexual problems.[27]

Further, when community institutions recognize violence as a problem, they can greatly influence strategies for reducing violence in their communities. An attitude of violence prevention in the community enhances the feeling of safety in a clinic, and the community may encourage minority patients to stick with a regular source and routine of health care. To have such an impact, however, the overall policy of the community institution has to support victimization screening, and implementation must be encouraged. Annual victimization updates are important for picking up new cases, but again, policy has to be introduced and enforced in order for staff to get involved and realize the intrinsic value of the screening. Finally, outcome studies of the impact of victimization screening on prevention need to be performed.

In conclusion, this study indicates that physicians should screen for victimization in medical clinics and advocate for policy supporting such efforts. Finally, while it appears that psychiatrically ill patients are more likely to suffer from sexual and physical victimization, medically ill patients still have a high prevalence of such victimization. Such patients should be identified so that secondary and tertiary prevention of future victimization can be provided and so that the morbidity and mortality associated with previous sexual and physical assaults can be reduced.

COMMENTARY

This article was our effort at doing work in a non-psychiatric patient population and represented a first step in another violence prevention initiative. The logic was that early identification of violence might allow for an intervention preventing future violence. We'd already proposed such a system for emergency rooms in "Black-on-Black Homicide: The National Medical Association's Responsibilities" (see Chapter 1). In this article, we were exploring how to begin the identification and referral system in not only emergency rooms but also outpatient medical clinics.

The CMHC's Victims' Services Program won the 1992 Gold Achievement Award from the Hospital and Community Psychiatry Service of the APA. We received the award because in addition to providing direct services, our research and advocacy activities had had a national influence. In 1991, the program staff had delivered 137 community education presentations on violence and victimization to a total of 7,559 participants. In that same year, the staff provided 43 professional training programs on how to counsel victims to 444 participants.

As with many of the articles in this book, this study's suggestion for victimization screening is still relevant today. I still study victimization, and I recently came across a very powerful study that reveals the disastrous effects on children who might have been helped with victimization screening (Felitti VJ, Anda RF, Nordenberg D, et al. Relationship of child abuse and household dysfunction to many of the leading causes of death in adults—the adverse childhood experiences [ACE] study." *Am J Preventive Med.* 1998;14:245–258). In the study, the authors pointed out the relationship between adverse childhood experiences (ACEs) and poor physical health outcome. This study examined seven ACEs: psychological abuse, physical abuse, sexual abuse, violence against mother, living with household members who were substance abusers, living with household members who were mentally ill or suicidal, living with household members who were imprisoned. Individuals who experienced four or more types of ACE had a significantly increased risk for alcoholism, drug abuse, depression, and suicide attempts. These individuals were also at higher risk for smoking, having poor self-related health, having fifty or more sexual partners, and contracting of STDs. In addition, respondents who experienced four or more types of ACE were at increased risk for physical inactivity, obesity, ischemic heart disease, cancer, chronic lung disease, skeletal fractures, and liver disease.

The message is simple: ACEs can cause children numerous problems later in life. The good news is that despite exposure to such experiences, there are factors that can protect children from the negative outcomes. One such factor is resiliency/learning resiliency. In a recent paper (Bell CC. Cultivating resiliency in youth. *J Adolescent Health.* 2001;29:375–381), I label characteristics of resiliency as (1) having curiosity and intellectual mastery, (2) having compassion, with detachment, (3) being able to conceptualize, (4) obtaining the conviction of one's right to survive, (5) possessing the ability to remember and invoke images of sustaining figures, (6) being able to be in touch with affects and not denying or suppressing major affects as they arise, (7) having a goal for which to live, (8) being able to attract and use support, (9) possessing a vision of the possibility and desirability of restoration civilized moral order, (10) having the need and ability to help others, (11) having an affective repertory, (12) being resourceful, (13) being altruistic toward others, (14) having the capacity to turn traumatic helplessness into learned helpfulness. There are also more esoteric characteristics of resiliency, such as kokoro, Atman, totems, and chi (see www.giftfromwithin.org for more information).

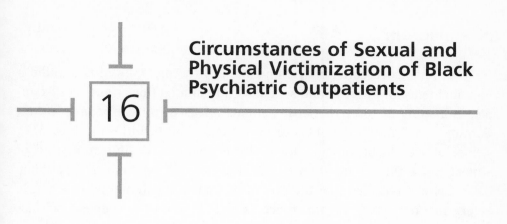

Circumstances of Sexual and Physical Victimization of Black Psychiatric Outpatients

16

A sample of 54 adult psychiatric outpatients, previously identified as victims of sexual or physical assault, were interviewed regarding their childhood and adult victimization experiences. Patients were questioned about the nature of the assaults, their relationship to the perpetrator(s), the number of assaults suffered in each relationship, and whether the assault(s) occurred before or after the onset of their mental illness. Eighty percent of the sample had experienced major physical assault as an adult and 59% had experienced major physical assault as a child; 37% and 31%, respectively, reported major sexual assault as a child and as an adult. Women were more likely than men to report physical and sexual assault as an adult and sexual assault as a child. Childhood assault most often occurred before the onset of the patient's mental illness; whereas adult sexual assault for women and physical and sexual assault for men was as likely to occur after the onset of the psychiatric disorder, suggesting an increased vulnerability to victimization for the adult mentally ill.

Originally printed as Jenkins Esther J, Bell Carl C, Taylor Julie, Walker Leslie. Circumstances of sexual and physical victimization of black psychiatric outpatients. *J Natl Med Assoc.* 1989;81:246–252. Presented at the 93rd Annual Convention and Scientific Assembly of the NMA, Los Angeles, CA, August 1, 1988.

INTRODUCTION

Previous research on victimization of the mentally ill has found a high incidence of physical and sexual assault among this group. For example, in a study of 188 psychiatric patients released from an inpatient unit, Carmen et al.[1] found that 43% of the patients had histories of physical or sexual abuse; Jacobson and Richardson[2] found a victimization rate of almost twice this figure (81%) in a study of 100 psychiatric inpatients. Hillard et al.[3] reported that the rate of homicidal death among psychiatric emergency room patients was twice as high as that of the general population.

The authors, recently reporting on a screening of patients at the Community Mental Health Council[4] (CMHC, an outpatient psychiatric facility with a 99% black, primarily poor patient population), found that 48% of the agency's patients had been sexually or physically assaulted. This study, one of the few on the victimization of black psychiatric patients, did not provide information about the circumstances of the patients' victimization. That is, the data revealed none of the following: whether the assault(s) occurred when the patient was a child or an adult, the number of assaults experienced by each patient, the patient's relationship to the perpetrator, whether the assault(s) occurred before or after the onset of the patient's mental illness. Such information is critical for understanding the impact of victimization and, even more important, for designing and implementing treatment and prevention strategies. The current study investigates the circumstances of victimization in a black, lower income sample of psychiatric outpatients.

METHODS

The sample consisted of 54 clients from the CMHC. This number represents one third of the adult patients who had been identified as victims of sexual molestation or assault, or physical assault at the time of the survey. All of the agency's patients are routinely screened for victimization as a part of the intake procedure (see Bell et al.[4]) The sample included 28 females and 26 males ranging in age from 19 to 65 years, with a median age of 35.

Sixty percent (N = 33) of the sample was in the agency's outpatient program (treating functional psychotic patients), 28% (N = 15) were in the community day-treatment program (providing structured programs for the most severely disturbed psychotic patients), and 11% (N = 6) were in the family systems program (providing psychotherapy to non-psychotic patients). In comparison with the agency's total patient population, community day-treatment patients were somewhat overrepresented, and family systems patients were somewhat underrepresented in the sample.

Fifty percent of the sample had been at the agency for two years or less at the time of the interview, although the median number of years for receiving mental health services was five to ten. Twenty percent of the sample had completed high school, and 40% (N = 22) had attended at least some college. Sixty-five percent of the sample reported an annual income of $10,000 or less.

Patients were contacted and interviewed by one of two second-year medical students. All patients were informed that their responses were strictly confidential and that their participation (or lack thereof) would in no way affect their privileges at the agency.

The interview instrument was a highly detailed, structured questionnaire developed by Jacobson and Richardson[2] for use with a psychiatric population. Four types of assault were assessed: physical assault as a child (PAC), experiences prior to age 16; physical assault as an adult (PAA); sexual assault as a child (SAC); and sexual assault as an adult (SAA). Physical assault varied in severity from being shot or stabbed to being threatened with hitting (ten separate acts). The twelve acts of sexual assault ranged from unwanted kissing and hugging to attempted and successful anal and vaginal intercourse. In addition, patients were asked if they had ever been asked to engage in any sexual acts before they were 16 years of age. Patients were instructed to exclude consensual acts with peers. When instructed to indicate the type of act they had experienced, patients were also asked to identify the frequency of the act and the identity of the perpetrator. Respondents could describe a maximum of four assault relationships per type of assault, i.e. respondents identified the perpetrator then identified the specific act(s) that they were subjected to for PAC, PAA, SAC, SAA. In addition to questions about the frequency of the incidents and the identity of the assailant, patients were asked to identify one of each of the four types of assault relationships that had an impact on them ("critical incident") and were asked a series of detailed questions about that specific relationship and its physical and emotional effects. Added to the original Jacobson and Richardson questionnaire was an item on the timing of the incident: the interviewer ascertained whether the critical incident occurred prior to, simultaneous with, or after the onset of the patient's mental illness.

RESULTS

The percentage of patients reporting assault is indicated in Table 1. Focusing on "major" assault (i.e., physical assault that involved at least hitting or kicking and sexual assault that involved at least genital touching, as well as attempted intercourse), well over half of the sample reported at least one major physical assault as a child, and 80% reported at least one major physical assault as an adult. Over one third of the patients (37%) reported that they had experienced at least one instance of major sexual assault prior to age 16, and 31% reported having experienced at least one major sexual assault as an adult.

Comparing the responses by gender, men were significantly more likely than were women to report PAC (x^2 [1] = 9.27, p < 0.005), although women were somewhat more likely to report PAA. Women were signifi-

TABLE 16.1. Prevalence of Major and Non-major Childhood and Adult Physical and Sexual Assault

Type of Assault	Men (N=26) N (%)	Women (N=28) N (%)	Total (N=54) N (%)
Physical Assault as a Child			
Major assault	21 (81)	11 (39)	32 (59)
Total assaults	23 (88)	20 (71)	43 (80)
Physical Assault as an Adult			
Major assault	19 (73)	24 (86)	43 (80)
Total assaults	23 (88)	25 (89)	48 (85)
Sexual Assault as a Child			
Major assault	7 (27)	13 (46)	20 (37)
Total assaults	8 (31)	16 (57)	24 (44)
Sexual Assault as an Adult			
Major assault	3 (12)	14 (50)	17 (31)
Total assaults	6 (23)	19 (68)	25 (46)

cantly more likely than men to report SAA (x^2 [1] = 5.57, p < 0.05) and were more likely, though not significantly so, to report SAC.

Many of the patients had experienced major sexual assault and physical assault as children and again as adults (see Table 2). Five women (18%) and one man (3%) had experienced all four types of assault. Almost one quarter of the men and one third of the women had experienced both major PAC and SAC. Two of the men and almost half of the women (43%) had experienced both major PAA and SAA. One third of the sample had experienced major PAC and PAA, and one quarter of the women and 11% of the men had experienced sexual assault as a child and again as an adult.

TABLE 16.2. Co-occurrence of Major and Non-major Assault

Type of Assault	Men (N=26) N (%)	Women (N=28) N (%)	Total (N=54) N (%)
Physical Assault as a Child and Sexual Assault as a Child			
Major assault	6 (23%)	9 (32%)	15 (28%)
Total assaults	6 (23%)	12 (43%)	18 (33%)
Physical Assault as an Adult and Sexual Assault and an Adult			
Major assault	2 (8%)	12 (43%)	14 (26%)
Total assaults	6 (23%)	18 (64%)	24 (44%)
Sexual Assault as a Child and Physical Assault as an Adult			
Major assault	9 (35%)	9 (32%)	18 (33%)
Total assaults	20 (77%)	18 (64%)	38 (70%)
Sexual Assault as a Child and Sexual Assault as an Adult			
Major assault	2 (8%)	7 (25%)	9 (17%)
Total assaults	4 (15%)	11 (39%)	15 (28%)

Women

Physical Assault as a Child (PAC). Twenty of the 28 women (71%) indicated that they had suffered physical assault (major and non-major) as a child. Twelve (60%) had experienced assault from one relationship, and eight reported assault from two to four such relationships, for a total of 30 different assailants across the 20 patients. The majority of the perpetrators were family members: mothers were listed eight times, fathers five times, and brothers five times. Only five of the 30 assaultive relationships occurred with non-family members—two boyfriends and three strangers. The most frequent assault consisted of beatings, although four of the situations involved threats with a weapon. The women also indicated that the relationships, more often than not, involved a high frequency of assaults. In 11 of the 30 relationships, patients indicated that an indeterminate number of assaults occurred; only six of the perpetrators committed the assault only once.

Nineteen of the 20 patients reporting PAC responded to the questions about the incident that affected them the most. One woman indicated that the assault occurred simultaneous with the onset of her mental illness; the remaining 18 indicated that this relationship occurred prior to their mental illness.

Physical Assault as an Adult (PAA). Twenty-five women (89%) reported at least one assaultive relationship as an adult. About half of this number (N = 12) reported one such relationship, and the remaining half (N = 13) reported two to four such relationships, for a total of 43 relationships. Six of these instances involved a shooting or stabbing. Unlike the physical assault that occurred when the patients were young, PAA was most likely perpetrated by a mate or stranger: 21 of the 43 relationships were with a husband or boyfriend, and 10 assaults occurred with strangers (three occurred with casual acquaintances). Three of the relationships were with a family member. Assault occurred once in over half of the 43 relationships (N = 23) and two to four times with six of the assailants. In 11 relationships, the perpetrator assaulted the patient over 20 times.

Ten of the 20 women responding to the questions on the critical incident indicated that medical attention was required as a result of that assault. The majority of these women indicated that this assaultive relationship occurred before the onset of mental illness. Of the 19 women for whom the information could be ascertained, 68% (N = 13) indicated that the relationship occurred before their mental illness, 20% (N = 4) reported that it occurred simultaneous with their illness, and 10% (N = 2) indicated that it occurred after the onset.

Sexual Assault as a Child (SAC). Sixteen of the 28 women (57%) indicated that they had been sexually assaulted or molested prior to age 16 and, as indicated previously, 13 of these involved major assault. Eleven (61%) indicated one such relationship and seven indicated two to four, for a total of 30 assaultive relationships. Almost half of these 30 relationships (N = 14) occurred with a family member (one father, four uncles, five brothers, four cousins). Three of the relationships involved a stranger, with the remainder involving friends, neighbors, and casual acquaintances. Seventeen of the 30 relationships were ones in which the assault occurred only once; five relationships involved two to four instances of assault; and eight involved five or more separate assaults by the same person. Half (N = 15) of the 30 instances involved intercourse.

When asked about their critical incident, three fourths (N = 12) of the women indicated that other children in the family had had similar experiences with this perpetrator. 75% of these critical incidents occurred prior to the onset of the victims' mental illness.

Sexual Assault as an Adult (SAA). Nineteen women had experienced at least one major or minor sexual assault as an adult. Twelve women had experienced one such relationship, and six had experienced two to four, for a total of 28 such relationships for the 19 women. Unlike the childhood experiences (SAC), the adult experiences were most likely to occur with a stranger (ten relationships) or casual acquaintance (seven relationships). One incident occurred with a family member (an uncle) and four occurred with mates. Most of the 28 relationships involved a single encounter—24, three involved two to four encounters with that individual, and 2 involved ten such encounters. Nineteen of the 28 incidents (68%) involved intercourse.

In response to the critical incident questions, 11 of the 19 women indicated that physical force was used, with nine being injured seriously enough to require medical attention. Unlike the previously reported instances of assault, SAA that had the greatest impact was somewhat more likely to occur after the onset of the woman's mental illness than before: ten women reported that victimization occurred after the development of their illness, one reported that the assault had occurred simultaneous with it, and six reported that the assault had occurred before.

Men

Physical Assault as a Child (PAC). Twenty-three of the 26 men in the sample (88%) reported having experienced some type of physical assault as a child. Seven (30% of those victimized) had been assaulted by one perpetrator, and 16 reported that they had been assaulted by two to four different assailants. The 23 male patients reported a total of 47 physically assaultive relationships. Twenty-nine of these relationships involved one instance of assault, five involved two to four instances of assault by the same individual, and ten involved eleven or more. The majority of the assaults involved beatings; however, four assaults involved a stabbing or shooting and 13 involved threats of such violence.

In comparison with the women, men were more likely to report that their childhood assault occurred at the hands of a non-family member. Of the 47 relationships described by the 23 men, only 10 were family members (three mothers, two uncles, two brothers, two sisters, one father). The most frequently listed perpetrator was a casual acquaintance (N = 11), followed by a stranger (N = 9). Six instances involved "multiple males," which quite possibly refers to a street gang.

Twenty of the 23 men responded to the critical incident questions, five of whom indicated that they received medical attention for injuries resulting from this assault. Consistent with the data on women, the majority of these patients indicated that this relationship occurred prior to the onset of their mental illness: three fourths of the men indicated that the incident(s) had occurred before their mental illness, two reported that it had occurred simultaneous with the illness, and three indicated that the assault relationship had occurred after they became ill.

Physical Assault as an Adult (PAA). Twenty-three men (88%) also reported physical assault as an adult, with 12 reporting one perpetrator, and 11 reporting two to four assault relationships. The 23 men reported a total of 44 different victimizers. As with their childhood physical assaults, the majority of the perpetrators were non-family members. Fourteen were strangers, nine were casual acquaintances, and nine were "multiple males," while only seven were family members (one father, one mother, three brothers, one sister, one wife). Thirty-six of the instances (81%) involved single occurrences, three involved two to four, and four involved five or more separate incidents with the assailant. In 8 of the 44 instances, a gun or knife was used on the patient, and in nine instances of assault such violence was threatened.

The seriousness of these encounters is suggested by the data on medical treatment: half of the 20 men responding to the critical incident questions reported that such treatment was necessary. This relationship was as likely to occur after the onset of the patient's mental illness as before: ten patients indicated that their illness began before their critical adult assault, whereas nine indicated that their illness began after the assaultive relationship.

Sexual Assault as a Child (SAC). Eight of the 26 men (31%) reported that they had been sexually assaulted as a child. Five reported one such relationship and three reported two different assailants. Only one of these eleven relationships involved a family member (a male cousin). Four involved strangers, four involved a casual acquaintance, one involved a neighbor, and one involved a friend. Six of the eleven relationships involved a single incident, and three involved two to four incidents. Two were apparently long-term abusive relationships involving over twenty instances of assault by the same perpetrator.

Of the seven men responding to the critical incident questions, six indicated that the SAC occurred prior to the onset of their mental illness.

Sexual Assault as an Adult (SAA). Six men (23%) reported SAA: five reported one such relationship and one patient reported sexual assault by four different perpetrators. Of the nine different perpetrators, three were strangers to the patients, four were casual acquaintances (all of whom apparently had assaulted the patient, indicating four victimizers), and two were "multiple male" incidents. One relationship involved two to four instances of assault, and the remaining eight involved a single encounter.

In response to the question on the assault relationship having the greatest impact, three of the six patients indicated that physical force had been used in the encounter, and one was injured seriously enough to need medical care.

Among the six victims, two indicated that the incident occurred prior to the onset of their mental illness, and four indicated that it had occurred after the onset of their psychiatric disorder.

DISCUSSION

Although the entire sample had been identified as victims of physical assault, sexual assault, or molestation in order to be included in the study, the high incidence of major physical and sexual assault reported by these psychiatric outpatients is still striking. Prevalence of major assault ranged from 80% of the sample reporting physical assault as an adult to between 31% and 37% reporting sexual assault as an adult and as a child, respectively. Physical assault as a child was reported by 59% of the sample.

The reported assaults were quite serious as well. The severity of the sexual assaults is indicated by the prevalence of actual rape (i.e., forced intercourse) that occurred: 68% of the women and 50% of the men reporting sexual assault as an adult reported having been raped, and 50% of the women reporting sexual assault as a child reported having been raped. In addition, 50% of both women and men who reported physical assault as adults had sought medical attention for their injuries, as did 25% of the men who were assaulted as children. Nearly one in five of the men who experienced physical assault as an adult were assaulted with a weapon. The violent nature of sexual assaults was also evident, as 50% and 17% of the women and men, respectively, who were sexually assaulted as adults had to seek medical attention due to the force used on them. The need for medical attention is an underestimation of assault severity, as patients were asked this question only in regard to one relationship in each of the four categories. It is quite possible that patients were injured severely enough to require medical attention on more than one occasion and in more than one relationship.

Consistent with other reports,[1,2] women were more likely than men to have suffered sexual victimization as a child or as an adult. They were equally as likely to suffer physical assault as an adult but were less likely to report having experienced physical assault as a child.

In terms of abuse patterns, men were more likely than women to report multiple perpetrators for physical assault as a child; primarily non-family members (acquaintances, strangers, and gangs) with whom they usually had only one encounter. On the other hand, women were more likely to report that their childhood abuse (both physical and sexual) was inflicted by a family member and that the assault had extended over time.

As adults, the pattern for physical assaults was similar to the patterns of childhood. Men tended to be assaulted by non-family members only once, and women tended to be assaulted over an extended period by a mate as adults and by a family member as children.

Although women were more frequently sexually assaulted as adults and children, it is important to compare the circumstances of these assaults. Two thirds of both men and women who were sexually assaulted as a child had one relationship in which the assault(s) occurred. The majority of the men were sexually assaulted by non-family members (over 90% were acquaintances and strangers), whereas about half of the women sexually assaulted as children were assaulted by a family member (27% by a secondary family member, 20% by a primary family member). Despite this difference, slightly over half of both men and women experienced only one assault per relationship as a child. Thus, the dynamic of being sexually assaulted by non-family members did not reduce the chances of being repeatedly assaulted by non-family members, as it happens in the case of physical assault as a child.

The different patterns and circumstances of assault are significant because to prevent victimization of different segments of the mentally ill population, approaches need to be tailored to the various segments. For example, the high incidence of physical assault as an adult reported by the women in the sample, usually at the hands of a mate, suggests that therapy with these patients should actively address spouse abuse to alleviate the trauma and prevent future victimization. To seek to prevent male adult physical assault victims by a similar strategy would be fruitless, because they are not assaulted in those same situations. Data indicate that men are more likely to be assaulted once by strangers, acquaintances, and gangs, so therapy should address safety outside the home setting.

The relationship of victimization to the onset of the patient's mental illness is difficult to interpret. The patients' victimization in childhood, which usually occurred prior to the onset of mental illness, may have predisposed these patients to developing their illness (as is suggested by much of the literature[5,6]), or their mental illness may have developed in the absence of the victimization as a result of other factors. On the other hand, the high frequency of adult assault after the onset of mental illness suggests that, in addition to victimization as a predisposing factor,[1,7] the mentally ill are more vulnerable to victimization because of their illness. Specifically, both adult men and women are at risk for sexual assault after the onset of their psychiatric disorder, and adult men seem equally as likely to be physically assaulted after the onset of their mental illness as before. It is interesting to note that the victimization that occurred after the onset of mental illness was most likely perpetrated by a stranger or casual acquaintance; whereas (with the exception of physical assault as a child for males) assaults that occurred prior to the illness were more likely to involve a family member.

CONCLUSION

This study is significant in that it describes the severity and circumstances of physical and sexual victimization in a sample of black psychiatric outpatients. These findings on the frequency of assault against this group may explain why some authors have found that being African American is significantly related to a higher score on phobia measures,[8] and may also lend insight into reports that black psychotic patients show more paranoia.[9] The severity of the victimization and circumstances (i.e., relationships) in which the victimization occurs needs to be addressed in treatment plans to resolve past psychic trauma and prevent future victimization.

COMMENTARY

This article's findings are still very relevant. The finding of repeated victimization from both sexual and physical assault during childhood and adulthood in so many patients continues to astound me. Quite often, I cite this article's findings while lecturing around the country. The article was useful to me in 1994 while I was serving on the American Academy of Pediatrics' Task Force on Adolescent Assault Victim Needs. The task force published a model protocol for addressing adolescent assault victim needs in their journal *Pediatrics* in late 1996. A major focus of the protocol was the finding that assaultive trauma is recurrent. Accordingly, any work with victims should focus on preventing their future victimization.

My colleagues and I designed this study to delve deeper into the victimization of black psychiatric outpatients reported in "Need for Victimization Screening in a Black Psychiatric Population" (see Chapter 14). We were quickly learning that victimization screening only uncovered the fact that there was a problem with victimization and didn't begin to reveal the depth of a patient's victimization experiences. What we found was nearly overwhelming. It also brought home a valuable lesson about how not to get "burnt out" doing community psychiatry or public health work: when faced with an insurmountable challenge, if you slowly chip away at the problem by trying to understand it, trying to put systems in place to fix the damage, and most importantly, trying to prevent the damage from occurring in the first place, then you'll be okay. On the other hand, if you sit around moaning and groaning about how bad the situation is and don't do something to lessen your sense of helplessness, which can become traumatic, then you're headed for a preventable psychological disaster.

The methodology of our research drew some heat from Ms. Debra A. Henry, a medical student in Nashville, Tennessee. In a letter to the editor of the JNMA (1990;82:80), the student identified what she felt to be several flaws in the study. She felt we needed to identify the period during which the data was collected. Further, she felt that besides its being too small, the study represented a selection bias due to a lack of randomization of participants. She also criticized our study because the lack of a control group made it impossible to tell if our findings were due to a random association. She concluded her letter by recommending that we use in the future "stronger research protocol." We wrote a reply to her (Jenkins E, Bell CC, Taylor J, Walker L. Letter to the editor, "Victimization of Black Psychiatric Patients." *J Natl Med Assoc.* 1990;82:80–81).

Ms. Henry's concerns point to a major problem in doing research in real-life community settings. For the past three years, I've been Co-Principle Investigator of the Chicago African-American Youth Health Behavior Project conducted by the Prevention Research Center at the University of Illinois. Despite a sophisticated multidisciplinary research team designing the research protocol, our research in a community setting continues to be very difficult. During a defense of the research project, Dr. Brian Flay, the principal investigator, made the following observations about the "messiness" of conducting prevention research in high-risk, real-life contexts. He noted, "For scientific purity, it would be desirable to conduct research in controlled, low-risk contexts." Further, he noted, "Some prevention research, by definition, however, must be conducted with high-risk populations in the uncontrolled settings of their chaotic everyday lives." These conditions challenge scientific purity because of several factors mentioned in Ms. Henry's letter and in our response. Because of population mobility, attrition will always be a problem when doing research on high-risk populations. There is always the risk of beginning a study with a sample large enough to draw valid conclusions from, but winding up with too few subjects for the findings to hold water. Because subjects have the freedom to participate or not participate in a clinic study, selection bias will always be a problem in such contexts. In intervention research, there will always be a threat to the integrity of the intervention because of all the factors in a subject's life or a community that could influence the outcome. Dr. Flay concluded, "These challenges can never be entirely eliminated. If they were, many of the risks to our subjects would also be reduced, and there would be less need for prevention research."

Prevention research rigor must be improved by (1) reducing the attrition of subjects and reducing the selection bias of subjects as much as reasonably possible; (2) pursuing missing data analytic methods to handle the selection bias and attrition that cannot be eliminated; (3) minimizing contamination of the treatment condition and maximizing treatment integrity as much as possible; (4) conducting extensive and intensive process evaluation to assess and allow for analysis of variations in the treatment and the context; (5) pilot testing both interventions and measures to ensure high integrity, reliability, and validity. However, as I've stated before, community-based organizations doing research will rarely have the kinds of resources found in academia. Ergo, we perform a kind of "bent nail" research. While not perfect, our work is extremely important. It flows out of high-volume, clinical experience in an underserved African-American population. It is based on observations that academic researchers are simply not privy to having. We at the CMHC have a partnership that brings together the best from my empirical, anecdotal, clinical worlds and the best from my colleague Dr. Esther Jenkins' research, social psychology world. This creates a combination of work that can be used for a community population and yet is rigorous enough to command respect in the scientific community. Consequently, our work has frequently led the way for academic scientists to do more sophisticated studies in areas in which we have been trailblazers.

Since getting a National Institute of Mental Health R-01 grant, I've been sanctioned as an official scientific researcher. The problem is that while rigorous science is required to get into the "scientist club," the impact of the sanctioned official scientist on practice is minimal in the behavioral science field. So, I'm beginning to feel that although my earlier studies were "bent nail" and not pure science, I had more impact and influence on the field than I'm having now as a "store-bought, straight nail" scientist.

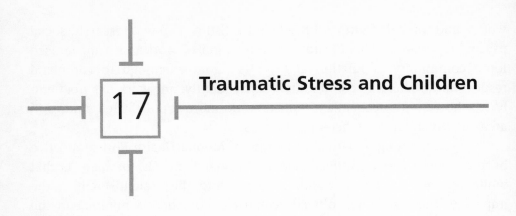

Traumatic Stress and Children

INTRODUCTION

News reports, official statistics, and research data indicate that a relatively large number of inner-city children are exposed to violence on a regular basis. Furthermore, the exposure occurs in such a manner that it and its pernicious effects are often subtle and underestimated. While child victims of violence elicit considerable concern, and rightfully so, many more children witness extreme acts of violence, often perpetrated against family and friends. This direct observation of the violent assault of another person, referred to as "co-victimization" by Shakoor and Chalmers,[1] is frequently accompanied by immersion in a violent milieu in which the child is in constant danger, even if never actually victimized. Such exposure to violence has serious consequences for the child's mental health, often resulting in post-traumatic stress disorder (PTSD) symptoms similar to those resulting from direct victimization. In the absence of understanding the symptoms and the circumstances under which they occur, the child's dysfunctional behavior, which often includes poor achievement and

Originally printed as Bell Carl C, Jenkins Esther J. Traumatic stress and children. *J Health Care Poor and Underserved.* 1991;2:175–188.

acting out, may be misinterpreted, inaccurately diagnosed, and inappropriately treated.

This paper discusses black youths' exposure to violence, the traumatic effects of such exposure, and some approaches to treating the effects and preventing the initial exposure. We conclude with research questions that need to be addressed in order to better serve these at-risk youth.

CHILDREN'S EXPOSURE TO VIOLENCE

Although very little data exists on the actual extent of children's witnessing of violence, there is evidence that such exposure is considerable, particularly for children in the inner city. For example, in Los Angeles county in 1982, 10–20% of the 2,000 homicides were witnessed by a dependent youngster.[2] An examination of one half of the homicide cases in Detroit in 1985 found that 17% were witnessed by a total of 136 youths aged 18 or younger.[3] In about one quarter of these cases, a family member was the victim. In an informal sample of ten mothers in a Chicago public housing development, Dubrow and Garbarino[4] found that "virtually all" of the children had had a first-hand encounter with a shooting by age five, and the majority of those incidents appeared to have involved witnessing someone get shot.

Our research at the Community Mental Health Council (CMHC), a comprehensive community mental health center on Chicago's Southside, provides further evidence of the extent of exposure and the types of incidents witnessed. Our first study surveyed 536 African-American schoolchildren in grades two, four, six, and eight.[5] A 32-item questionnaire asked about background, involvement in fights and arguments, and exposure to violence and asked whether the child had seen someone shot or stabbed. While the study contained many of the flaws (most notably that the measures were self-reports) that have characterized similar studies,[6] it revealed that a disturbing number of these children had in fact witnessed violence in their environment. Approximately one quarter (26%) of these children reported that they had seen a person get shot, and 29% indicated that they had seen an actual stabbing.

A subsequent screening of over 1,000 middle and high school students found very similar results.[1,7] Among those students from relatively high crime areas on Chicago's Southside, 35% had witnessed a stabbing, 39% had seen a shooting, and almost one quarter (24%) had seen someone get killed. In the majority of cases, the students reported that they knew the victims, and about half (47%) of the victims were known as friends, family members, classmates, or neighbors. In addition, 46% of the sample reported that they had personally been the victim of at least one of eight violent crimes, ranging from having a weapon pulled on them to being robbed, raped, shot, or stabbed.

Homicide statistics and data on the epidemiology of violence in the black community also suggest that a considerable number of black children will be exposed to life-threatening violence. After an extended period of decline, the homicide rate among African Americans has increased dramatically and consistently since 1985.[8,9] Currently, the homicide rate for black males is seven times that of white males; homicide is the leading cause of death for black men and women aged 15–34,[10] showing a 39% increase for black males since 1984.[11] These statistics will probably worsen. Estimates based on the number of homicides in the first six months of 1990 suggest that 1990 killings will exceed those of the previous year by 2,000 victims, making it, in the words of one national politician, the "bloodiest year in American history."[12] Even more disturbing, the factors fueling this killing frenzy—joblessness, family disruption, drug use—show no sign of abating.

Blacks are more likely than whites or Hispanics to be killed by a friend or acquaintance in the home with a handgun during a verbal argument.[13] This kind of killing—in a residence, unpremeditated, resulting from an emotional outburst—seems quite likely to be observed by family members, including children. In addition, the increase in gang/drug killings, which in many cities is accounting for the dramatic increase in homicides among young black males, points to greater exposure for children as witnesses and increases the chances that the victim will be one of their peers. In Chicago in 1989, one of every five homicide victims was between the ages of 11 and 20, an increase of 22% over the previous year, and one that police attributed to gangs and drugs.[14]

What is not captured in the statistics on homicide is the public, random nature of violence that pervades many inner-city communities, turning them into veritable war zones where citizens live under chronic threat.

A recent *Wall Street Journal* article chronicled the day-to-day violence in an inner-city housing project, most of it from gang shootouts outdoors, with bystanders caught in the middle and literally running for their lives:

> Once again the sound of gunfire fills the air. They catch glimpses through the windows of young gunmen waving their pistols about. One youth totes a submachine gun. In an apartment upstairs, other gang members blast away at rivals in a building across the street. In the middle of the battle, the elementary school across the street lets out.[15]

In the previously mentioned Dubrow and Garbarino[4] study at a Chicago housing development, all ten of the mothers listed shootings when asked to name the most serious danger confronting them. On the contrary, kidnapping was the most serious concern of a matched sample of people residing outside the city.

While most killings still occur indoors as a result of arguments between family and acquaintances, a distressing amount of unpredictable, life-threatening violence occurs in public places, exposing innocent bystanders. Although statistics indicate that the involvement of bystanders is the exception rather than the rule, bystanders are killed in the crossfire and occasionally inside their homes, as gang/drug wars are waged with increasingly powerful weapons that penetrate doors and walls.

EFFECTS OF EXPOSURE TO VIOLENCE

Research and clinical experience indicate that children who witness and are otherwise exposed to violence are deeply affected by the events, often showing symptoms of PTSD. Pynoos and Nader's work with children who witnessed the murder of a parent and who were exposed to community violence[16] found that the youngsters displayed the following classic PTSD symptoms: re-experiencing the event in play, dreams, or intrusive images and sounds associated with the event; psychic numbing characterized by subdued behavior and inactivity; constricted affect and diminished interest in activities; sleep disorders, avoidance behaviors, and startle reactions. In addition, the children are frequently plagued by fears that the violence will reoccur, guilt over their behavior during the incident, a pessimistic future orientation, and difficulty forming interpersonal relationships. These latter symptoms can manifest in a sense of futurelessness,[17] characterized by children's belief that they will not reach adulthood, and can manifest in difficulty with close interpersonal relationships, as they hesitate to establish bonds they fear will be broken.

Children exposed to violence may have lowered self-esteem[18] and show a decline in cognitive performance and school achievement. These school difficulties, which are so easily misdiagnosed in inner-city children, may be a result of the child being distracted by the intrusion of thoughts related to the trauma, making it impossible to concentrate on school material; the development of a cognitive style of deliberate memory lapses to help control these spontaneous reminders of the event; or simple fatigue from sleepless nights.[16] In a more psychoanalytical oriented explanation, Gardner[19] argues that exposure to chronic violence inhibits development of precision learning by leading to an avoidance of the aggressive-assertive behavior necessary for problem-solving. Indeed, a frequently noted characteristic of children exposed to violence is a passive-aggressiveness—difficulty controlling aggressive impulses[20] but also emotional withdrawal and passivity.

While children may experience any or all of the PTSD symptoms, the specific manifestations of PTSD are a function of the age and developmental level of the child, and the event itself may impact on the developmental process.[2,16,21] Preschool children are more likely to display passive reactions and regressive symptoms such as enuresis (bed-wetting), decreased verbalizations, and clinging behavior. In comparison, school-age children tend to be more aggressive and more inhibited, have somatic complaints such as stomachaches, and have cognitive distortions and deficits that show up as learning difficulties. Adolescent trauma reactions more closely resemble those of adults and, as Pynoos and Eth[2] note, are characterized by a "premature entrance into adulthood or a premature close on identity formation." Children of this age who have witnessed or been exposed to violence may engage in acting out and self-destructive behaviors such as substance abuse, delinquency, promiscuity, life-threatening reenactments, and other aggressive acts.[2,16,20] The aggression and other destructive behaviors are viewed as an attempt to protect the self from anxiety and to prevent its fragmentation.[2]

Exposure to violence can be particularly problematic when the violence results in the death of a family member or close friend; personal reactions to trauma clash with grief and mourning.[16,21] The trauma/grief connection is most severe when the death is sudden or grisly.[22] Reminiscing about the deceased is necessary for grief resolution, but the survivors may avoid memories because they trigger anxiety surrounding the event. The grieving may also be complicated or impeded by the child's intense rage and desire to punish the perpetrator.[21]

An issue of considerable concern to those working with inner-city children is the impact of chronic exposure to violence. Whereas seeing even one act of life-threatening violence is a traumatic event that requires intervention, many inner-city children have experienced multiple losses due to traumatic violence and are themselves exposed to shootings and other mayhem on a regular basis. After listening to her young classmates in a "grief class" describe the deaths of close family members, one of whom had lost seven relatives, an 8-year-old remarked that "just" three folks in her family had died violently.[23] Lafayette, the 12-year-old subject of Kotlowitz's[15] description of life in Chicago housing projects, personally witnessed three shootings during his lifetime and lost two acquaintances during the three months that the reporter observed him and his family. In two case studies of black adolescent males referred for behavioral problems, a Chicago social worker[20] found that one youth had experienced the violent death of an uncle, cousin, and brother, and the second youngster had lost two aunts, an uncle, and his mother.

One may argue that repeated exposure will produce an adaptation to the violence; however, the evidence more strongly suggests an overload. Pynoos suggests that the "effects of each episode can be additive and seriously deplete the child's inner resources."[16] Lenore Terr, a psychiatrist who treated child victims of the Chowchilla kidnappings,[24] noted that while brief traumas have only limited effects on the individual, repeated trauma may lead to anger, despair, and severe psychic numbing resulting in major personality changes.[17]

Violence that touches children has consequences far beyond the individual victim, eventually having an impact on the quality of life in the black community. In addition to losing resources from a fully functioning member with a healthy mind and body, exposure to violence creates an individual more likely to engage in future violence and other antisocial acts. The PTSD symptoms include such behavior. In addition, social learning theory predicts that observing violence may lead to an acquisition of that behavior, depending on the child's identification with the perpetrator and the outcome of the violence.[25] At the least, violence may be perceived as an appropriate response in a very broad range of situations. Many children in a violent milieu may resort to violence in order to avoid victimization or in retaliation for prior victimization of self or close others. Eventually, children who are exposed to a steady diet of violence will themselves feed into the cycle of violence, victimization, and fear that paralyzes many inner-city neighborhoods.

TREATMENT OPTIONS

Growing awareness of the extent of violence among black youth has led to the development of numerous approaches and programs. Because most of the concern surrounds homicide and violent victimization, much of the activity has been directed at violence prevention, thereby indirectly affecting violence exposure. While anything that reduces violence in the black community (e.g., control of firearms, strengthening black families and improving parenting skills, reducing head injury[9]) will necessarily reduce youth involvement in violence, there are a number of programs designed specifically for the young. Currently, a number of school-based programs[26,27] teach conflict resolution skills in an attempt to alter behaviors and norms that contribute to the violent encounters in which the role of victim and perpetrator is almost decided by chance. A variety of community-based programs are aimed at reducing youth involvement in gangs, drugs, and violence by enhancing self-esteem, improving conflict resolution skills, and encouraging or providing education and job training.[28]

While programs to prevent violence are much more prevalent, some programs address the impact of witnessing violence. In an elementary school in South Central Los Angeles, children who have experienced losses through violence attend a "grief class" in which they explore their feelings about life, death, and their loss.[23] On Chicago's Southside, Johnnie Dyson, a school social worker, began traditional group and individual therapy sessions with her "behavioral problem" referrals after finding that all those students who had experienced the violent death of at least one close family member reported a marked improvement in emotional health at the end of the semester.[20]

Detroit's Family Bereavement Center provides treatment to child witnesses of homicide based on a model developed by Robert Pynoos and associates at the Prevention Intervention Program in Trauma, Violence, and Sudden Bereavement in Childhood at UCLA.[16,21,29] The Pynoos model is one of the most developed approaches to the treatment of childhood trauma. It is based on the principle that the consequences of a violent event (e.g., endangerment of a child's life, witnessing of injury or death, loss of significant other, worry about the safety of another, reminders of some previous traumatic event) will determine the child's symptoms (PTSD, grief, separation anxiety, renewal of old symptoms) and the treatment. An initial assessment examines factors that mediate the impact of the trauma (e.g., degree of exposure, relationship to victim, presence of other stressors). The intervention can occur at the individual, family, classroom, group, or community level, addressing level-specific goals. Workers in this area agree that a key to successful treatment is intervention soon after the trauma occurs; even if the child is not showing obvious signs of post-traumatic stress, symptoms will probably eventually emerge, and delayed intervention carries the risk that so-called maladaptive trauma resolution will have occurred in response to the overwhelming anxiety.[17,21]

At issue in the treatment of children exposed to violence is the identification of these silent victims. While sensational events, such as the 1988 shooting of six children in a Winnetka, Illinois, classroom[30] and the 1989 slaying of five children on a Compton, California, playground, [31] have created enormous concern for those children, children in inner cities face chronic violence but often do not receive such attention.[32] Many observers may assume that since violence is such a part of these children's lives, they are no longer affected by murder and mayhem. This position, as we noted previously, is not accurate. Inner-city school systems and communities may simply have fewer resources to commit to the problem. Less than a year before the Winnetka incident, a high school student in Chicago was shot in the hallway as classes were changing. Crisis workers visited for one day. No crisis workers visited a Southside elementary school when a 15-

year-old student was killed on the street, even though teachers and students were quite shaken by the incident.[32]

Witnesses of family and community violence can be expected to receive even less attention. In most instances, these crimes are handled by law enforcement professionals whose concern is the event and the actual victim and who care little about the others present unless they have a bearing on the case. When violence occurs in a public or quasi-public place, professionals may not even be aware of the number of witnesses. That a violent event is witnessed by so many contributes to the perception that the trauma is shared and thus has less impact on the individual than if that person alone had been present when the incident occurred.

An additional complicating factor in the treatment of inner-city victims exposed to violence is that many PTSD symptoms are considered endemic to the inner city. In many such neighborhoods, poor school achievement, aggression, and the self-destructive behaviors of substance abuse, delinquency, and promiscuity occur with such frequency and in close linkage with other destabilizing factors (e.g., family disruption, poverty, poor schools) that the contribution of violence exposure is overlooked. In such instances, the diagnosis of the child's difficulties is inadequate and treatment may be inappropriate or misdirected.

One approach to identifying violence-traumatized children who need mental health services is to screen at-risk children for their exposure to violence.[1,33,34] Schools in high-crime areas would be appropriate places to conduct such a routine screening, since they would allow one to reach a large number of children. In addition, physicians and mental health workers are encouraged to collect this information as part of their patients' medical history and to provide the appropriate referrals or treatment. Our research,[34] as well as that of others with psychiatric patients,[35] suggests that individuals do not volunteer such information regarding these violent incidents but will respond honestly if asked directly. In screening for exposure to violence, one needs to examine not only witnessing violence and identity of the victims, but also victimization and perpetration. These factors seem to be related, with exposure and victimization predicting perpetration.[7] All of these three experiences suggest a need for intervention.

The most direct way to identify children who have witnessed violence is to gather this information from police homicide records. The advantage of this approach is that it targets the most severely affected children—those physically close enough to a killing, to be listed as a witness. In many instances, the victim will be related to the child witness. This approach will also yield a smaller pool of children in need of services, which for many agencies will be more manageable given their often-limited resources.

Regardless of how these young co-victims are identified, steps must be taken to make sure that appropriate and adequate services are available for them. Currently, few direct service organizations provide victims' services, and even fewer provide these services for children. Most are geared toward adult female victims of sexual assault. Moreover, few professionals are trained in this area. Establishing treatment centers can satisfy both of these needs by providing service and training opportunities for professionals via workshops and internships. Such training centers should grow out of a collaborative effort between institutions (police, schools, child welfare agencies) that can identify co-victims; academics who can provide expertise in grantsmanship, research, and treatment approaches; and service agencies from which the professionals are drawn, which can provide a site for the programs.

RESEARCH NEEDS

While there has been some encouraging progress regarding the identification and treatment of children who witness violence, there is much more to be learned about and done for the silent victims. There is a desperate need for more research on the circumstances and extent of exposure and research on factors that mediate the impact of exposure. There is a need as well to understand the prevalence of children's exposure to violence against family, friends, and strangers. More needs to be known about the impact of witnessing the victimization of close others as opposed to strangers. Very little is known about the impact on witnesses differs whether they know or do not know the perpetrator; how the identity of the perpetrator and victim may interact (the impact of a family member killing another family member versus killing a stranger); and how the circumstances surrounding the violence affect the extent or severity of traumatic reaction. Do children respond differently to expressive violence marked by anger and impulsivity, and to instrumental violence more calculated toward achieving some specific goal? Do they respond differently if the violence is perceived as provoked and justified?

More research needs to be conducted on the impact of multiple, chronic exposure to violence and the interaction of violence exposure and other stressors in the lives of poor inner-city children. What effect will the recent incidents of bystanders killed by stray bullets *inside* their apartments and houses have on the emotional health of children who can no longer count on their families and the four walls of their homes to shield them from street violence?

Clearly, all children exposed to violence do not sustain psychological damage. It is important to discover who the exceptions are. What buffers them against the deleterious effects of violence and victimization? Age and developmental level appear to be important variables. One report on psychiatric patients found that those experiencing their initial trauma before age ten were about three times more likely than teens to develop post-traumatic symptoms.[36] What about family characteristics and relationships and the child's personal values?[37] Does the extended family buffer the child from or facilitate the child's working through the trauma by providing additional adult nurturing? Are middle-class children, who have fewer stresses from poverty and have a greater sense of control over their environment,[38] better able to cope with violence than are children from poorer backgrounds? Does a strong ethnic identity or belief in religious values buffer African-American children against the impact of victimization or co-victimization, as it apparently does for substance abuse?[36] Similarly, does a rural Southern background, with its attendant sense of family cohesion, traditionalism, and conservative attitudes,[39] buffer children from the impact of witnessing violence?

There is a need for continued research on the symptoms that occur as a result of trauma. Given the relationship between school phobia and anxiety disorders, are children with a history of school phobia at greater risk for PTSD from exposure to violence via victimization or witnessing? Does witnessing or being a victim of violence in childhood or adolescence increase the risk of attempted or successful suicide as the individual matures without having resolved the anxiety associated with earlier trauma?

Gender differences in responses to violence are a fascinating area of study. In a study[34] of victimization of black psychiatric patients, we found that while young patients (age 17 and under) did not differ significantly in their degree of personal victimization, girls were five times more likely to report knowing of close others having been victimized. Replication and comparison with a medically ill sample found comparable results.[33] In the latter study, both the mentally ill and medically ill male youngsters were less likely than girls in these groups to report that a relative or acquaintance had been murdered. These findings raise interesting questions about denial and other responses of young black males to threatening events, and may have implications for their risk-taking and occasionally nihilistic behavior.

There is much to be done regarding the treatment of and research on children who have been exposed to violence. Physicians, mental health workers, law enforcement officers, and educators should be aware of the circumstances and symptoms of PTSD and of the necessity for quick referrals and intervention. Data needs to be collected uniformly so that researchers can make cross-study comparisons. Collaboration among front-line service organizations, universities, and public institutions that can identify co-victims is essential in creating programs that effectively address this problem.

COMMENTARY

On October 2, 1990, we presented this article at the "Children at Risk" Third National Conference on Health Care for the Poor and Underserved, held by Meharry Medical College. The conference gave CMHC's research team the opportunity to highlight our continued work on the issue of traumatic stress in children. The children we studied had caught the attention of Ms. Johnnie Dyson in 1989. As a practicing clinical social worker who was working in a school we surveyed, Ms. Dyson saw first hand the results of the violence we had been accenting. She went on to publish "The Effect of Family Violence on Children's Academic Performance and Behavior" in the January 1990 JNMA. She presented two

cases of six students, all of whom had extensive histories of family violence, including a murder of a close family member. These cases illustrated the extreme impact of violence in the lives of African-American children.

"Traumatic Stress and Children" also highlighted a previous CMHC
research team study on over 1,000 schoolchildren aged 10–19 years, com-
pleted during the 1987–1988 school year. The results from this study were
published in two articles: "Co-victimization of African-American Children
Who Witness Violence: Effects on Cognitive, Emotional and Behavioral
Development" (Shakoor B, Chalmers D. *J Natl Med Assoc*. 1991) and
"African-American Youth Encounters with Violence: Results From the
Community Mental Health Council Violence Screening Project" (Uehara E,
Chalmers D, Jenkins E, Shakoor B. *J Black Studies*. 1996;26). When we
began this work in the early 1980s, we had no idea how great an impact it
would have.

Dr. Jenkins, who, like me, has continued to refine efforts in the
area, designed in 1992 a study of 203 African-American students from a
public high school on Chicago's Southside. After refining some National
Institute of Mental Health Child and Adolescent Disorders Research Branch
survey instruments, we replicated the study Dr. Richters and his group had
done a few years prior. Nearly two thirds of the adolescents surveyed
reported they had seen a shooting, and 45% reported having seen someone killed. This research was published in *Anxiety Disorders in African-
Americans* (New York: Springer Publications; 1994) in a chapter entitled
"Post-traumatic Stress Disorder and Violence among Inner City High
School Students." This research also formed the basis for another chapter
entitled "Exposure and Response to Community Violence among Children
and Adolescents" (In: Osofsky J, ed. *Children in a Violent Society*. New
York: Guilford Publications; 1997:9–31). I alluded to this study in the intro-
duction of "Stress-Related Disorders in African-American Children" (see
Chapter 3). It aided in our realizing that youth could develop other types
of stress-related disorders in response to trauma. Our work has recently
come to the attention of the American Psychoanalytic Association, providing me with the opportunity to present "Impact of Violence on African-
American Youth" at their Public Forum, "Creation of a Self: Color and
Trauma in the Life of a Child" in New York, December 19, 1997. My hopes

are that this association will realize the practical value of Freud's empirical work on traumatic stress and begin to apply some psychoanalytic principles toward working with children exposed to traumatic stress.

A more recent development in this line of inquiry deserves special mention. The Anxiety Prevention and Treatment Research Center (Department of Psychiatry and Behavioral Sciences, Medical University of South Carolina) in Charleston has been advancing our understanding of exposure to violence in children. Doctors Michelle Cooley, Samuel Turner, and Deborah C. Beidel have written about the difference in reported emotional distress symptoms between high-exposure and low-exposure community violence groups. These authors point out that the "literature on acute (non-recurring) violent incidents suggest that children exposed to community violence manifest psychological disorders, fear and anxiety, depression, helplessness and hopelessness, emotional withdrawal, and somatic symptoms (features associated with internalizing disorders)" (Cooley-Quille MR, Turner SM, Beidel, DC. Emotional impact of children's exposure to community violence: a preliminary study. *J Am Academy Child and Adolescent Psychiatry*. 1995;34:1362–1368). However, when children are exposed to a high level of community violence (which was the case in the authors' study and in our "Post-traumatic Stress Disorder and Violence Among Inner City High School Students"), "the focus should be on a broad array of areas including measures of academic, interpersonal, and social adjustment" (Jenkins EJ, Bell CC. Violence exposure, psychological distress and high risk behaviors among inner-city high school students. In: Friedman S, ed. *Anxiety Disorders in African-Americans*. New York: Springer Publishing; 1994:76–88). Simply put, exposure to one event of traumatic violence may cause post-traumatic stress disorder, while exposure to multiple events of traumatic violence may cause academic, interpersonal, or behavioral problems.

As a result of my work, I participated in the Strategy Session on Children, Violence, and Responsibility with President Clinton and Vice President Gore at the White House, May 10, 1999. This was a very interesting meeting, as there were only about thirty experts in the room with the first and second families. After the children present had a chance to speak, Mrs. Hillary Clinton introduced Dr. James Garbarino, Dr. Robert Pynoos, and myself as experts on children who where exposed to violence.

Dr. Garbarino did a great job of emphasizing that although the recent mass-murder school shootings taking place in white suburban schools were tragic, we needed to be mindful that the traumatic stress of community violence had been occurring in inner-city schools for some time. I then talked about the fact that mass murder/suicide was essentially a white male phenomenon similar to what Dr. Chester Pierce called a "white male entitlement dysfunction."

Right after the Columbine school shootings, I made the observation that mainly European-American males are responsible for anger/revenge mass murders/suicides, serial killings, presidential assassination attempts, and murder sprees. When I referred to this phenomenon as "white male entitlement dysfunction," needless to say, several European-American male reporters accused me of "white-male bashing" and became quite hostile. The European-American female reporters seemed to be more understanding, explaining to me that they could relate to what I was talking about because they had frequently been victims of "white male entitlement dysfunction." I remember outlining those dynamics to a *Newsweek* reporter, but when the article was published, my observations were "conveniently" left out. A couple of weeks later, I was at the 1999 American Psychiatric Association meeting in Washington, DC. During a think-tank on juvenile violence, I remarked to several colleagues that I found it interesting that most of the reporters had neglected mentioning the suicide component of all the recent white mass murders. About two weeks later, *Time* put out a story citing a white colleague who underscored the suicide/depression component of all the recent mass murders. That colleague had been in the room with me during the think-tank. I guess the moral of the story is that if an African-American psychiatrist is critical of European-Americans, it's not acceptable, but if a European-American psychiatrist says the same thing about European-American, it's okay. I guess the reverse is also true, but isn't truth always truth, regardless of the politics of who says it?

At the White House meeting in May 1999, I also talked about my work within the Chicago Public Schools on violence prevention. As soon as I left the White House, I bummed a ride to the Reno/Shalala "Violence against Women" meeting with Secretary Shalala. We had a very interesting talk on the way to the meeting. Because of my insight, I was invited back to the White House Conference on Mental Health with President Clinton and Vice President Gore on June 7, 1999.

Section Four

STATES

OF

CONSCIOUSNESS

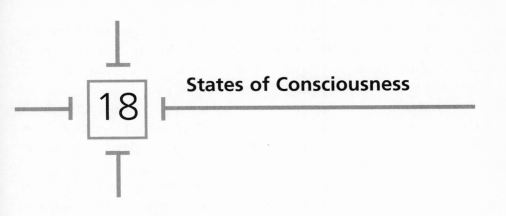

States of Consciousness

18

The art of psychiatry offers many different viewpoints from which to catalog behavior and thinking styles; therefore, many physicians tend to have difficulty in conceptualizing features of behavioral medicine. A classification of states of consciousness, with clinical examples of such states, is presented to aid in a more clear understanding of human behavior.

INTRODUCTION

The art of psychiatry offers many different viewpoints regarding the conceptualization of the medical aspects of behavior. As a result, physicians tend to be somewhat perplexed regarding the diagnostic categories of behavioral medicine. The confusion regarding the assessment of behavior is due not to the unscientific nature of psychiatry but rather to the nature of the knowledge. Unlike physical medicine, behavioral medicine has few objective reference points upon which to communicate observations. As behavioral scientists, psychiatrists are not able to state that because a patient's "schizophrenic enzyme" is 360 units, his illness has begun to remit, whereas physicians who practice physical medicine can use enzyme

Originally printed as Bell Carl C. States of consciousness. *J Natl Med Assoc.* 1980;72:331–334.

levels, white blood cell counts, x-ray photos, etc., to determine the patient's physical state. As a result, the knowledge of physical medicine tends toward empirical knowledge while the knowledge of behavioral medicine tends to be metaphoric and thus more subjective. Therefore, the confusion concerning the assessment of behavior is due to the difficulty of standardizing metaphoric knowledge, as different individuals favor different symbolic representations of subjective phenomena, depending on their own personal experiences.

As pointed out by Butts, "The search for altered states of consciousness is as old as human thought and human behavior."[1] Many different people from many different cultures have attempted, and still attempt, to alter consciousness by using drugs, meditative practices, religion, biofeedback, psychotherapy, etc. The quality of a person's consciousness varies from moment to moment depending on that individual's state of being. While a normal range in intensity of these various states of consciousness tends to be present in most persons, some individuals experience greater intensity and thus demonstrate behavioral abnormalities. The purpose of this article is to give the physician subjective reference points for the conceptualization of various states of consciousness, which are overtly expressed by the patient's behavior and by a verbal report of how he thinks and feels. While the concepts may aid in a diagnostic assessment, they are mainly presented to aid in understanding patients to better manage their treatment.

"State of consciousness" as presented here has been generally defined by Stanley Krippner as "a mental state which can be subjectively recognized by an individual (or by an objective observer of the individual) as representing a *difference* in psychological functioning from that individual's 'normal,' alert, waking state."[2] Some objective differences can be demonstrated by electroencephalogram (EEG).

Normal Waking State. This state of consciousness is most familiar to most individuals and is characterized by reflective thinking, rational thought, an awareness of self, goal-directed behavior, and cause-and-effect thinking. It tends to give one the illusion of being in control of one's thought processes; while it is usually known as "awake," it is jokingly referred to by some as "asleep."

Dreaming. This state of consciousness is characterized by rapid eye movements (REM); an EEG showing a low voltage and relatively fast, mixed frequency pattern; and a tonic inhibitory influence on motor output. Upon being awakened from dreaming, or REM sleep, patients often report complex dream experiences. Clinically, difficulties in this state of consciousness come from frightening dreams and produce insomnia, which may be an indication of psychopathologic functioning.

Narcolepsy is an illness characterized by overwhelming sleep attacks, cataplexy, sleep paralysis, or hypnogogic hallucinations. The sleep attacks are actually episodes of total REM sleep. The occurrence of REM sleep at the onset of sleep is pathological relative to the rhythm of normal sleep.[3]

Deep Sleep. This level of sleep is differentiated from dreaming, or REM, sleep by the absence of REM; thus, it is also known as non-rapid eye movement (NREM) sleep. NREM sleep also differs from REM sleep in that tendon reflexes can be elicited and the EEG shows high-amplitude, slow waves. On being awakened from this phase of sleep, subjects may give a brief report indicating that there is some minimal mental activity. Sleepwalking and bed-wetting (in children) occur in this state, as does pavor nocturnus ("night terrors").

Hypnopompic and Hypnogogic Hallucinations. These states of consciousness occur between the "normal awake" state of consciousness and sleep. Hypnopompic states occur just before awakening, while hypnogogic states occur just before one falls asleep. These two states are felt to be similar in that while they occur at different phases of the sleep cycle, they are related to Stage 4 of deep sleep. They are characterized by visual imagery and occasionally by auditory impressions with the subjective feeling that one is awake. These states may occur as normal phenomena (probably related to an altered sleeping pattern) or may be induced by antidepressant medication, which increases Stage 4 phenomena.[4] It is clear that these hallucinations need to be differentiated from those occurring in psychosis, as one is indicative of a disorder of the sleep-related state of consciousness, and the other is a disorder of the state of consciousness involving fragmentation.

Daydreaming. Also known as engaging in fantasy, this state is characterized by a fabricated mental picture or rapidly occurring thoughts that have little to do with the external environment. Daydreaming may serve as the basis for creativity or neurotic distortions and can occur with the eyes opened or closed. It may be induced by boredom, wish-fulfillment needs, or dream-sleep deprivation, or can occur spontaneously. It might be referred to as a "Walter Mitty" experience.

Repressed Memory. This state of consciousness involves past experience that is not directly available to an individual's reflective awareness. Freud observed that this phenomenon caused fragmented states in the dissociative states of hysteria.[5] Using psychoanalysis, Freud found that these memories could be brought to consciousness, resulting in the cure of certain types of mental illness. The content of this area of consciousness has also been observed to influence the nature of daydreams as well as dreaming sleep. The state of consciousness in which the repressed memory is recollected may be induced by meditation or drugs (such as LSD), or may occur spontaneously.

Trance States. Trance is characterized by the absence of continuous alpha waves on the EEG, attention focused on a single object, hyper-suggestibility, and alertness. It can be induced by hypnosis (first used by Charcot to induce hysterical paralysis and later by Freud to recover repressed memories before he used psychoanalysis). Other means of inducing this phenomenon are chants, rituals, dramatic presentations, or performing a task requiring attentiveness but little variation in response. "Highway hypnosis" is a trance state where subjects find themselves having driven far past their destination with no recollection of having done so. Trance is common among participants in black churches, Shamanism, and voodoo ceremonies.[6,7]

Meditative States. Meditation is self-induced and characterized by minimal mental activity, usually with the presence of continuous alpha waves on the EEG[8] (other types of waves may be produced by different types of meditation[9]), a lowering of cortical and autonomic arousal during a wakeful state, and in certain meditation forms, a lack of visual imagery. There are many modes of meditation, among them Transcendental Meditation, various forms of Yoga and Buddhism (including Zen), and Christian and Islamic practices. Meditation may be either positive and psychotherapeutic[10] or harmful, in some cases causing depersonalization[11] or hallucinations.[12] By techniques such as "bare attention" or "mindfulness," one may be able to reach another state of consciousness called "enlighten-ment." The practice of meditation allows the practitioner to experience var-ied states of consciousness.

Internal Scanning. An awareness of sensory input regarding the bodily functions may be heightened through this state of consciousness. Most individuals are able to get in touch with their physiological sensations (some more than others, depending on amount of practice). The process of "selective inattention" usually makes one unaware of such sensations. However, when physiologic processes are intensified through tachycardia or hunger, one may be spontaneously involved in internal scanning. Individuals who tend to be hypochondriacal involve themselves in a great deal of preoccupation with internal scanning. It may be a useful process, as knowledge of physiologic feelings can lead to some degree of control over processes like those seen in some meditative masters or persons engaging in biofeedback, the electronically aided internal scanning.

Regressive States. Regression occurs when the individual's thinking processes resemble earlier styles of thinking that are age-inappropriate to the subject's present circumstances. These states may be temporary, as seen in mental illness, during physical sickness, or when induced by hyp-nosis. They may be permanent, as seen in chronic organic brain syn-dromes such as senile dementia. Regression may also be helpful in the cre-ative process, as it involves letting go of one coping style and leaving a vacancy that may be filled by a more adaptive method.

States of Fragmentation. There are several types of fragmentation, all of which may be said to show a lack of integration between important aspects of thinking, feeling, or personality. One major split is characteris-tic of schizophrenia, in which the emotions felt are not in concert with the thoughts. In one form of hysteria, a portion of the personality is split off from consciousness by the process of dissociation.[5] Fragmented states may also be produced by drugs, trauma, stress, sensory deprivation, or meditation.

Stupor and Coma. Both of these states involve a limited degree of ability to perceive incoming stimuli. This ability is greatly reduced in stu-por, and in coma, there is a total inability to perceive incoming stimuli. A simple way to remember the various etiologic agents causing such states is remembering AEIOU TIPS: A-Alcohol, E-Epilepsy, I-Infection, O-Opium and other drugs, U-Uremia, T-Trauma, I-Insulin (too much or too little), P-Poisons, and S-Shock.

Lethargic State. This state is characterized by dulled, sluggish, slowed mental activity. It may present in an extreme form in patients with depression. It may be induced by drugs, sleep deprivation, fatigue, mood disturbances, anxiety, or metabolic imbalances such as hypoglycemia and anemia.

Hyperalert State. Hyperalertness is the opposite of lethargy and as such, is characterized by crisp mental activity and vigilance. It is seen in an extreme form in manic states or paranoia; however, it may also be a positive state of consciousness, experienced when a person is really "hot." It may be induced by drugs, by increased concentration due to a danger in the environment, by problem-solving needs, or by clearing up the thoughts that clutter the mind via meditation.

States of Frenzy. These states are characterized by negative emotional storms in which the subject experiences an overpowering emotion that is subjectively evaluated as unpleasant. Frenzy may be induced by rage, panic, fear, anxiety, terror, drugs, mobs, pain, suffering, etc. Clearly, the frenzied patient requires a form of management that reestablishes controls, whether through environmental methods, medication such as tranquilizers, or interpersonal methods such as "talking someone down."

States of Rapture. Rapture differs from frenzy in that the overpowering emotion is subjectively experienced as positive or pleasurable. It may well be seen clinically as the mood of the manic-depressive patient in the manic phase. It may be induced by religious rituals, sex, chanting, singing, whirling or dancing (dervish), drugs, jumping up and down, religious conversion, or fervent prayer.

Expanded States of Consciousness. The act of expanding one's state of consciousness can be found in every culture and religion. There is a surprising conformity in the descriptions of the expanded state of consciousness, regardless if the author is a practitioner of Zen, Christian mysticism, Islamic mysticism, shamanism, Taoism, or Buddhism. In such states, practitioners report a subjective alteration of space, time, body image, and sensory input. Practitioners often mentioned the subjective experience of being "one with God" or being in a state of "satori," "samadhi," or "cosmic consciousness." There are additional experiences of a subjective light, moral elevation, loss of fear of death, sense of immortality, intellectual illumination, and loss of feelings of sin.

The reactions of others to a subject in such a state may be a feeling of strong attraction to the subject and a feeling that the subject is manifesting something quite different from an ordinary state of consciousness.[13] Such states may occur spontaneously or through meditation or drugs. Expanded states of consciousness have also been called "peak experiences."[14] On the road to this state of consciousness, some may experience states of fragmentation, rapture, frenzy, and trance.

DISCUSSION

It is felt that this catalog of states of consciousness aids in the structuring of very subjective experiences. With this schema, readers may identify such states as they occur in themselves and others. Individuals have varying propensities for developing different states of consciousness; however, most obvious are those who produce behavior that is difficult to overlook, such as fragmentation, frenzy, and narcoleptic sleep.

Generally, people tend to believe what they think, without realizing that what and how they think is strongly affected by their state of consciousness and without realizing that these states are produced by factors that they rarely examine or seek to control. As a result, believing what one thinks is a double-edged sword. On one hand, it may lead to a creative fantasy that can be actualized into productive invention; on the other, it may lead to believing a fantasy that becomes a delusion or a neurotic expectation which is never actualized, leading to unnecessary frustration.

In conclusion, some states of consciousness may have been omitted here due to ignorance of their existence; however, it is clear that other states will become known only through the process observing self and others. Hopefully, as psychiatry becomes more sophisticated, more objective means for describing and measuring the various states of consciousness will be found. Until that time, a metaphoric understanding must suffice.

COMMENTARY

A good physician has to be compassionate. However, to practice psychiatric medicine, you have to keep clear boundaries between yourself and the patient. It doesn't help to get over-involved, because this can make you lose perspective. It doesn't help either to share too much of your private life with them because this blurs boundaries between the patient-doctor relationship. As a result, I've always been a very private person with my patients. I have learned that fortunately, I can be very interpersonal without being personal. Because of this philosophy, this article (as well as "Endurance, Strength, and Coordination Exercises without Cardiovascular or Respiratory Stress," see Chapter 34, which I was working on at the same time) proved very difficult for me to write. Both articles revealed a very personal side of me, exposing some extremely valuable lessons I'd learned in my private life. For one, some form of meditation training is required for martial arts training. It is necessary to develop "internal scanning" and "bare attention," or "mindfulness," because these skills help the mind control the body in ways necessary for performing internal martial arts techniques. The more proficient I became at meditating, the more I became aware of several states of consciousness, and they became more clearly defined and sharpened in my mind. Because I wanted to share my insight with the African-American medical community, I wrote this article. It would later become a foundation for some of my best work.

After I'd identified as many states of consciousness as I could, I realized that whenever I was under stress, I would alter my state of consciousness to manage my tension. Shortly after I wrote this article, I exposed my newly found insight that people cope with stress by changing their states of consciousness in the article "How Blacks Can Overcome 'Combat Fatigue,'" which appeared in the *Chicago Sun Times Views* (November 14, 1981). This article stressed the four basic things people should do to cope with stress. First, they should prepare for stress (this simple idea would later form the foundation for my interest in how various Non-white cultures prepare for stress by cultivating resiliency or resistance). Second, most people should take a break, as this helps in distancing themselves from the stress and gain some perspective on solving the problem and possibly removing the stressor. Third, if it is possible, the source of the stress should be addressed in a constructive manner. I have always found it amazing that many people under stress do things to make their situation worse! Finally, if you cannot change the outside source of the stress, you should work on your perspective about the stress and try to deal with it internally. The interesting thing for me was that each of these stress-coping components involved altering states of consciousness. I then understood that all the various treatments designed to help mentally ill patients were based on techniques to alter state of consciousness.

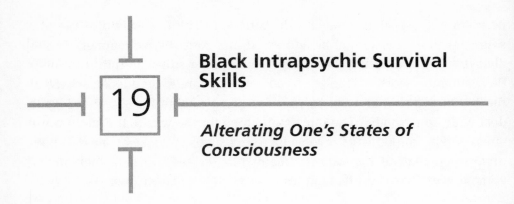

Black Intrapsychic Survival Skills

19

Alterating One's States of Consciousness

Psychiatry tends to be interested only in states of consciousness as they relate to psychopathology. In this paper, the author presents the thesis that the ability to alter one's state of consciousness is a survival skill useful for coping with the physiologic and psychological effects of stress. Furthermore, he discusses techniques indigenous to black culture for altering states of consciousness and gives phenomenologic transcultural evidence that black culture is quite sophisticated in its knowledge and use of intrapsychic survival skills.

INTRODUCTION

In a previous chapter, the present author described 17 states of consciousness[1] (see Chapter 18). It is of interest that Freud in his *Interpretation of Dreams*[2] mentions each of these states of consciousness several times but tends to focus on the *content* of various states (what a person is thinking) as opposed to the *process* (how a person is thinking) or the mechanisms of *altering* the states (why a person is thinking with a cer-

Originally printed as Bell Carl C. Black intrapsychic survival skills: alteration of states of consciousness. *J Natl Med Assoc.* 1982;74:1017–1020. Presented at "Black Survival Skills: Past, Present, and Future," the Fourth Annual Transcultural Seminar of the BPA, Montego Bay, Jamaica, West Indies, November 15, 1981.

tain quality of thought and when this quality of thinking appears). One finds Freud's works focusing on the content of repressed memories and their relation to fragmented states of neurotic patients[3] and to the content of dreams. This is not to imply that Freud did not regularly indulge in exploring methods of altering states of consciousness such as hypnosis, free association, etc.; it seems fair, however, to state that his attention was focused not on the states themselves but on their derivatives. Furthermore, he was preoccupied with psychopathic derivatives and tended to cast aspersions on the validity of states such as internal scanning and expanded states of consciousness. Finally, Freud tended not to focus on the psycho-creative aspects involved in altering one's state of consciousness. Kohut, on the other hand, places great emphasis on introspection[4] (psychological internal scanning). He began his work on narcissism with an observation of states of rapture in a paper about the enjoyment of listening to music.[5] In addition, he emphasizes the vulnerability of narcissistic patients to fall victim to states of frenzy, in which the overpowering emotion is rage.[6] Rarely in psychiatric literature does one find a focus on the qualities of states of consciousness as they relate to human adaptation and survival. Very little attention has been paid to the human ability to navigate between states of consciousness as a means of managing stress. Yet, amongst blacks, this skill is utilized daily to help black people manage stress. This research seeks to outline some sources of stress for blacks and discuss their mastery of stress, and will focus on some methods blacks use in altering their states of consciousness to master their daily stress and avoid "survival fatigue."

SURVIVAL FATIGUE

During World War II, the existence of a "traumatic neurosis" resulting from combat fatigue became well documented. Fenichel[7] gives an excellent definition of this phenomenon as one occurring during a quite stressful life circumstance, in which the ego takes steps to protect the organism from overpowering dysphoric experiences by implementing techniques like fainting, depersonalization, amnesia, or other psychiatric symptoms. While these psychiatric illnesses were generated in a combat setting during war, it is the author's contention that given the stress and chronic trauma blacks face daily while attempting to survive in the inner city, blacks are likely to develop a similar illness, conceptualized as "survival fatigue." This chronic trauma comes to blacks in response to severely burdensome life events producing loss and major threat to integrity and valued goals. Such events are (1) prolonged separation from parents in childhood, (2) experiences of rejection, (3) illness and death of parents, (4) severe illness and injuries throughout life, (5) change of school or residence, (6) loss of job, (7) divorce, (8) complications of pregnancy, and (9) experiences of war or natural disaster. All of these are overwhelmingly represented in an inner-city environment,[8] along with its attendant high death rate, crime, unemployment, illness, and discrimination, as well as its inadequate housing, nutrition,[9] education, and health and mental health care.[10]

We find that often a stressful event is so upsetting that it inhibits an individual's attentiveness, information collecting, relevant memory retrieval, judgment, planning, etc., all of which are skills necessary for actively reducing the stress. In addition, a stressful situation erodes the self-concept. This makes it even more difficult for the stressed individuals to remember who they are and to remember that they have survived other similar situations, a memory that makes one think, "this too shall pass," or "I'll survive." We find that the stressful event often calls for creative, active solutions to seemingly unsolvable problems. Finally, the stressful event reminds one of the need to be prepared for unexpected hardships. This stimulates the need for education and training in generic skills that will enable one to operate more effectively during any situation of frustration and confusion, to which one must respond for survival. Such preparation develops expectations of an increased range of discomforts the individual can tolerate, thus inducing the capacity to persevere—despite one's suffering—in finding a solution to a problem.

MASTERY OF STRESS

Taking this into consideration, Caplan[11] defines mastery of stress as behavior by the individual that (1) results in reducing to tolerable limits physiological and psychological manifestations of emotional arousal during and shortly after the stressful event, and (2) mobilizes the individual's internal and external resources and develops new capabilities in him that lead to changing his environment or his relation to it, so that he reduces the threat or finds alternative sources of satisfaction for what is lost.

Caplan outlines four interrelated facets of an individual's response to a stressful event: (1) behavior that changes the stressful environment or enables the individual to escape from it, (2) behavior to acquire new capabilities for action to change the external circumstances and their aftermath, (3) intrapsychic behavior to defend against dysphoric emotional arousal: anxiety, anger, grief, depression, and excitement and their attendant defenses of denial, selective inattention, isolation, etc., (4) intrapsychic behavior to come to terms with the event and its sequelae by internal readjustment, i.e., grief work. In looking at these facets useful in navigating the mastery of stress, the ability to alter one's consciousness is clearly useful in facets three and four. In facet two, daydreaming, i.e., the preparation for stressful events, is useful. In addition, the behavior in facet one often calls for creative action. The creative act is very much involved in altered states of consciousness, as demonstrated by Koestler's[12] statement: "The creative act, insofar as it depends upon unconscious resources, presupposes a relaxing of the controls and a regression to modes of ideation which are indifferent to the rules of verbal logic...At the decisive stage of discovery the code of disciplined reasoning is suspended." This is often thought of as an incubation process with features of thinking through and imagining solutions that follow the preparation and information gathering of the creative act and which can be accomplished by dream work.

ALTERING STATES OF CONSCIOUSNESS

In more recent psychiatric literature, one finds much more attention being placed on altered states of consciousness and the adaptive functions contained therein. Butts[13] makes it clear that drugs, religion, and sex—three vehicles for altering states of consciousness—are "all valid attempts to gain temporary release from daily living via an excursion into an altered state of consciousness." There has been a great bulk of work investigating psychotherapy, meditation, and states of consciousness,[14] with resultant beliefs that meditation produces relaxation, global desensitization, lowering of cortical and autonomic arousal,[15] and clearer conceptual thinking in both normal and mentally retarded persons.[16]

In looking at blacks' cosmology, one finds that blacks from many different countries have similar beliefs about the structure of their world and have similar techniques for altering their states of consciousness for them to navigate through stress of their intrapsychic, interpersonal, and environmental interactions. Sow, in his *Anthropological Structures of Madness in Black Africa*,[17] notes that persecution has a prominent position in the anthropological system of Africa and as such, colors all of African psychiatry, as it is a socialized, firmly institutionalized intra-community defense. Persecution has as its base a view that the world is composed of three worlds: (1) microcosmos, the immediate perceptible social world; (2) mesocosmos, having genies, spirits, and good and bad forces; (3) the world of ancestors and God, beyond all human senses. It is the mesocosmos (like a nocturnal world with an inexhaustible source of collective imagery; a structured and organized parallel or replica of the microcosmos) where conflicts are transposed, develop, and unfold to yield persecution, thus stimulating one's need to get un-persecuted or un-hexed or un-hoodooed, which requires a healer to heal. One finds such healers in all facets of black culture in the form of root workers,[18] readers, voodoo priests,[19] witches,[20] mojo-ers, spiritualists,[21] conjure doctors, and the two-headed.[22] This healing process involves attaining an altered state of consciousness to aid in survival and mastery of stress. Involving one's self in traditional black cultural healing reduces the dysphoric psychological aspects of stress as well as the physiologic reactions to stress and mobilizes the individual's resources by aiding in collection information, focusing attention, strengthening self-concept, and giving a fresh perspective from which to problem-solve. Healing practitioners provide reassurance and seek to restore confidence while strengthening social bonds. In Africa, the best way to get to the heart of the relationships between man, God, and the world is through mythology. One finds that these myths about the microcosmos, mesocosmos, and the macrocosmos often cause regressive states of consciousness, which are open to the metaphoric wisdom contained in the story. Thus, one learns skills that will enable more effective operation when a calamity strikes.

In keeping with the notion that unnatural acts exist, black folklore understands that there are natural acts that are the work of "all being right in God's world." As a result, one finds that black cultural techniques for altering states of consciousness are an attempt to remain in harmony with one's universe and prevent harm from downfall. In Africa, we find the art of divination by either the interpretation of signs or by possession. This too comprises measures to ensure the correct balance of nature and proper decisions. Christian black culture has a technique of altering one's state of consciousness to an expanded state by letting the spirit of God, in the form of the Holy Ghost, enter and heal the body of all its woes. Griffith describes this method in his exposition of a prayer meeting in which participants sang (a form of breath control and thus meditation), entered trance states, shouted, and testified.[23] Blacks seek to alter their consciousness also through various rhythms such as those from dancing, music, and singing in attempt to gain harmony with their universe. In addition, physical exertion aids in developing internal scanning skills, which allows for greater physiologic control over responses to stress and provides a practice ground for performing under stress and developing skills of concentration. In some instances, it stimulates mental imagery and problem-solving capabilities. This form of altering one's consciousness is found as well in Sufism, the mystical sect of the Moslem religion, and takes the form of dancing and whirling one's body beyond the point of physical exhaustion. It is interesting to note that linkages may exist between the Moslem mystical teachings and the Catholic mysticism that developed and flourished in 16th- and early 17th-century Spain.[24] There are other techniques found in black culture for altering states of consciousness (e.g., masks, drugs, and fasting) not discussed here, as the goal of this paper is not to be an exposition on all techniques used by blacks in altering their states of consciousness to enable them to adapt to life, but rather to point out that blacks do use certain techniques to alter their consciousness to enhance their survival potential.

CONCLUSIONS

It seems that one of life's universal principles is to try and heal whatever ails it, and one method man has developed to aid in his survival is discovering and using techniques to alter states of consciousness. Blacks have historically used altered states of consciousness to (1) help reestablish harmony with their environment, (2) protect themsleves from harmful forces, both spiritual and natural, in their universe, (3) help themselves develop creative solutions for problems they face and alleviate dysphoric effects of stress, thus rendering them better able to eliminate the source of stress, (4) help themselves redirect their life's path toward a more rewarding future. It may not be true that all blacks use traditional black cultural techniques of altering consciousness. Some may in fact borrow consciousness-altering techniques from many other cultures, leading to a more eclectic approach to consciousness, depending on how the individual was acculturated. However, it is true that black people are culturally, historically, and spiritually using altered states of consciousness to better survive their life circumstances.

COMMENTARY

Early insights I had about black intrapsychic survival skills would serve as a theoretical construct from which my work has evolved. This article continues to guide my own coping with stress and my efforts in helping patients who have stress or anxiety disorders. I emphasize that altering these states is key for coping with stress (I suggest this only for normal or anxious patients, not for patients with psychotic disorder, as their grasp on reality is too tenuous). The problem with this coping method is keeping it in the forefront of the mind. When we're under stress, our state of consciousness more often gets altered—perhaps to one negative for the situation we're in—without our realization. This can cause problems. For example, having stress and inducing the state of consciousness of "intoxication" for 30 years isn't very constructive! Clearly, we need to shift from a negative, stress-induced state of consciousness to a positive state of consciousness. If our stress is causing the state of "frenzy" and we seek to alter that state through excess sleeping, we might never address the real-life situation causing our problem. On the other hand, if we respond to the stress by changing our state of consciousness to "hyperalert," we might see a solution to the problem. In order for such states of consciousness techniques to work, we have to practice them repeatedly. Unfortunately, many people don't invest in being proactive.

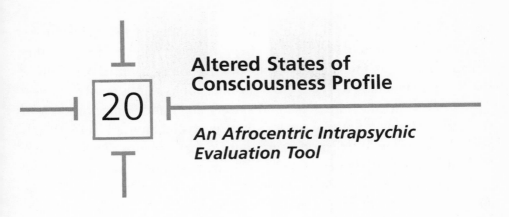

Altered States of Consciousness Profile

An Afrocentric Intrapsychic Evaluation Tool

In an effort to develop an Afrocentric intrapsychic evaluation tool, the CMHC, Inc., Altered States of Consciousness Research Team, developed a structured interview used to quantify and qualify the seventeen states of consciousness[1] that occurred in black control, pre-care, and aftercare subjects. Differences were noted in the three groups as to the incidence, prevalence, and quality of the various states of consciousness. It was also noted that the profile obtained from the interviews yielded a sharp clinical picture of the subjects' total intrapsychic propensities.

INTRODUCTION

While it is important to realize that blacks differ from one another in attitudes, values, folkways, mores, ethnic identity, religious beliefs, diet, language, social class, family history, and other distinguishing characteristics of groups of people,[2] it is also apparent that the ethnic aspects of black American lifestyles show a richness and diversity that is quite different from other ethnic groups in America. One example of how black Americans may differ from other American ethnic groups can be found in

Originally printed as Bell Carl C, Thompson Belinda, Shorter-Gooden Kumea, Mays Raymond, Shakoor Bambade. Altered states of consciousness profile: an Afro-centric intrapsychic evaluation tool. *J Natl Med Assoc.* 1985;77:715–728.

various beliefs and behaviors that form the body of black folk medicine.[3-8] In addition to differences in belief systems about illness, other readily available examples include diet (soul food),[9] music (soul music, blues, jazz),[10] and language.[11] There are clear indications that a number of vestiges of black African culture[12,13] and slavery are found in black American ethnic groups today. Despite the fact that "everyone knows blacks are different" from other American ethnic groups, what constitutes these differences and how they influence the psychiatric evaluation and treatment of blacks has not been rigorously investigated. This paper discusses a model of intrapsychic functioning designed to investigate the uniqueness of blackness and how it differs from characteristics of other American ethnic groups.

BACKGROUND

Blacks have been evaluated with theories and models of the mind and with psychological evaluation tools originally developed by members of other ethnic groups, who did not take into consideration black cultural differences. "The assumption that these theories and psychological requisites are applicable to all groups of people, regardless of ethnic or cultural differences, has not been adequately evaluated or assessed."[14] Based on Freud's clinical observations and treatments of patients from middle-class, white, European, and Jewish backgrounds, many have found his theories of questionable value in treating black American patients. It has been hypothesized that Freud's theories are applicable to other ethnic and cultural groups, but the way in which the theories are applied reduces their functional utility.[14-16]

Recently, psychiatry has been moving away from using psychodynamic theories and models of the mind as the basis of assessment and diagnosis; it has begun to focus instead on descriptive aspects of emotion, thinking, and behavior. In addition, there is a growing database that indicates a lack of an adequate, accurate assessment of the psychiatric disorders of blacks.[14,17-32]

One proposed explanation for the cause of misdiagnosis of black patients is that clinical presentations of black patients are significantly different from those of other ethnic groups. Evidence of this difference is found in the literature, which reports that blacks have a greater frequency of hallucinations and delusions.[13,22,24,33-38]

Moreover, there have been reports that blacks and other ethnic groups have differing symptomatology of depression.[20-23] Jones et al.[39] have proposed that the "precise expression of a particular symptom may assume any of a potential number of allomorphic forms, with the exact selection possibly being influenced by a number of factors, including culture and economics." Spurlock[40] has also discussed how culture may influence the symptoms that black patients present when coming for evaluations. Finally, others have written about the different drinking patterns displayed by blacks[41] and the possible influences these patterns may have on symptom formation in black patients.[42] At the other end of the spectrum are hypotheses that there may be some basic genetic or biologic differences responsible for the speculated differences in how blacks and other ethnic groups exhibit symptoms of the same mental illness.[35]

Related to the possibility that blacks present with significantly different symptoms of mental illnesses is the potential for diagnostic tools standardized on non-black populations to result in a biased test result, causing an inaccurate assessment of the black patient. In the early 1970s, black psychologists began to question the use of existing IQ tests, which they asserted had been culturally biased against blacks and yet were being used to determine a black child's educational placement within the school system.[43,44] Adebimpe[45] points out that the Minnesota Multiphasic Personality Inventory (MMPI), widely used in psychiatric research and practice, is also biased toward blacks, who tend to obtain higher baseline scores on a number of scales, including the schizophrenic scale.

Another proposed explanation for the cause of misdiagnosis of black patients is that the descriptive diagnostic criteria, used in determining the presence or absence of psychiatric disorders, are applicable across ethnic groups, but clinicians may not be consistent when using the criteria to diagnose black patients. This has been documented in several studies.[18-21,29-31,39,46] Pinderhughes[47-49] and others[14,24,28,50] have attributed this lack of consistency to the tendency mental health professionals have in stereotyping the black patient. Adebimpe[24] and others[30,33] have said that part of the problem is the social and cultural distance between the patient and clinician. He cites differences in vocabulary, modes of communication, value systems, the expression of distress, and a breakdown in rapport as factors that increase diagnostic errors. Others assert that racism is in part responsible for the problem because of clinicians' racist attitudes[32] and dynamics of institutional racism.[14,18,19,27,28,40,51–58]

It was hoped with the advent of the *Diagnostic and Statistic Manual* (DSM-III)[59] that bias resulting in misdiagnosis of black patients would decrease. However, DSM-III has problems in that it does not take into account differences in ethnic and cultural patterns, which may cause differences in the epidemiology of certain illnesses. For example, DSM-III descriptions of alcohol-related, organic-brain syndromes report that the typical age of onset of these disorders is about age 35–40 and occurs after ten or more years of heavy drinking. Yet, there is no mention of the fact that while alcoholism is an illness of middle-aged whites, it is an illness of adolescence in blacks[41,60]; therefore, the age of onset of organic-brain syndromes associated with heavy drinking is likely to occur earlier in blacks.[42] Nor is there any mention of black alcoholics having more hallucinations than white alcoholics,[61] which could lead clinicians to possibly misdiagnose black alcoholics with schizophrenia.[24,42] Another example of bias can be found in the DSM-III *Case Book*,[62] in which the one and only clearly identified black patient (out of a total of 214 cases presented) was diagnosed with "adult antisocial behavior." This case was originally used as the jumping-off point of a lengthy discussion on morality, historical and cultural contexts, racism, and conceptual ambiguity.[63] There was very little indication of how much the case had been taken out of its original context.[64]

The likelihood of misdiagnosis of black patients carries with it grave consequences. Once misdiagnosed, the patient may begin a lifetime of mistreatment with varying degrees of iatrogenic consequences, including poor compliance with treatment,[18,19] excessive relapses, correctional institutionalization rather than hospitalization,[29] excessive side effects from somatic treatments, decreased recognition of rehabilitation potential,[42] and demoralization. More significantly, misdiagnosis perpetuates stereotypes and tolerates the provision of inadequate mental health services.[15] Misdiagnosis further provides inaccurate and unreliable epidemiologic data upon which to make incidence and prevalence assumptions and plan the delivery of mental health services.

The remedy to the problem of misdiagnosis is slowly developing as several authors address the issue of trans-ethnic and transcultural psychiatry and address where such knowledge and skills are best placed in the curriculum of psychiatric residency training.[14,65-67] Most psychiatrists have undergone a fairly standardized training curriculum maintaining the basic premises of the dominant culture and omitting curricula significant to trans-ethnic or transcultural psychiatry. This leaves a psychiatric resident (regardless of cultural or ethnic identity) to investigate these areas on his or her own.[14] Some have reported that black psychiatrists are equally prone to misdiagnosing the black patient as psychiatrists from other ethnic groups.[22] However, the propensity for a black psychiatrist to misdiagnose a black patient is a multivariant phenomenon. Certain factors significantly influence the psychiatrist's awareness of factors responsible for the misdiagnosis of blacks: the psychiatrist's ethnic identity, whether trained at a black medical school or not, whether trained alone or with other black psychiatric residents,[53,68] whether training took place under white or black supervisors.

Black psychiatrists are beginning to be more concerned about misdiagnosis, as this issue has appeared increasingly in the literature in the past decades. The BPA, the NMA section on Psychiatry and Behavioral Sciences, the black medical schools, the Center for the Study of Minority Group Mental Health, and others continue to stimulate research in these areas. This results in an impact being made on how accurately black psychiatrists diagnose black patients in comparison to white psychiatrists.[25]

In summary, bias in the assessment of black patients, resulting in misdiagnosis and mistreatment of black patients, stems from the majority of American psychiatry's continued selective inattention to racial, ethnic, and cultural differences, and how these factors affect assessment, diagnosis, and treatment. For these reasons, the authors decided to develop the Altered States of Consciousness Questionnaire, an evaluation tool that would investigate the full parameters of black intrapsychic life. This tool was designed to investigate incidence and prevalence of altered states of consciousness (dreaming, deep sleep, daydreaming, recovery of repressed memory, trance, meditation, internal scanning, regression, fragmentation, intoxication, coma, lethargy, hyperalertness, frenzy, rapture, and expanded states of consciousness) in black subjects. The tool was tested on subjects from the following three groups: controls, those who had never been treated for psychiatric illness; "pre-cares," those who had been treated for psychiatric illness only as outpatients; "aftercares," those who had been treated both as inpatients and outpatients.

This approach was taken by blacks with blacks in mind. One result of this study has been reported in an earlier article (see Chapter 21). The intriguing finding there was that sleep paralysis occurs in blacks at a rate more than twice that in whites.[35] It was further found that 45% of the study cohort had had experience with the state of coma.[69] There is clear evidence that a fresh approach to black intrapsychic dynamics can yield results heretofore unconsidered. The object of this paper is to demonstrate how this approach yields a "states of consciousness profile" for assessing the total range of intrapsychic phenomena that can occur in black individuals, and how this profile can be useful in better evaluating black patients and help them to acquire intrapsychic insight as well.

PROCEDURES

Thirty-six control subjects were selected from the research team's nominations of individuals known to them personally; 36 pre-care and 36 aftercare subjects were taken from volunteers from the CMHC's patient population. During an individual interview, a trained interviewer read to the subjects the definition of each state of consciousness (see glossary at end of chapter) and followed the standardized interview format for each state of consciousness (see Questionnaire).

The first question was designed to ensure that the subjects understood the nature of the state of consciousness being investigated and that their reported experience matched the definition given. Once it was determined that the subject had experienced the state, the subsequent questions were designed to determine the quality and quantity of these altered states of consciousness. The interviews were audio taped and reviewed by the principal investigator to check for consistency in the interviewing technique and the validity of the subjects' reports.

QUESTIONNAIRE. States of Consciousness Interview Schedule

Read brief description of _____ (insert state of consciousness).
   1. Have you ever experienced _____ (insert state of consciousness)?
      ( ) Yes: Tell me about it:
      ( ) No: Do you know anyone who has ever experienced _____ (insert state of consciousness)?
         ( ) Yes: Tell me about their experience.
         ( ) No: Go on to the next state of consciousness.
   2. Are you able to bring this state on by yourself? ( ) No ( ) Yes: How?
   3. Can other people or situations bring on this state in you? ( ) No ( ) Yes: How?
   4. Are you able to bring yourself out of this state? ( ) No ( ) Yes: How?
   5. Can other people or situations bring you out of this state? ( ) No ( ) Yes: How?
   6. Do you feel that you have control over this state? ( ) No ( ) Yes
   7. Would you like to experience _____ (insert state of consciousness) more often?
      ( ) Yes: Why?
      ( ) No: Why not?
I'm going to ask you some questions concerning how many times you have had states of _____ (insert state of consciousness) and approximately how long each state lasts.
   8. In general, do you experience _____ (insert state of consciousness)
      ( ) never ( ) rarely ( ) occasionally ( ) frequently ( ) always?
   9. What is the shortest amount of time that this state has lasted?
  10. What is the greatest amount of time that this state has lasted?
  11. How long does the average experience last?
  12. On the average, how often do you experience _____ (insert state of consciousness)? _____ (insert number/time. Example: twice a day, once weekly, once monthly, once yearly, once in my life)
I have a few more questions about _____ (insert state of consciousness).
  13. Are you usually comfortable or uncomfortable when you are in this state? Explain.
  14. Has this state ever caused you any difficulties or gotten you into trouble?
      ( ) No ( ) Yes: How?
  15. Does this state of consciousness help you cope? ( ) No ( ) Yes: How?
  16. Has your experience of this state of consciousness changed with age?
      ( ) No ( ) Yes: How?

RESULTS

Table 1 reveals that there were differences in the reported incidence of various states of consciousness among control, pre-care, and aftercare subjects. A closer look at sleep paralysis (see Chapter 22), intoxication, and coma (see Chapter 24) were reported earlier.[35,42,69] A profile was developed in order to produce an overview of the reported incidence and prevalence of the states of consciousness in each subject. Incidence rates were determined from responses to Question 1 on the states of consciousness interview schedule, which asked if the subject had experienced the state of consciousness being asked about. Prevalence rates were based on responses to interview Question 12, which asked the frequency of experiencing the state. Examples of three control, pre-care, and aftercare profiles are to be found in Figures 2 through 10.

TABLE 20.1. Incidence of Altered States of Consciousness

	Control No. (%)	Pre-care No. (%)	Aftercare No. (%)	Total No. (%)
Dreaming	36 (100)	36 (100)	35 (100)	108 (100)
Sleeping	30 (83)	30 (83)	29 (81)	89 (82)
Sleep paralysis	14 (39)	18 (50)	12 (33)	44 (41)
Hyperalert	32 (89)	31 (86)	31 (86)	94 (87)
Lethargic	32 (89)	32 (89)	34 (94)	98 (91)
Rapture	34 (94)	31 (86)	29 (81)	94 (87)
Frenzy	31 (86)	33 (94)	30 (83)	94 (87)
Fragmentation	2 (6)	10 (28)	30 (83)	42 (39)
Regressive	16 (44)	22 (61)	26 (72)	64 (59)
Meditative	28 (78)	19 (53)	23 (64)	70 (65)
Trance	11 (31)	6 (7)	5 (14)	22 (20)
Daydreaming	36 (100)	36 (100)	33 (94)	105 (98)
Internal scanning	32 (89)	31 (86)	31 (86)	94 (87)
Coma	19 (53)	26 (72)	23 (64)	68 (63)
Intoxication	32 (89)	34 (94)	35 (97)	101 (94)
Recovery of repressed memory	2 (6)	5 (14)	6 (17)	13 (12)
Expanded consciousness	14 (39)	5 (14)	8 (22)	27 (25)

DISCUSSION

All of the population had experienced states of dreaming, and most of them (over 80%) reported some recognition of having had deep sleep. Forty-one percent of the population reported having had sleep paralysis; chi-square analysis demonstrated that there was no significant difference among the three groups when the incidence and the prevalence of sleep paralysis were considered[35] (see Chapter 21). The incidence of hyperalert states that occurred in the three subject groups was not significantly different (all were between 85% and 90%); however, in considering how often each group reported hyperalert states, the use of chi-square analysis revealed that the groups were found to be different (significant at the 0.01 level).[70]

Approximately 90% of the three subject groups reported personal experience with lethargic states of consciousness. The control population reported the greatest incidence of states of rapture, and the aftercare subjects reported the least. This will be subjected to further scrutiny, as it may indicate that the use of rapture is a coping strategy. The absence of rapture in the seriously mentally ill may indicate an intervention point for treatment. It was found that the control, pre-care, and aftercare populations demonstrated a difference in the prevalence and the incidence of states of frenzy when examined by chi-square analysis (significant at the 0.05 level).[70]

As expected, the aftercare subjects reported the greater incidence of fragmentation (83%), while the pre-care and control subjects only reported states of fragmentation occasionally and rarely (28% and 6%, respectively). Three subjects in the pre-care population were psychotic but had never been severely ill enough to warrant hospitalization. In addition, there were pre-care subjects who, on occasion, had extreme amounts of stress that caused them to temporarily fragment; such reports raised the incidence of fragmentation in the pre-care group.

Incidence of regression, like that of fragmentation, was found to increase with the severity of the subject group's psychiatric condition (i.e., controls had the lowest incidence, aftercares had the highest incidence of regression, and pre-cares were in the middle). The controls described using regression as a restorative function that was temporary; the aftercare subjects talked about the inability to function properly with no expectations of immediate restoration; and the pre-care subjects reported regression in connection with dependency.

The control population reported an incidence of meditative states at 78%. This was higher than the pre-care population's report of 53%, even though the pre-care population used relaxation techniques taught at CMHC to help them to learn to relax. There is some evidence that the aftercare subjects' report on meditative states was based on the cognitive slippage these patients experienced due to their psychotic experiences, and it was felt this accounted for a "decrease in mental responsiveness" by this group.

In view of the phenomenon of "getting the Holy Ghost" found in black churches,[71] there was some surprise that there was not a greater incidence of trance in this population. The control subjects reported trance states twice as often as did the pre-care or aftercare patients. The significance of this has not yet been evaluated. It was found that all of the control and pre-care groups reported experiencing daydreaming, but not all aftercare subjects reported daydream; this is consistent with previous reports on fantasy in nonpsychotic vs. psychotic patients.[72]

Most of the subjects (86%) were able to "get in touch" with their bodily processes by using internal scanning, which indicates the possible utility of this state to help various kinds of patients learn relaxation techniques to calm their psychophysiologic anxiety processes.

More than half of each subject group reported having experienced a coma (coma induced by surgical anesthetics and other factors were counted in this report). Only two subjects reported stupor (not represented in Table 2). A more detailed analysis of this state of consciousness is reported elsewhere,[69] but it is important to note that 45.5% of the total population reported experiencing a coma unrelated to surgery.

The interview on intoxication revealed that the vast majority of the study population had experienced this state; chi-square analysis revealed there was no significant difference regarding prevalence among the three subject groups. Excessive drinking patterns are a serious problem in the black community and may be related to the reason blacks report more hallucinations[42] and sleep paralysis.[35]

The recovery of repressed memory was highest in the aftercare population. It seems that the state of fragmentation these patients experienced weakened psychic defenses that had kept certain memories repressed. The reports of the pre-care population regarding recovery of repressed memory were in the context of psychotherapy, and the reports of the control subjects were associated with practices of meditation and the experience of expanded states of consciousness. It is apparent that the controls engaged in more meditative states that were reported useful to them in coping with stress, and through this practice, they experienced the expanded state. The aftercare population reports on this state of consciousness were contaminated with content related to psychotic delusions. More work regarding the incidence, prevalence, quality, and coping usefulness of the states of consciousness will be investigated in later reports.

CASE REPORTS

Figures 1 through 9 give a clear picture of selected individuals' intrapsychic experiences using the states of consciousness profile. Figure 1 illustrates a control subject who regularly experiences dreaming and deep sleep but who has never had sleep paralysis. This individual reported daily meditation, internal scanning, and daydreaming associated with the reports of expanded consciousness, the recovery of repressed memories, and rare incidences of intoxication. The subject denied ever having been in a coma, trance, or a state of fragmentation. States of frenzy and regression

FIGURE 20.1. States of Consciousness for Control Group, Subject 1

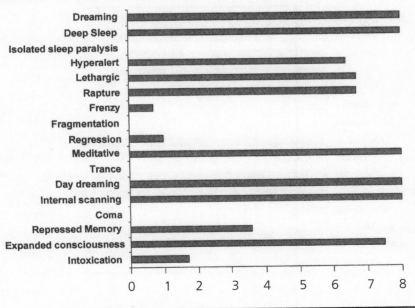

0 = None
1 = Twice in a lifetime
2 = Six times in a lifetime
3 = Once every three years
4 = Once a year

5 = Once every six months
6 = Once a month
7 = Once a week
8 = Daily

were reported to have occurred rarely, and the subject experienced states of being enraptured, lethargic, and hyperalert more than once a month.

Figure 2 illustrates another control who has similar sleeping patterns, but with less deep sleep (at least once a week). Another similarity is the prevalence of meditative states, internal scanning, and daydreaming. This subject, however, had not yet experienced expanded consciousness or recovery of repressed memories as a result of her practices, but her prevalence of intoxication was only once every two years. There was one episode of coma from surgery and no reports of sleep paralysis, frenzy, fragmentation, regression, or trance. This subject experienced hyperalert, lethargic, and enraptured states about once a month.

The third control, a student in a demanding graduate program, reported daily dreaming and deep sleep (Figure 3). Earlier in his life, he

FIGURE 20.2. States of Consciousness for Control Group, Subject 2

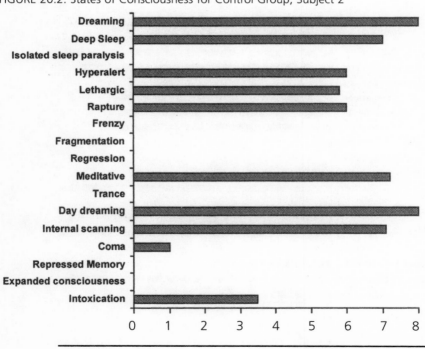

0 = None
1 = Twice in a lifetime
2 = Six times in a lifetime
3 = Once every three years
4 = Once a year

5 = Once every six months
6 = Once a month
7 = Once a week
8 = Daily

had two episodes of sleep paralysis. The reported states of frenzy, regression, and intoxication were associated with the waxing and waning of taking tests important to staying in school. This subject reported trance states to be related to intense concentration while studying, often to the exclusion of external stimuli. There were no reports of meditation, fragmentation, recovery of repressed memory, or expanded consciousness. The subject reported one incident of surgery. Hyperalert, lethargic, and enraptured states were reported similar to the reported incidence in the other two control subjects.

Figure 4 illustrates the profile of a pre-care subject who reported nightly dreaming and daily daydreaming with an active fantasy life that often resulted in the patient falling into a "hypnoid state." The contents of these states were analyzed, with the subsequent recovery of two repressed

FIGURE 20.3. States of Consciousness for Control Group, Subject 3

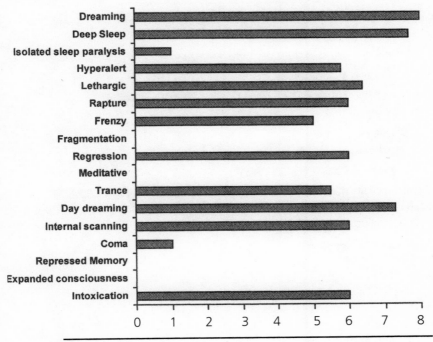

0 = None
1 = Twice in a lifetime
2 = Six times in a lifetime
3 = Once every three years
4 = Once a year

5 = Once every six months
6 = Once a month
7 = Once a week
8 = Daily

memories instrumental in reducing the patient's frequency of states of frenzy to about once weekly and in decreased intensity from the patient's initial treatment. The subject reported one episode of coma due to a head injury during childhood; it lasted only for a few minutes. The subject reported several episodes of surgery. There were no reports of sleep paralysis, fragmentation, regression, meditation, internal scanning, expanded consciousness, or intoxication and reported only rare episodes of rapture. This makes for interesting speculation on possible therapeutic effects, should the patient consciously alter some of these states of consciousness. This subject reported only occasional hyperalert and lethargic states, a further indication of limited flexibility in altering his states of consciousness.

FIGURE 20.4. States of Consciousness for Pre-care Group, Subject 1

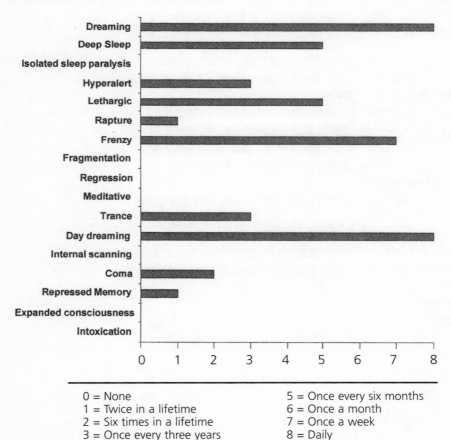

0 = None
1 = Twice in a lifetime
2 = Six times in a lifetime
3 = Once every three years
4 = Once a year

5 = Once every six months
6 = Once a month
7 = Once a week
8 = Daily

The possibility remains that increasing his capacity to alter his state of consciousness might also increase his coping skills.

The pre-care profile in Figure 5 reveals an individual who dreams nightly, who is aware of a deep sleep about once a week, and for whom sleep paralysis occurs once every three months. This patient reported daily states of being hyperalert and had frenzy once a week that was primarily due to agoraphobia and panic attacks. This patient was treated with tricyclic antidepressants, and was given meditation and internal scanning exercises to help him reduce stress. Guided visual imagery (structured daydreaming) was also used to help desensitize him to frightening situations. Through this process of treatment, the recovery of repressed memories occurred that were related to the psychotraumatic experiences at the root of his disorder. The patient denied having states of fragmentation,

FIGURE 20.5. States of Consciousness for Pre-care Group, Subject 2

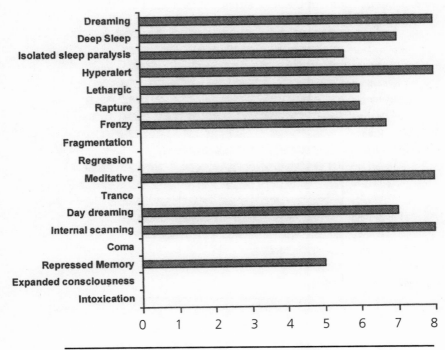

0 = None
1 = Twice in a lifetime
2 = Six times in a lifetime
3 = Once every three years
4 = Once a year
5 = Once every six months
6 = Once a month
7 = Once a week
8 = Daily

regression, coma, trance, intoxication, or expanded consciousness, but reported monthly states of rapture and lethargy.

The final example of a pre-care intrapsychic profile reveals an individual in severe neurotic distress (Figure 6). The patient reported deep sleep and sleep paralysis only once a month, raising the question of whether sleep paralysis and deep sleep may be inversely related (i.e., the less deep sleep an individual gets, the more likely he or she will be to having sleep paralysis). This is a likely possibility, as it seems that sleep paralysis is related to rapid-eye-movement sleep,[35] which is at the opposite end of the spectrum from deep sleep. The patient also reported hyperalert states and intoxication once a week, which may also contribute to the prevalence of the sleep paralysis and lack of deep sleep. This subject also reported fragmentation in the form of being so overwhelmed from stress

FIGURE 20.6. States of Consciousness for Pre-care Group, Subject 3

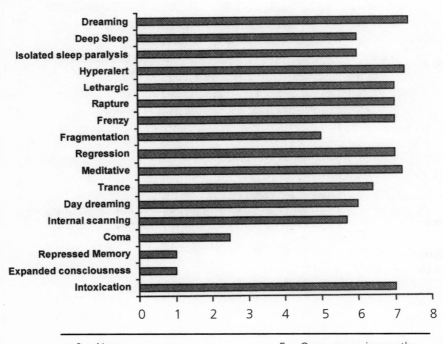

0 = None
1 = Twice in a lifetime
2 = Six times in a lifetime
3 = Once every three years
4 = Once a year
5 = Once every six months
6 = Once a month
7 = Once a week
8 = Daily

that she subjectively experienced a loss of contact from reality; her week-ly regression and lethargic states were related to these episodes of being overwhelmed. The patient had attempted to use meditation, hypnosis, day-dreaming (with the aid of guided imagery), and internal scanning to try to gain control of her severe anxiety disorder. She reported one brief coma due to trauma during childhood and several episodes of surgery. The rare recovery of repressed memories and an expanded consciousness were related to the meditative experience. It is to be hoped that continued prac-tice in altering her state of consciousness will give this subject more intrapsychic control over her condition.

The aftercare patient represented by Figure 7 had an intrapsychic profile that indicated having experienced dreaming but having little recog-nition of deep sleep. This is most likely related to the six episodes of frag-mentation the patient reported, as sleeping disorders are frequent compo-

FIGURE 20.7. States of Consciousness for Aftercare Group, Subject 1

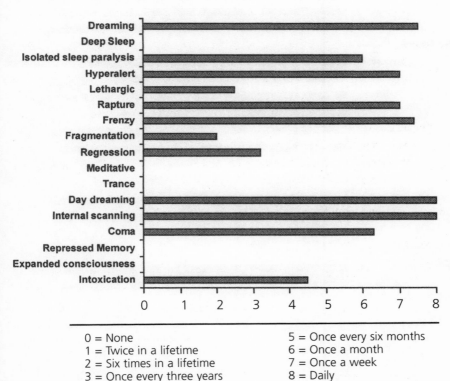

0 = None
1 = Twice in a lifetime
2 = Six times in a lifetime
3 = Once every three years
4 = Once a year

5 = Once every six months
6 = Once a month
7 = Once a week
8 = Daily

nents of psychotic states. This is also true of the regression the patient reported, and these episodes were associated with the patient's "nervous breakdowns." The daily daydreaming was related to the subject's efforts to "tune people out" if they bothered her. Her daily internal scanning was related to somatic preoccupations. The patient reported a lack of deep sleep, as well as monthly sleep paralysis and weekly states of being hyper-alert, enraptured, and frenzied, indicating a possible connection among these states as well. The state of intoxication was reported to have been induced to obtain better sleep. The subject reported one episode of trau-matic coma from a train accident and six episodes of surgery; there were no reports of meditation, trance, recovery of repressed memory, or expand-ed consciousness.

FIGURE 20.8. States of Consciousness for Aftercare Group, Subject 2

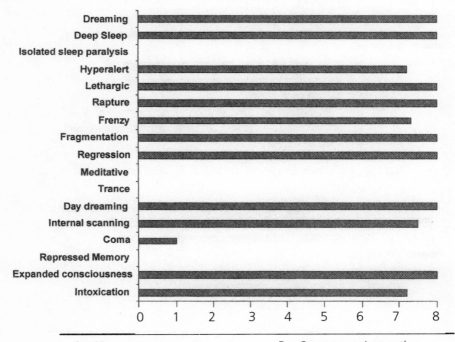

0 = None
1 = Twice in a lifetime
2 = Six times in a lifetime
3 = Once every three years
4 = Once a year

5 = Once every six months
6 = Once a month
7 = Once a week
8 = Daily

The aftercare patient represented in Figure 8 reported daily dreaming, deep sleep, lethargic states, enraptured states, fragmentation, regression, daydreaming, and expanded states of consciousness. In fact, the subject was fragmented when interviewed, which caused him to interpret his intrapsychic milieu in a very loose and incoherent fashion. His report regarding his expanded state of consciousness had a delusional content of a religious nature. He denied sleep paralysis, meditation, trance, and recovery of repressed memory, and he reported two episodes of surgery. The weekly intoxication was induced to help the patient relax and to "stop the voices"; the frequent frenzy and hyperalert states were also related to his current psychotic state.

The profile of the final aftercare patient (see Figure 9) reveals a similar lack of deep sleep that was present in Figure 8, but this subject denied

FIGURE 20.9. States of Consciousness for Aftercare Group, Subject 3

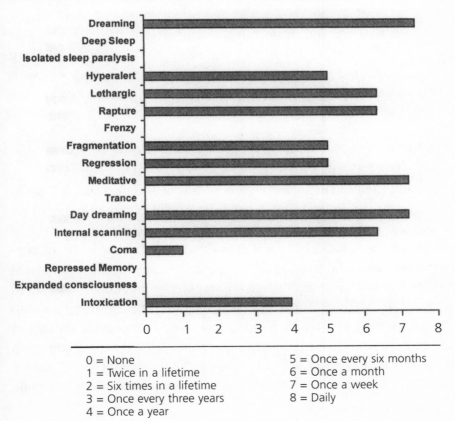

0 = None
1 = Twice in a lifetime
2 = Six times in a lifetime
3 = Once every three years
4 = Once a year

5 = Once every six months
6 = Once a month
7 = Once a week
8 = Daily

having sleep paralysis. The subject also denied frenzy, trance, recovery of repressed memory, and expanded consciousness. The patient reported a childhood incident of coma that lasted for more than 30 minutes after being hit by a car. The reports of fragmentation and regression that occurred twice a year were associated, and the twice-weekly episodes of meditation and daydreaming were induced to "take troubles off of my mind." There were reports of states of lethargy, rapture, and internal scanning about once a month, which were also used to relieve the patient from thinking about her problems. This patient reported intoxication once a year (Figure 9).

From the examination of the altered states of consciousness profile on each of these nine subjects (three each from the control, pre-care, and aftercare groups), it is apparent that the profile gives a clear indication of the subjects' intrapsychic milieu. Further, the process used to develop the profile yielded a helpful approach to the intrapsychic dynamics of black patients, as it gives a comprehensive view of the subjects' intrapsychic capacities in a way different from the standard psychiatric mental status examination. As a result, discoveries regarding high incidence of sleep paralysis and coma experienced by black populations were made,[5,69] with indications that this approach may be useful in investigating other aspects of black life.[42,70]

CONCLUSIONS

The examination of states of consciousness as a research vehicle to explore the intrapsychic life of black subjects has been shown to be a useful methodology because it has revealed several previously uninvestigated intrapsychic phenomena in blacks. It is felt that by using the states of consciousness interview and making a states of conscious profile, one is able to get a clear picture of an individual's intrapsychic functions. The states of consciousness approach is useful in teaching subjects a vocabulary with which to understand how stressful situations affect intrapsychic status and how altering states of consciousness may be helpful in coping with stress.[73] Participation in the states of consciousness interview encourages subjects to further engage in that introspection so vital to healthy, adequate functioning.

GLOSSARY: ALTERED STATES OF CONSCIOUSNESS

Dreaming. A state of consciousness that occurs periodically during the night while one is asleep. It is characterized by visual images, which may or may not be felt to represent a story. Dreams may be experienced as nightmares or pleasant experiences. Most people can remember their dreams if they pay attention.

Stupor and Coma. These two states involve a limited ability to perceive incoming stimuli. In stupor there is a clouding of the awake state, and the levels of alertness and arousability are low. In coma there is a total inability to perceive incoming stimuli. Coma is commonly known as being unconscious.

Daydreaming. Also known as engaging in fantasy, this state of consciousness occurs while awake and is characterized by an imagined mental picture or rapidly occurring thoughts that have little to do with what is going on at the time. Usually while daydreaming, the person has only a vague awareness of what is going on around him.

Meditative States. These states are characterized by lowered mental activity with a relaxed, calm feeling. There is a decrease in mental responsiveness. It is also known as "bare attention" or "mindfulness." There are many ways to induce a state of meditation.

Deep Sleep. A state of consciousness that occurs periodically during the night while one is asleep. Most people are not aware of themselves while in deep sleep but recognize the absence of deep sleep when they miss it at night. Usually missing deep sleep is felt as getting sleep that was not very restful or that was very light. Another characteristic of deep sleep is difficulty being awakened or aroused while in this state.

Lethargic States. These states of consciousness are characterized by dulled, sluggish, and slowed thinking. They may be experienced as mental fatigue or mental exhaustion. It is commonly referred to as the "blahs."

States of Frenzy. These states are characterized by negative emotional storms that the individual experiences as an overpowering and unpleasant emotion. The overpowering emotion may be experienced as rage, panic, fear, anxiety, and terror. The behavior is erratic and frantic, but the person does not "lose touch" with what is happening.

States of Fragmentation. There are several types of fragmentation, all of which show a lack of balance between important aspects of thinking, feeling, or personality. Accompanying this lack of balance may be hallucinations (seeing or hearing things that are not there), confused and incoherent thinking, and the inability to know what is real and what is not real.

Trance States. These states are characterized by the attention being focused on a single object or idea, by intense mental activity and concentration, and by alertness. Following trance states, there is no recollection of what occurred. A common example occurs in black churches where people "get the Holy Ghost," after which they have no recollection of what they did. A less obvious example is people becoming so engaged in and heavily concentrated on a single activity that time slips by extremely quickly but unnoticed. The most common example of a trance state is hypnosis. Trances are induced by activities that require attention but little variation in response.

Regressive States. Regression occurs when the individual's thinking processes resemble earlier styles of thinking that are age-inappropriate to the individual's present circumstances. It is often temporary. A common example of regression occurs when some people get ill and demand to be taken care of as though they were helpless infants. Another common example is adults playing with or relating to children, on the children's level.

Hyperalert States. These states are characterized by crisp thinking, alertness, and awareness. They are experienced as one being really "on top of things" and being "really hot." Thoughts may be accelerated and very sharp. Inability to slow down may also be experienced.

Intoxication. A state of consciousness in which one's coordination or speech is impaired. Drunkenness and the drug "high" are examples.

Sleep Paralysis. This state is experienced either while falling asleep or waking up from sleep. It is characterized by an experience of waking up or falling asleep and being unable to move for several seconds or minutes. Often people see or hear things that are not really there. For example, one may hear someone breaking into the house, or see someone standing over the bed, but despite this sense of danger, the individual is unable to move or respond. After this state of consciousness passes, the individual often sits up with a start and has feelings of anxiety, only to realize that perceptions of danger were false. An old Southern expression is that when people are in this state, "a witch is riding them."

Internal Scanning. This state involves a focused awareness of how the body feels. Through this state of consciousness, most individuals are able to get in touch with the feelings from their bodies. Usually, the process of "selective inattention" makes one unaware of such sensations. However, when feelings from the body are intensified through hunger or increased heart rate, one may become automatically involved in internal scanning.

Repressed Memory. A repressed memory refers to a past experience that is not easily remembered. It may prompt behaviors that are not easily explained or understood. Once a repressed memory is recovered (i.e., remembered), persons may gain greater awareness of themselves and their behavior. One such example could be seen in a person with an extreme dislike for strawberry soda pop, who does not remember the reason for such a strong dislike. One day while discussing an unpleasant childhood experience of being beaten up by the school bully, the person remembers that the bully threw strawberry soda pop on him and made him drink some after he beat him up—a memory the individual had not had in years. With the recovery of the repressed memory, he is able to enjoy strawberry soda pop.

States of Rapture. These states are characterized by positive emotional storms, which the individual experiences as an overpowering and pleasant emotion. The overpowering emotion may be experienced as euphoria or elation.

Expanded States of Consciousness. During such states, there is a change in the way the individual thinks and feels about space, time, or her body. There is also a feeling and understanding of being a part of something bigger than one's self, a sense of being in tune with the universe. There are additional experiences of "seeing the light," moral purity, loss of fear of death, sense of immortality, revelation, and a loss of feelings of sin. When others meet a person in an expanded state of consciousness, they often sense the person is manifesting something quite different from an ordinary state of consciousness.

COMMENTARY

I've always wanted to devise a true African-American-centered psychology. In many ways, the states of consciousness model qualifies. The model of altering states of consciousness to cope with stress was appropriate for the African-American experience. Although it was far from original, the states of consciousness approach sprang from my own personal experience, and as such, I thought it might qualify. When I became the medical director of the CMHC, I made sure I would get some time to pursue my research interests in African-American mental health issues. I worked with the CMHC research team, and the Altered States of Consciousness Questionnaire was born. The Altered States of Consciousness Profile led us to some very important original observations of African-American mental life. We published a series of articles on "isolated sleep paralysis" (originally called "hypnopomic and hypnogogic hallucinations" in the "States of Consciousness" article—see Chapter 18). We also published a paper, "The Prevalence of Coma in Black Subjects" (see Chapter 24). To date, this approach has led to the biggest discovery about African-American mental health I've made.

To have greater value, the Afrocentric intrapsychic evaluation tool we developed needed much more refinement. Unfortunately, we have never had enough resources to do so. Instead, we pursued the heuristic lessons we learned from our exploration of African Americans' states of consciousness—we used our scant resources to study isolated sleep paralysis and coma in African Americans. I hope that science will one day be better developed for qualifying and quantifying the various states of consciousness. When that happens, I plan to revisit our model and work at further refining it, since I still think it could be a very useful way of exploring the mental life of African Americans.

As my work has begun to focus more on African-American strengths rather than deficits, I've found that this earlier work on states of consciousness forms a firm foundation for my theories on how individuals cultivate resiliency or, as Dr. Chester Pierce would say, "resistance." Based on my experience, I've found that there were two types of people when confronted with trauma: those who play funeral music deep inside and those who play adventure music. In 2002 during the 9/11 symposium of the Carter Center's Mental Health Program, who I'd been working with for a few years, I had the opportunity to interact with the former mayor of New York. As he talked about his response to the terrorist attack, I pointed out to him my observation about "trauma music." I asked him which did he have. He knew exactly what I was talking about, because he responded with the name of an Italian opera. I wasn't familiar with it, but the opera clearly represented adventure music for this man of Italian heritage. A Latino woman I met during the symposium noted that her music was African drums and Spanish guitar. She underscored the point that the music in each of us is culture-bound. I completely agreed. Much of my "trauma music" is black gospel and always underscores that "joy comes in the morning." It's clear to see, then, that if a healer is not culturally sensitive, for example, and suggests that an African American listen to Italian opera to be strengthened against adversity, this healer might have a disconnect and accordingly might not be very effective in that situation.

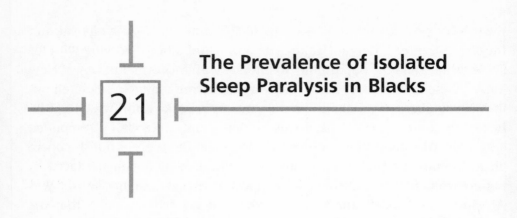

The Prevalence of Isolated Sleep Paralysis in Blacks

21

Sleep paralysis is a state of consciousness experienced while waking from sleep or falling asleep. It is characterized by an experience of being unable to move for several seconds or minutes. This study represents the first survey to measure the incidence of this disorder in a black population of healthy subjects and psychiatric patients.

INTRODUCTION

Sleep paralysis has been described as an unusual neurologic phenomenon and is normally considered a component of the narcolepsy tetrad (sleep attacks, cataplexy, sleep paralysis, and hypnogenic hallucinations).[1] Sleep paralysis is a state of consciousness experienced either while waking up or falling asleep, characterized by feeling unable to move for several seconds or minutes. The individual who experiences this state has full awareness during the episode and has complete recall of it. Vivid and terrifying hallucinations often accompany this state of consciousness, and a sense of acute danger may be felt. Once the episode passes, the individual

Originally printed as Bell Carl C, Shakoor Bambade, Thompson Belinda, Dew Donald, Hughley Eugene, Mays Raymond, Shorter-Gooden Kumea. The prevalence of isolated sleep paralysis in blacks. *J Natl Med Assoc.* 1984;76:501–508.

often sits up with a start and experiences symptoms of anxiety (e.g., tachycardia, hyperventilation, fear), only to realize that the perceptions of danger were false.

The first definite case of sleep paralysis was reported by Binns in describing a patient's "daymare."[3] Cases were next reported in 1876 by Mitchell[4,5] who referred to his patients' experiences as "nocturnal hemiplegia," "night palsy," "nocturnal paralysis," and "sleep numbness." In *Interpretation of Dreams*,[2] Freud mentions hypnagogic hallucinations, citing Johannes Muller's 1826 term for this experience, "imaginative visual phenomena." It is not clear, however, that Muller's phenomena occurred in conjunction with sleep paralysis. Other authors have called this state of consciousness "delayed psychomotor awakening"[6] or "cataplexy of awakening,"[7,8] "postdormital chalastic fits,"[9] "hypnapompic or hypnagogic hallucinations,"[10] and "predormital or hypnagogic sleep paralysis and postdormital or hypnapompic sleep paralysis."[11] Wilson[12] in 1925 was first to call the phenomenon "sleep paralysis," which has become the most accepted term for this state of consciousness. He noted that it was a "transient physiologic disorder, a physiological cataplexy."[12]

The great majority of incidences of sleep paralysis have been associated with narcolepsy. Sleep paralysis in patients with narcolepsy has been reported at 24% by Yoss and Daly,[13] 8% by Levin,[14] and 18% by Goode.[15] However, there has been increasing recognition that sleep paralysis occurs as an isolated entity and not in association with narcolepsy or cataplexy.[12,16–18] Schneck reports 14 such cases in his extensive writing on the subject.[19–22]

Two studies were done to ascertain the incidence of sleep paralysis in a generally healthy population. Goode[15] found that the incidence of sleep paralysis in four studied populations (163 medical students, 68 junior and senior medical students 53 nursing students, and 75 hospital private inpatients—67 medical and 8 open-ward psychiatric) was 6.1%, 7.8%, 0%, and 2.7%, respectively. Out of an 80% male total population of 359 individuals, 17 (4.7%) experienced sleep paralysis, with one reporting narcolepsy. Of these 17 subjects, five had experienced sleep paralysis only once, eight had had less than six episodes per year, and four had had approximately one episode each month. Everett[23] studied a first-year class of 52 medical students and found that 7 of the 47 men and 1 of the 5 women reported having had isolated sleep paralysis (a total of 15.4%).

Finally, there was a report about two families that had a severe form of isolated sleep paralysis.[24] In one family, 14 persons over four generations had suffered from sleep paralysis, and in the second, four persons over three generations had been affected. This finding supports the heredofamilial trend that Goode[15] noted in some of the subjects he studied.

In the majority of case histories reported and in both surveys referenced here, the issue of ethnicity was not addressed. Considering that the surveys focused on the early 1960s medical and nursing students at Duke Medical School and School of Nursing, the University of Oklahoma Medical School, and the Johns Hopkins School of Medicine, it is likely that the two populations surveyed were predominately white.

The present study is the first to measure the incidence of isolated sleep paralysis in a black population of generally healthy subjects and psychiatric patients.

METHODS

In response to the lack of basic research on the psychodynamics of black populations, CMHC began a research project to qualify and quantify the states of consciousness experienced by blacks. The three groups studied were black control subjects who had never suffered a mental illness; black pre-care patients who had been treated for a mental illness only as outpatients; and black aftercare patients who had received both inpatient and outpatient treatment for mental illness. The research team selected its control subjects based on nominations of individuals known to them personally. The pre-care and aftercare subjects were chosen from CMHC patients who volunteered to participate in the study. Thirty-six individuals in each of the three groups were studied. Out of the total population of 108 subjects, 52 were men and 56 were women.

A structured interview was designed in which a trained interviewer read the definition of sleep paralysis to the research subjects. Next, the subjects were asked to decide if they had experienced this state of consciousness and if so, tell the interviewer about it. Subjects who had not experienced sleep paralysis were asked if they had heard of it or known someone who had experienced it. This part of the questionnaire was designed to ensure that the subjects understood the nature of sleep paralysis. Once it was established that the subject had experienced the defined state, a standard series of questions was asked to determine whether this state could be self-induced or self-terminated, induced or terminated by others, or whether the subject had any control over the state of isolated sleep paralysis. Subjects were asked if they wanted to experience this state more often and to explain why they did or did not wish to do so. They were asked about the frequency and duration of the state. Subjects were asked to explain why this state made them either comfortable or uncomfortable; to explain if it ever got them into trouble or difficulty; and to explain if it ever helped them to cope. Finally, they were asked whether this state of consciousness had changed with age, and if so, how. The subjects were also asked about their experience with dreaming, deep sleep, daydreaming, repressed memory, trance, meditation, internal scanning, regression, fragmentation, coma, stupor, intoxication, lethargy, hyperalertness, frenzy, rapture, and expanded states of consciousness.[10]

The interviews were audio taped and reviewed by the principal investigator to check for consistency in the interviewing technique and in the validity of the subjects' reports. In addition to the structured interview about states of consciousness, subjects were given the following objective written tests: Holmes-Rahe Social Readjustment Scale, Saafir Stress-Anxiety Diagnostic Scale, Millon Clinical Multiaxial Inventory (MCMI). The data was tabulated and certain correlations became evident.

RESULTS

It was discovered that out of the total population of 108 black subjects (52 males and 56 females), 44 (41.0%) had experienced at least one episode of isolated sleep paralysis. This group was composed of 14 (39.0%) of the 36 controls, 18 (50.0%) of the 36 pre-care subjects, and 12 (33.3%) of the 36 aftercare subjects (see Table 1). Of the 44 subjects who had experienced sleep paralysis, 18 (40.9%) were male and 26 (59.1%) were female. Isolated sleep paralysis had been experienced by 34.6% of the total male population and by 46.4% of the total female population.

TABLE 21.1. Episodes of Sleep Paralysis

	Control (%)	Pre-care (%)	Aftercare (%)	Total (%)
None	22 (61.1)	18(50.0)	24 (66.7)	64 (59.3)
Less than one yearly	7 (19.4)	4 (11.1)	6 (16.7)	17 (15.7)
One or more yearly	5 (13.9)	8 (22.2)	2 (5.6)	15 (13.9)
One or more monthly	2 (5.6)	4 (11.1)	2 (5.6)	8 (7.4)
One or more weekly	0 (0.0)	2 (5.6)	2 (5.6)	4 (3.7)
Total	36 (100)	36 (100)	36 (100)	108 (100)

X^2 analysis—not significant

Because all of the subjects were around the same age (31.3 years), no definite conclusions could be made about the relation between age and absence or presence of sleep paralysis. In comparing number of years of formal education, it was found that the control subjects had an average of 15.4, the pre-care subjects had an average of 13.6, and the aftercare subjects had an average of 12.5. Controls with and without sleep paralysis had a similar number of years of formal education, and the same pattern was present amongst both the pre-care and aftercare populations. When considering marital status, 41.7% of the control subjects were living with a spouse, compared with 11.1% of the pre-care and aftercare subjects. It did not appear that marital status was related to the absence or presence of sleep paralysis.

Owing to the bulk of data and results, the findings on the other states of consciousness will be reported in a future paper. It was of interest, however, to find that isolated sleep paralysis was correlated with frenzy in the aftercare subjects ($r = 0.307$, significant at the 0.06 level) and was negatively correlated with meditation in the controls ($r = -0.319$, significant at the 0.058 level).

The Holmes-Rahe Social Readjustment Scale scores indicated that 34.3% of the total population, with scores above 300, had a major life change during the year prior to the survey and indicated that only 19.4%, scoring below 149, experienced very little life change (see Table 2). Subjects reporting sleep paralysis ($N = 44$) had an average Holmes-Rahe score of 310 and those not reporting sleep paralysis ($N = 63$) had an average score of 248. Control subjects reporting sleep paralysis ($N = 14$) had an average Holmes-Rahe score of 303, compared with controls not reporting sleep paralysis ($N = 22$), who had an average score of 230. A similar trend was seen with the pre-care subjects: those with sleep paralysis (N = 18) had an average score of 327, while those without (N = 18) had an average score of 205. Aftercare subjects with sleep paralysis (N = 12) had an average score of 292 and those without (N = 24) had an average score of 297. The correlation coefficient between sleep paralysis and Holmes-Rahe scores was significant at the 0.01 level ($r = 0.398$) in the pre-care subjects but was not significant in the control and aftercare subjects.

TABLE 21.2. Holmes-Rahe Social Readjustment Scale Scores[29]

Score Range	Interpretation	Control (%)	Pre-care (%)	Aftercare (%)	Total (%)
300+	Major life change	11 (31.6)	14 (38.)	12 (33.3)	37 (34.3)
250–299	Serious life change	2 (5.6)	4 (11.1)	8 (22.2)	14 (13.0)
200–249	Moderate life change	8 (22.2)	2 (5.6)	5 (13.9)	15 (13.9)
150–199	Mild life change	6 (16.7)	9 (25.0)	6 (16.7)	21 (19.4)
0–149	Very little life change	9 (25.0)	7 (19.4)	5 (13.9)	21 (19.4)
Total		36 (100)	36 (100)	36 (100)	108 (100)

X^2 analysis—not significant

Results of the Saafir Stress-Anxiety Diagnostic Scale revealed that no control subjects, 6 pre-care subjects, and 13 aftercare subjects had scores above 100, indicating clinically significant stress and anxiety. When considering sleep paralysis and the Saafir scores in the pre-care subjects, r was 0.331, significant at the 0.06 level. The MCMI disclosed no single particular personality pattern in the subjects who had experienced sleep paralysis. It was found, however, that sleep paralysis and MCMI symptom scale scores for hypomania were associated in the control subjects ($r = 0.324$, significant at the 0.06 level).

DISCUSSION

Of the total population of 108 black subjects, 44, or 41.0%, had experienced at least one episode of isolated sleep paralysis. The vast majority of subjects who had experienced sleep paralysis responded with conviction (many had the "aha!" experience) when asked about this state of consciousness. This gave a strong subjective impression about the validity and reliability of their reports.

Unfortunately, the incidence of isolated sleep paralysis in white pre-care and aftercare patients has never been studied, so the authors are unable to compare the incidence for these two groups with this study's black pre-care and aftercare populations (50% and 33.3%, respectively). However, American psychiatric literature does report fewer than 100 cases from 1842 to present, which gives the distinct impression that white pre-care and aftercare populations do not experience sleep paralysis nearly as often as did the black patients in this study. The literature[15,23] reports the incidence of isolated sleep paralysis in a presumably "normal" or control white population as 4–15%, whereas this study's black control population had isolated sleep paralysis occurring in 14 of 36 black subjects (39%), at least twice that reported in whites. This finding should be thoroughly investigated by sleep paralysis surveys of white and black control, pre-care, and aftercare populations. Should the results of the present study be verified, the psychiatric and neurologic professions would have a puzzle: "What causes blacks' incidence of isolated sleep paralysis to be at least two times that of whites'?"

The mechanism for sleep paralysis is at present unknown; however, the work on the sleep-dream cycle by Hobson et al.[25] and McCarley and Hobson[26] may hold some answers. These authors maintain that an interaction between the neurons of the raphe and locus ceruleus (aminergic level setters) and the neurons of the gigantocellular tegmental field (cholinergic generators) of the pontine brainstem is the mechanism for sleep-dream cycle generation. In awake consciousness, perception is vivid and externally generated; thought is logical and rational; and movement is voluntary with high muscle tone. The electroencephalographs (EEGs) taken during this state show a desynchronized pattern of low-voltage fast waves, and the eye movements are voluntary. In the awake state, the aminergic, locus ceruleus neurons are maximally active, whereas the cholinergic, giant pontine neurons are minimally active. In deep sleep, perception is dull or absent; thought is repetitious or absent; and movement is infrequent but possible, with medium muscle tone. EEGs taken in this state show a synchronized pattern of high-voltage slow waves, and the eye movements are slow. In the deep-sleep state, the aminergic, locus ceruleus neurons have diminished activity, whereas the cholinergic, giant pontine neurons become progressively more active. In dreaming, perception is vivid and internally generated; thought is illogical and delusional; and movement is impossible, with muscle tone absent (i.e., the body is paralyzed). EEGs taken during this state show the desynchronized mode, and eye movements occur automatically and rapidly, without relationship to the visual field. In this state, the aminergic, locus ceruleus neurons are minimally active, whereas the cholinergic, giant pontine neurons are maximally active. Sleep paralysis is a state of consciousness characterized by a dysrhythmia of the sleep-dream cycle, in which the aminergic, locus ceruleus neurons and the cholinergic, giant pontine neurons are maximally active. This would account for perception being vivid and both internally and externally generated; thought being logical and rational but at the same time panicky and delusional; and movement being impossible because of absent muscle tone. The EEG in this state shows a pattern of low-voltage, mixed-frequency waves with bursts of rapid eye movements—characteristic of dreaming sleep.[27] Implicated in the etiology of sleep paralysis because of its role in the sleep-dream cycle, the locus ceruleus is also involved. Stimulation of the locus ceruleus has been found to be associated with fear responses,[28] the essential emotional response in sleep paralysis.

If blacks experience significantly more isolated sleep paralysis than whites and the etiology of this prevalence lies in an overactive locus ceruleus, what would cause blacks to have a more active locus ceruleus than whites? The answer to this question may lie in part in the findings of Vander Heide and Weinberg,[18] who found a connection between sleep paralysis and combat fatigue. Recent studies of Vietnam veterans suggests that post-traumatic stress disorder involves an abnormal arousal of the central adrenergic system and responds to adrenergic blockers like clonidine, which blocks the alpha$_2$-adrenergic receptors in the locus ceruleus. Post-traumatic stress syndrome is accompanied by frequent episodes of frenzy and is manifested in hyperalertness or an exaggerated startle response, explosiveness, nightmares, intrusive thoughts, and sleep disturbance. This information suggests that there may be a connection between the frequency of sleep paralysis, the frequency of frenzy, and the presence of stress. The association of sleep paralysis with hypomania in this study's controls, life changes and stress-anxiety in the pre-care subjects, and frenzy in the aftercare subjects supports this hypothesis. However, to confirm or refute this hypothesis, other factors that mediate response to life changes and stress must be taken into account by further analysis of the data. For example, states of meditation, which have been shown to lower cortical and autonomic arousal during a wakeful state, were demonstrated to have been negatively correlated with sleep paralysis in the controls. Certainly all three groups, as indicated by the Holmes-Rahe scores, had undergone considerable life change over the year prior to the study.

Interpretation of the scores for this study's total population indicates that in the coming year, 34.3% will be susceptible to a major illness, 13% will have lowered resistance to diseases, and 13.9% will be susceptible to depression.[29] Although the incidence of sleep paralysis among the three populations (39% in control, 50% in pre-care, and 33.3% in aftercare) was not found to be statistically different, the difference in incidence of frenzy reported amongst them was statistically significant. There is the possibility that homicide, sometimes referred to as a "crime of passion," could also be thought of as a state of frenzy.[30] All three groups experienced basically the same degree of life change in the year preceding the survey, yet showed a significant difference in their reports of frenzy. This may indicate a difference in how the control, pre-care, and aftercare populations cope with change, which might influence a manifestation of stress like sleep paralysis or frenzy.

The results presented thus far support the previously published concept[31-33] that being black in this society is associated with stress due to racism, with its attendant lack of parity in housing, health care, employment, nutrition, education, and opportunity. This stress is best described not as a "traumatic neurosis"[34] or "combat fatigue" (occurring during battle), but as "survival fatigue"—stress that results from the tremendous effort necessary for survival in a harsh environment. A great number of black persons suffer from "survival fatigue," a situational predicament that may result in an overaroused adrenergic central neurobiologic system and leading to a variety of behaviors, attitudes, and psychophysiologic diseases. It may well be that the high occurrence of sleep paralysis seen amongst the blacks studied here is the result of "survival fatigue." This may also hold true for the amount of frenzy reported.

With the exception of surveys by Goode[15] and Everett,[13] previous cases of isolated sleep paralysis have been reported in case history, anecdotal fashion. These occurrences were also psychoanalytically interpreted as an actualization of a passive-aggressive conflict present in the patient's personality makeup. Therefore, the patient experiencing an episode of isolated sleep paralysis was diagnosed as wanting to move (being aggressive) but unable (remaining passive). Vander Heide and Weinberg[18] noted in their twelve patients aggressive intent with docile action, as well as indecisiveness and lack of goal-directed behavior. Schneck,[35] in a number of cases he treated, also noted a parallel amongst sleep paralysis and conflicts between active, aggressive functioning and inactive, passive behavior. Payn[36] reported a case of a black female patient who felt she needed to inhibit her aggressive feelings because of guilt and thus remained passive. After her sleep paralysis was interpreted as a sign of inhibition against hostility, she was reported to have improved. Levin[37] discusses sleep paralysis and cataplexy from the standpoint of conditioned inhibition. The stereotypes held about blacks (regarding their need to keep their rage and aggressiveness in check and remain passive[38]) may offer a way to explain the prevalence of isolated sleep paralysis in blacks. However, the results from the MCMI personality profiles, which revealed a wide range of personality types, suggest that no single personality type or intrapsychic conflict underlies sleep paralysis.

In addition to psychoanalytic factors being implicated in the occurrence of isolated sleep paralysis, the reports of both Goode[15] and Roth[24] indicate heredofamilial predisposition. It is conceivable that blacks, in addition to being at high risk for excessive life change, have a genetic predisposition to high occurrence of sleep paralysis, possibly because of a more sensitive central adrenergic system. One also finds cultural evidence of blacks' high incidence of sleep paralysis in black American folklore, with references to "the witch riding you." This might refer to sleep paralysis victims' common report of feeling as if someone is sitting on their chest or standing over their bed. Certainly, a genetic predisposition to sleep paralysis would help explain the finding that black African cultural cosmology is in part based on the existence of genies and spirits.[32] There is some evidence that North Africans have more daydreams than Westerners, which might indicate that blacks have generally greater access to various states of consciousness.[39]

More investigation and inquiry into these issues is needed. Indications are that such will be fruitful.

PROPOSALS

The hypothesized neurologic model for sleep paralysis could be tested by animal studies using electrodes to stimulate the locus ceruleus and doing sleep studies on the subjects. An over-stimulated locus ceruleus etiology for sleep paralysis could be confirmed also in a study of patients withdrawing from opiates. Since it has been shown that withdrawal syndrome is produced by excess locus ceruleus activity,[40] this raises the possibility of high amounts of sleep paralysis in such patients. This hypothesis could be verified if administration of clonidine (an anti-hypertensive medication shown to reduce over-stimulation of the locus ceruleus neuropharmacologically through agonistic alpha$_2$-adrenergic activity) to such patients suffering frequent sleep paralysis attacks eliminates these attacks. It is of interest that tricyclic antidepressants, used in treating sleep paralysis[27,41-43] and panic attacks,[44] also decrease locus ceruleus arousal[45] (possibly by preventing adrenergic neurotransmitters from re-entering the nerve cells of the locus ceruleus nucleus). There is evidence of a brain norepinephrine system being involved in the production of anxiety,[46] and a study of sleep paralysis may well confirm this hypothesis.

The finding that hypnosis is useful in treating sleep paralysis[47] is not surprising. The present study revealed that sleep paralysis and meditation were negatively correlated. Both hypnosis and meditation might be used, then, as non-pharmacological treatments to lower cortical and autonomic arousal and decrease locus ceruleus activity.

Studying the difference in isolated sleep paralysis prevalence between white and black patients with post-traumatic stress syndrome may help delineate if the etiology of sleep paralysis is rooted in a contrasting central adrenergic system sensitivity or in a contrasting amount of daily stress. The finding of sleep paralysis in the present study's aftercare patients may indicate an overaroused adrenergic central system superimposed upon a graver neurochemical disorder responsible for the aftercare patients' fragmentation. The current trend is to treat fragmentation with antipsychotics and hope the patient's anxiety will abate along with the psychosis. The treatment of an overaroused central adrenergic system might benefit patients who are fragmented and report anxiety.

The significant possibility that sleep paralysis indicates a difference in whites' and blacks' neurobiology should be proven and properly interpreted. A racial difference in neurochemistry might greatly influence how racial groups respond to medication or drugs. This has been demonstrated, for example, in the ways different racial groups respond to the pharmacokinetics of lithium[48] and alcohol.[49,50]

Sleep paralysis may be an early warning sign for the development of an overaroused central adrenergic system. This should be considered, as it may be a useful clinical marker of a patient's potential for developing other proposed hyperadrenergic syndromes, such as frenzy, post-traumatic stress syndrome, and hypertension.

Finally, sleep paralysis frequently accompanied by hypnogenic hallucinations may possibly indicate that blacks have more hallucinatory experiences than do whites and that blacks are more predisposed to the hallucinatory phenomena reported in the literature.[51,52] This should be considered as well. The difference might be partly responsible for the misdiagnosis of black patients with manic depressive illness[53,54] or other disorders.[55]

COMMENTARY

When the CMHC research team decided to do some basic empirical research on the quality and quantity of African-American states of consciousness, we had absolutely no idea what we'd find. Essentially, after we on the research team shared with each other our experiences with altered states of consciousness, we thought we had a very interesting model to catalogue human behavior. It seemed more African-American-user friendly than the disjointed, un-encompassing Western method of categorizing mentation.

A few of us on the CMHC research team had had episodes of isolated sleep paralysis, but we'd never really talked about it to anyone before. I confessed to the team that in medical school, a fellow student named

Ronald Banks asked me about his experience with the state since he knew my interest in psychiatry. I didn't have a clue what he was talking about but was intrigued by the mysterious state he explained. I later read about sleep paralysis studying neurology, since it is usually associated with the neurologic disorder narcolepsy. I had not experienced it, though, so it was just an intellectual point to file. It wasn't until I had my first experience that I personally understood the phenomenon. I was in the Navy at the time and had gone to sleep one day after a 24-hour period of being on call and awake. I remember waking up completely paralyzed and having a sleep hallucination—I thought I heard three hoodlums breaking down my front door to do me some bodily harm! I recall being wide awake and knowing were I was. I was struggling to get up and defend myself, but I couldn't move! Finally, I could sit up. My heart was racing and I was scared, breathing fast, and sweating, only, there were no home invaders. It was the sleep paralysis that Banks had told me about years before.

We at the CMHC were surprised to find that 41% of the African-American population we studied had at least one episode of this disorder, considering that studies of European-Americans reported the phenomena at a rate of 15%. We had discovered something new and unusual about black people that had never before been reported. It seemed to be related to the levels of stress that black people experienced, but we couldn't be sure. I remember telling Dr. William Dement, the father of sleep research, about my discovery. He blew me off and told me my finding was nothing to get excited about, as European-Americans had it more frequently than the literature reported. I learned of Dr. David Hufford, the world's leading expert on isolated sleep paralysis, and wrote him about my findings. In his response, he indicated that the incidence isolated sleep paralysis we were recording was more extreme than he'd seen. I had also been in contract with Dr. Loudell Snow, an expert of US folk medicine. She informed me that the phenomenon of isolated sleep paralysis is known in the African-American community as "the witch is riding you" or "the haint is after you." She sent me numerous African-American folk cures. One such was putting a broom by the door at night. This way, the witch coming to "ride" the sleepers in the house would get so caught up in counting broom straws that morning would be upon her and she'd have to flee. This information was quite handy as we refined our work in the area.

After we published this article, we received some interesting feedback. Dr. K. Fukuda in Japan sent me an article he had written describing a Japanese population that had experienced isolated sleep paralysis at a rate of 40% (Fukuda K, Miyasita A, Inugami M, Ishihara K. High prevalence of isolated sleep paralysis: Kanashibari phenomena in Japan. *Sleep.* 10:279–286). In this article, he and his colleagues discussed my findings and compared theirs. As a result, we communicated about our work for some years. My correspondence with him paid off, since his sleep laboratory later confirmed that isolated sleep paralysis was associated with anxiety (Fukuda F, Hozumi N. Some aspects of Kanashibari phenomena (sleep paralysis) may have minor association with some variable concerning anxiety within a sample of psychiatric outpatients. *Bull Faculty of Ed Fukushima Univ.* 1989;47:45–53). The Japanese researchers also added a big piece to the puzzle when they discovered that the interruption of sleep—a frequent occurrence in individuals under stress—could elicit isolated sleep paralysis (Takeuchi T, Miyasita A, Sasaki Y, Inugami M, Fukuda K. Isolated sleep paralysis elicited by sleep interruption. *Sleep.* 1992;15:217–225).

I had the opportunity to present my research on isolated sleep paralysis during an international conference co-sponsored by the BPA, the African Psychiatric Society, and the APA entitled "Psychiatry in Africa and the Americas Today" (Nairobi, Kenya, August 4–15, 1986). While there, I was able to encourage Dr. A. O. Odejide, a Nigerian psychiatrist, to replicate my study in Nigeria. I was very proud to see his work published (Ohaeri JU, Odejide AO, Ikuesan BA, Adeyemi JD. The pattern of isolated sleep paralysis among Nigerian medical students. *J Natl Med Assoc.* 1989;81:805–808). Despite a different rate of isolated sleep paralysis found in his subjects, the research confirmed that the myths behind the phenomenon in Nigeria were similar to those amongst African Americans. Another Nigerian psychiatrist, Dr. J. U. Ohaeri produced several papers with his colleagues as well (Ohaeri JU. Experience of isolated sleep paralysis in clinical practice in Nigeria. *J Natl Med Assoc.* 1992;84:521–523, and Ohaeri JU, Adelekan MF, Odejide AO, Ikuesan BA. The pattern of isolated sleep paralysis among Nigerian nursing students. *J Natl Med Assoc.* 1992;84:67–70).

The CMHC's research was being recognized primarily in the international scientific community. It wasn't until Doctors Angela M. Neal and

Samuel M. Turner published the article, "Anxiety Disorders Research with African Americans: Current Status" (*Psych Bull.* 1991;109:400–410), that the US scientific community began to notice our work. In this article, Doctors Neal and Turner reviewed the "available literature on anxiety disorders in African Americans." CMHC's research was given a great deal of exposure and covered in great detail, as our research team had been one of the country's few to focus on panic disorder in African Americans.

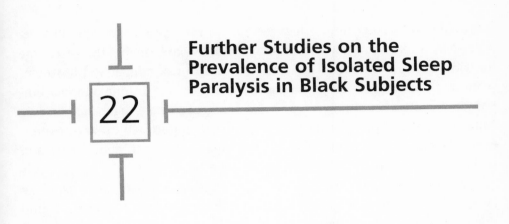

Further Studies on the Prevalence of Isolated Sleep Paralysis in Black Subjects

22

In a previous study, one of the authors (Carl C. Bell) found that isolated sleep paralysis was common in blacks. In this study, conducted by interviews, a recurrent pattern (one or more episodes per month) of isolated sleep paralysis episodes in blacks was described by at least 25% of the afflicted sample studied. Frequent episodes were associated with stress, and subjects with isolated sleep paralysis had an unusually high prevalence of panic disorder (15.5%). The genetic transmission of sleep paralysis was studied in a large black family, and in addition to stressful environmental factors being associated with the condition, there appears to be a dominant genetic factor associated with predisposition for developing sleep paralysis. The implications of these findings for stress, anxiety, sleep, and psychophysiologic disorders are discussed.

INTRODUCTION

In a previous paper, Bell et al.[1] reported findings from their first survey measuring the prevalence of isolated sleep paralysis in a black population of healthy subjects and psychiatric patients. The authors defined sleep paralysis as a state of consciousness[2] occurring upon falling asleep

---

Originally printed as Bell Carl C, Dixie-Bell Dora D, Thompson Belinda. Further studies on the prevalence of isolated sleep paralysis in black subjects. *J Natl Med Assoc.* 1986;78:649–659.

or awakening, lasting from a few seconds to several minutes, and characterized by a feeling of inability to move. While experiencing this state, the individual is fully aware of the condition and surroundings and has complete recall of the episode. Vivid and terrifying hallucinations often accompany this state of consciousness, and a sense of acute danger may be felt. Once the episode passes, the individual often sits up with a start, experiencing symptoms of panic (e.g., tachycardia, hyperventilation, fear) and realizing that the perceptions of danger were false.

In reviewing the existing literature on isolated sleep paralysis, some interesting patterns emerge. With regard to its prevalence, Bell et al.[1] found that 41% of the total sample (N = 108) had experienced the state. Goode[3] and Everett[4] studied white populations and determined isolated sleep paralysis rates of 4.7% and 15.4%, respectively. Hufford's[5] work on isolated sleep paralysis, spanning more than a decade, began with a study of a college student population in Newfoundland, in which 23% of the 93 students reported having experienced sleep paralysis (known as the "Old Hag" in Newfoundland). Hufford's research has led him to assert that the phenomenon is found in various cultural settings. He documents this with case histories of Eskimos and Filipinos who had experienced the state. Hufford estimates that in the general population, 15% or more have had at least one recognizable episode of isolated sleep paralysis.

Hufford made a significant contribution in his observation about recurrence of isolated sleep paralysis:

> The recurrence of the event repeatedly during a single night is uncommon but not unique. Most frequently there is a single attack, either never repeated or repeated infrequently at intervals of months, or more often, years. In other cases a series of attacks may occur frequently, even nightly, for a period of a week or two. Multiple attacks during a single night are most likely during one of these runs. A victim may experience one such run and no more, or a number of these sequences may recur separated by months or years. Least common is the individual who experiences the attacks frequently over a period of years.[5]

Bell et al.,[1] however, found that recurrence of frequent episodes over a period of years was not uncommon among the black population they studied. Specifically, 27.3% of the subjects reported experiencing isolated sleep paralysis once or more monthly. It would seem that the findings from this study are unique, since the prevalence of isolated sleep paralysis in blacks appears to be higher than in other populations studied and since recurrence of isolated sleep paralysis episodes is prevalent in blacks but least common in whites (i.e., the individual who experiences the episodes frequently over a period of years).

These discrepancies led the authors to further investigate isolated sleep paralysis amongst blacks. Of particular interest from the previous study was that 50% of the pre-care subjects (anxious patients) experienced isolated sleep paralysis, indicating a possible correlation between sleep paralysis and stress. Other indications of such a correlation were the close relationship between sleep paralysis and Holmes-Rahe Social Readjustment Scale scores in the pre-care subjects ($r = 0.398$; $p < 0.01$) and panic-attack-like symptoms that occur immediately after an isolated sleep paralysis episode.[1] Another connection between stress and sleep paralysis is suggested by the finding that "combat fatigue" is the only social phenomenon associated with sleep paralysis.[8] The overaroused central adrenergic system,[6,7] hypothesized to cause both sleep paralysis and anxiety, was of interest to the authors as well. Finally, the authors investigated the relationship between sleep paralysis and hypertension (both hypothesized to be caused by an overaroused central adrenergic system), as well as the proposed heredofamilial trend reported by others.[3,9]

METHOD

To solicit subjects for the study, the CMHC mailed flyers to 962 people on its mailing list and asked them to call CMHC to participate in a 10–15-minute confidential phone interview. The flyer contained a description of sleep paralysis and informed that the study purported to answer some questions about it (e.g., if it runs in families, if it is caused by stress, if it is associated with high blood pressure). In addition, an article on the research project advertising the need for callers appeared in the *Chicago Defender*, a black newspaper. One of the authors (D. D. Dixie-Bell) made herself available for three weeks from noon to 4:30 pm, Monday through Friday, to interview subjects by phone. In addition to the call-in study, a family study was done by selecting proband with isolated sleep paralysis. Every available family member took a structured interview, developed by the authors, on isolated sleep paralysis.

The interview, which provided the subjects with a definition of sleep paralysis, collected demographic variables (e.g., age, sex, ethnicity, occupation, annual income, marital status, education) and probed for a complete description of the subjects' experiences with the state. Once the callers gave a phenomenologic report of their experience with sleep paralysis, the interviewer determined if further probing should take place. The interview included questions on the subjects' control over the state and the intensity and nature of it, precipitating events (e.g., stress and heavy meals), and knowledge of folk medicine cures. The subjects were also asked if about their comfort level during an episode and whether sleep paralysis episodes got them into trouble. Finally, to probe biological relationships and heredofamilial trends, subjects were asked questions regarding family history of high blood pressure, panic attacks, mental illness, and sleep paralysis.

RESULTS

Callers

Twenty-five black subjects called in and were interviewed about their episodes of sleep paralysis. Their average age was 38. They had about 15 years of education and an average annual income of $19,480. Nineteen subjects were female and six were male. Eleven were single, 12 were married, 1 was divorced, and 1 was widowed. Table 1 catalogues the responses given to general questions regarding the callers' episodes of isolated sleep paralysis. With regard to voodoo and folk cures, 14 had heard that sleep paralysis was due to voodoo or a hex, and 7 had heard of folk cures for it. Only three felt they could have either controlled the state (e.g., preventing episodes by following an anti-hypertensive diet) or brought themselves out of the state. Three wanted sleep paralysis to happen more often, primarily to figure out what was happening to them.

The questions regarding frequency and intensity provided the patterns seen in Table 2. Five of the 25 subjects no longer had sleep paralysis

TABLE 22.1. Causes and Control of Sleep Paralysis in Callers

	Yes	No	Do not Know
Causes			
Self (i.e., can you cause it?)	4	21	0
Other people or other situations	8	17	0
Stress	9	13	3
Irregular sleep habits	7	15	3
Heavy meal before sleeping	3	21	1
Drinking alcohol	2	21	2
Control			
Self (i.e., can you end it?)	9	16	0
Others (i.e., can others end your episode?)	4	21	0

episodes. On the average, their episodes had not recurred in 5.4 years. Four of those five had experienced the state only a few times in their lives and one had episodes weekly. Nine subjects said it seemed they grew out of having episodes, eleven said they had not, and five were not sure. Only 5 of the 25 subjects reported that they were comfortable during their episodes, and only 4 of 25 reported that sleep paralysis had caused difficulties (mostly embarrassment and fear of going back to sleep). Seven participants felt their episodes increased with age, 17 did not, and one did not know.

TABLE 22.2. Episodes of Sleep Paralysis

	Callers	Family Members with Sleep Paralysis	Total
Frequency			
Daily	1	2	3
Weekly	2	1	3
Monthly	8	5	13
Semi-annually	4	5	9
Yearly	0	3	3
Every 3 years	1	2	3
A few times in lifetime	4	9	13
Never anymore	5	6	11
Totals	25	33	58
Duration			
1 minute or less	5	7	12
1–3 minutes	6	2	8
3–5 minutes	2	4	6
10–15 minutes	1	1	2
15 minutes or longer	1	0	1
Do not know	10	19	29

Responses to the questions designed to probe for biological and heredofamilial relationships showed that sleep paralysis ran in the families of seven subjects (three reported mother had it, one reported mother and aunt, and one each reported sister, grandmother, or grandfather). Eight of 25 subjects (32%) reported having been diagnosed with high blood pressure. Of these who were treated for high blood pressure, five said that after treatment the frequency of their sleep paralysis stayed the same, two said the frequency decreased, and one was not sure if there had been a change. Twenty-one of the 25 subjects (84%) reported that hypertension ran in their families. Twelve mothers, nine fathers, seven brothers, five sisters, three aunts, two uncles, five grandmothers, and one grandfather were reported as having hypertension. Six of the subjects reported family members who had both sleep paralysis and hypertension; two reported their mothers were dually afflicted, two reported their fathers, one reported a sister and aunt, and one reported a grandmother. Twenty-one subjects reported they had never been treated for a mental illness or nervous condition, three reported treatment as outpatients, and one reported treatment as an inpatient.

The information gathered relating to panic attacks is especially interesting: 9 subjects reported at least 4 of the 12 symptoms listed in DSM-III criteria[10] for panic attacks. Of these subjects, two reported that they used to have weekly attacks, which stopped a year ago for one and 27 years ago for the other; one reported having attacks once daily; one reported weekly attacks; one reported attacks twice yearly; two reported yearly attacks; one reported having only one such attack in his life; and one did not respond to the question. Thus, 4 of 25 subjects (16%) at some point in their lives had panic attacks frequently enough to qualify for a diagnosis of panic disorder according to DSM-III criteria.

Family Study

The family that was studied consisted of a proband whose grandmother and grandfather (first generation) both had sleep paralysis (Figure 1). The proband's grandparents had 13 offspring (second generation, six male and seven female). Of these, seven subjects (53.8%, three men and four women) reported having had sleep paralysis. The proband's mother, aunts, and uncles (third generation) had 50 offspring (18 male and 32 female). Of these, 20 (40%, 5 men and 15 women) reported having sleep paralysis. The proband, her sisters, and cousins (fourth generation) had nine offspring (three male and six female). Of these, five subjects (55.6%, two men and three women) reported having sleep paralysis.

FIGURE 22.1. Family Tree

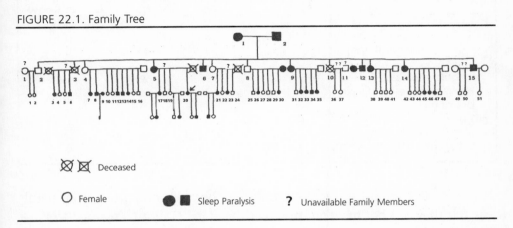

⊠ ⊠ Deceased

○ Female   ●■ Sleep Paralysis   ? Unavailable Family Members

Of the 64 family members who were interviewed, a total of 33 (51.6%) reported having had at least one episode of sleep paralysis. Their average age was 32.7, and they had about 13.2 years of education and an average annual income of $13,495. Twenty-two were female and eleven were male. Fifteen were single, fifteen were married, two were divorced, and one was widowed. The average age of the 31 family members who denied ever having sleep paralysis was 29.7, and they had about 12.9 years of education and an average annual income of $10,829. Eighteen of these subjects were female, and thirteen were male. Fifteen were single, twelve were married, and four were divorced.

The family members' responses to questions concerning frequency and intensity of their sleep paralysis episodes can be found in Table 2. Six members reported that the episodes had ceased, and on the average, the episodes had not recurred in 11.8 years. One of the six reported that the episodes had occurred monthly; one reported semi-annual occurrences; three reported it occurred only a few times in their lives; and one did not respond to the question. The responses in Table 3 were given to the general questions that were asked regarding the family members' episodes of

isolated sleep paralysis. Thirteen had heard of sleep paralysis being related to voodoo or hex, and 20 had not. Only three reported that they had
heard of folk cures for sleep paralysis.

TABLE 22.3. Causes and Control of Sleep Paralysis in Family Members

	Yes	No	Do not Know
Causes			
Self (i.e., can you cause it?)	3	30	0
Other people or other situations	9	24	0
Stress	14	16	3
Irregular sleep habits	97	23	1
Heavy meal before sleeping	3	29	1
Drinking alcohol	3	30	0
Control			
Self (i.e., can you end it?)	17	6	0
Others (i.e., can others end your episode?)	13	20	0

Most (N = 26) of the 33 family members who reported sleep paralysis felt they did not have control over the state. Only two wanted to have
the episode more often. Fourteen subjects said it seemed they grew out of
having episodes, and 19 said they had not. Only three of 33 reported they
were comfortable during their episodes, and only two of 33 reported that
sleep paralysis had caused difficulties. Nine felt their episodes increased
with age, compared with 24 who did not.

Eight of 33 subjects (24.2%) reported that they had been diagnosed
with high blood pressure. Of these, six said the frequency of their sleep
paralysis stayed the same, one said the frequency decreased following
treatment, and one was not sure. Since all of these subjects are related, it
is apparent that hypertension runs in the family. Among the 64 total family members (with and without sleep paralysis), 15 reported having hypertension (23.4%), and 8 reported having both sleep paralysis and hypertension (12.5%).

Sixty family members reported that they had never been treated for
a mental illness, three reported treatment as outpatients (two of whom had
sleep paralysis), and one reported treatment as an inpatient (did not have
sleep paralysis). Twenty members (31%) reported symptoms of panic
attacks (13 with sleep paralysis and 7 without). Of the seven subjects who
did not have sleep paralysis, one reported that his panic attacks, which

stopped two years ago, used to occur once monthly; one reported he was currently having panic attacks monthly; four reported having them twice yearly; and one reported having them once a year. Due to the infrequency of the panic attacks, none of the 31 family members without sleep paralysis has ever qualified for a panic disorder diagnosis as defined by DSM-III criteria.[10] Of the 13 subjects who have sleep paralysis, two reported they were having panic attacks once daily, three reported having them once weekly, three reported having them once monthly, two reported having them twice yearly, and three reported having them once a year. Thus, five (15.2%) of the 33 family members who had sleep paralysis had panic attacks frequently enough to qualify for a panic disorder diagnosis according to DSM-III criteria.[10] In all, five of the 64 total family members (7.8%) qualified for a diagnosis of panic disorder at some point in their lives.

STATISTICAL RESULTS

Callers with sleep paralysis and the family members with sleep paralysis were not significantly different in frequency of experiencing sleep paralysis episodes. This was determined by comparing the ratio of individuals in both groups who have one or more sleep paralysis episodes per month with individuals who have episodes less often. Twelve of 25 callers (48%) and 9 of the 33 family members (27.3%) reported having one or more sleep paralysis episodes per month, and these subjects were designated as having sleep paralysis disorder. Thirteen of the 25 callers (52%) and 24 of the 33 family members (72.7%) reported having fewer than one episode of sleep paralysis per month and were designated as having sleep paralysis attacks. All of the subjects (callers and the family members) with sleep paralysis disorder were more likely than those with sleep paralysis attacks to report that sleep paralysis was caused by stress. The difference between these two groups in this regard was significant at the 0.5 level ($x^2 = 3.98$; df = 1). All of the subjects (callers and the family members) with both sleep paralysis and panic attacks were also more likely than the subjects with sleep paralysis and no panic attacks to report that stress caused sleep paralysis. The difference between these two groups was significant at the 0.05 level ($x^2 = 4.2$; df = 1). All of the subjects (callers and family members) with sleep paralysis disorder were more likely than those who had sleep paralysis less frequently (i.e., those with sleep paralysis attacks) to report that they had had panic attacks. The difference between these two groups was significant at the 0.05 level ($x^2 = 5.2$; df = 1).

The family members with sleep paralysis were more likely than family members without sleep paralysis to report having had panic attacks. The difference between these two groups was significant at the 0.01 level ($x^2 = 15.04$; df = 1).

There was no significant difference between the callers, the family members with sleep paralysis, and the family members without sleep paralysis regarding their having hypertension.

DISCUSSION

In the previous study[1] of 108 black subjects and patients, 27.3% had sleep paralysis disorder (one or more episodes of sleep paralysis per month). In the current study, 48% of the callers and 27.3% of the family members with sleep paralysis are classified as having sleep paralysis disorder. Initially, the authors thought the callers had possibly been motivated to call because of the frequency of their sleep paralysis episodes, thereby accounting for the greater percentage of subjects with sleep paralysis disorder in the caller sample. Statistical analysis, however, discounts this explanation, as the ratio of sleep paralysis disorder to sleep paralysis attacks (less than one episode per month) was not significantly different in the three groups. Although the populations in the current study were not randomly sampled, it again appears that at least one fourth of the black population have the pattern of isolated sleep paralysis recurrence that Hufford reports as the least common: "experienc[ing] the attacks frequently over a period of years."[5]

Another indication that the epidemiology of sleep paralysis is different in blacks is evident when comparing the prevalence of sleep paralysis in the two white families studied by Roth et al.[9] and the black family in the current study. Specifically, the two white families had 14 of 56 (25%) and 4 of 19 (21.1%) family members who experienced sleep paralysis, compared with 33 of 64 (51.6%) members of the black family in the current study.

The low number of callers (25) responding to the large number of mailed flyers (962) might lead one to question the authors' hypothesis that sleep paralysis is more common among blacks. The authors reason that the low response to research participation is similar to the explanation offered by Pierce[11] regarding the difficulty of getting black subjects to volunteer for research on hypertension. In the past, research findings have been interpreted in ways that have been damaging to blacks, and many blacks feel that when they volunteer for research, they may risk getting involved in experimentation similar to the infamous Tuskegee experiment on syphilis. These factors make blacks reluctant to volunteer for research, even if it is being done by blacks to benefit blacks. However, it seems that the answer to getting black research volunteers depends more on the presentation than the worth of the project; most of the callers in the present study reported they had responded because of the *Chicago Defender* article.

The characteristics of sleep paralysis episodes were similar in both the callers and family members with sleep paralysis. There were, however, three times as many female as male subjects who had sleep paralysis episodes in the call-in group and twice as many women in the family group. At first glance, this supported the observations of Roth et al.[9] that the prevalence of sleep paralysis was greater in women, and was contrary to those of Goode,[3] who found that men outnumbered women 4:1. However, in considering that the callers did not constitute a random sample and that more females were born to the black family studied; and considering the difficulties involved in recruiting black men for research studies, the predominance of women in these two cohorts is not a significant indicator of females being more at risk for having sleep paralysis. Moreover, the authors' previous work,[1] which had more randomly selected sample populations, and Hufford's work[5] revealed approximately the same percentages of men and women with sleep paralysis.

For both the callers and family members, sleep paralysis seems to be a paroxysmal phenomenon in which the afflicted have little control over the inducement or termination of the episodes. In general, neither the callers nor family members with sleep paralysis felt it was caused by irregular sleeping habits, heavy meals, or drinking. Callers were nearly equally divided about stress being a cause of sleep paralysis. Of the family members with sleep paralysis, more (2:1) felt that stress caused it. When the callers and the family members with sleep paralysis were divided into those with sleep paralysis disorder (more frequent episodes) vs. those with sleep paralysis attacks (less frequent episodes), it became apparent that those with sleep paralysis disorder felt stress caused their episodes. This finding was consistent with the preliminary findings in the previous study[1] that sleep paralysis and stress may be correlated.

As with the callers, half of the family members with sleep paralysis had heard of supernatural causes of sleep paralysis. While one third of the callers had heard of folk cures, less than 10% of the family members with sleep paralysis had heard of such cures. Hyatt[12] reports folklore cures like putting a Bible under the head of the bed; catching "the hag" in a bottle; laying a broom at your door; putting a fork under your pillow; tying horsehair on your wrist; putting a horseshoe over your door; saying, "Lord, have mercy"; putting mustard seeds, red pepper, or salt on the floor; and using a sifter in various places. Hufford[5] notes similar folklore cures, and the subjects of the current study had knowledge of folk cures similar to those outlined by Hyatt.[12] Since the body of black folk medicine includes cures for sleep paralysis (also known as "the witch is riding you") and since blacks may be more afflicted with sleep paralysis than whites, questions arise regarding the availability of African folk medicine cures and the prevalence of sleep paralysis in black Africans. Further, if there is a similar phenomenon in Africa, is there any relationship between the two (i.e., are black American folk cures for sleep paralysis cultural vestiges of African ones?)?

The majority of subjects with sleep paralysis (callers and family members) do not wish for recurrences, and most feel uncomfortable during their episodes. This is most likely due to the panic-attack-like symptoms that are experienced after the paralysis ceases. The callers and family members were also similar in that there seemed to be two divergent groups of sleep paralysis victims—one with subjects feeling the frequency of their sleep paralysis episodes decreased with age and one with subjects feeling the frequency increased with age. The meaning of this finding remains unclear and will take further study to unravel.

Thirty-two percent of the callers reported having hypertension, and 84% reported that hypertension ran in their families. The family members with sleep paralysis reported having hypertension at a rate of 24.2%, which was nearly identical to the family members without sleep paralysis with a rate of 22.6%. Since 11 family members were younger than 20 years (five with sleep paralysis and six without), the prevalence might increase as these younger members get older. Twenty-four percent of the callers reported having relatives with both hypertension and sleep paralysis. Of the black family studied, 12.5% actually had sleep paralysis and hypertension. Unfortunately, this information does not shed much light on the possible connection between sleep paralysis and hypertension. The range of the prevalence of hypertension in blacks is 18% to 37%[13]; neither the callers nor family members with sleep paralysis had a greater-than-average prevalence of hypertension.

The relationship between hypertension and sleep paralysis, however, cannot be excluded. Perhaps a better method of studying this relationship would be to compare the prevalence of sleep paralysis in hypertensives and normotensives. There were not enough subjects with sleep paralysis who had been treated for hypertension to determine whether there was a concomitant decrease in sleep paralysis episodes with treatment designed to reduce hypertension via central nervous system neurotransmitter alterations. Such a finding would support the hypothesis that an overaroused central adrenergic system is a significant factor in the development of both sleep paralysis and hypertension. Again, it may be better to study this relationship by looking at hypertensive subjects with sleep paralysis to see if anti-hypertensive medication (acting via central nervous system neurotransmitter alteration) reduces the frequency of their sleep paralysis while controlling their blood pressure.

The family members with sleep paralysis were more likely to report having had panic attacks than the family members without sleep paralysis, and the difference between these two groups was statistically significant. Sixteen percent of the callers and 15.2% of the family members with sleep paralysis reported frequent enough panic attacks to have been diagnosed with panic disorder. Significantly, none of the family members without sleep paralysis reported frequent enough panic attacks frequently to have been diagnosed with panic disorder. The morbidity risk for developing panic disorder in the black family studied was 7.8%. These percentages are much higher than those reported for the general population. Anxiety disorders in the general population have a prevalence between 2% and 5%.[14] Weissman et al.[15] reported generalized anxiety disorder having a prevalence of 2.5%; panic disorders, 0.4%; and simple phobias, 1.4%—a total prevalence of about 4.3%, using DSM-III criteria. Uhlenhuth et al.[16] found the prevalence of agoraphobia and panic disorder to be 1.2%; for other phobias, 2.3%; and for generalized anxiety disorder, 6.4%. It appears that subjects with isolated sleep paralysis may be more at risk for developing panic disorder than individuals in the general population, and the two syndromes may be different clinical manifestations of the same disorder. Certainly, subjects report panic-attack symptoms during and following an episode of sleep paralysis.

It is the authors' clinical experience that patients with panic disorder who report isolated sleep paralysis episodes note a concomitant decrease in panic attacks and sleep paralysis episodes when treated with antidepressant medication. Additional support of a relationship between sleep paralysis and panic disorder comes from the finding that subjects with sleep paralysis disorder (both callers and family members) were more likely than those who had sleep paralysis attacks to report they had panic attacks. Clinical experience with patients who have depressive disorders and who report both panic attacks and sleep paralysis episodes or report sleep paralysis episodes alone also reveals that treatment with antidepressant medication relieves symptoms of all three.

Family studies of probands with panic disorders reveal that the morbidity risk of first-degree relatives (parents and siblings) for developing panic disorder is several times higher than in control subjects who do not suffer from panic disorders. Noyes et al.[17] found that morbidity risks for first-degree relatives of patients with anxiety neurosis (panic disorder) was 19.1%. Crowe et al.[18] found morbidity risks for first-degree relatives of probands with panic disorder to be 17.3% but only 1.8% for the first-degree relatives of normal control subjects. Harris et al.[19] found that morbidity risks for panic disorder was 20.5%, compared with only 4.2% in first-degree relatives of normal control subjects. Pauls et al.[20] found that the morbidity risks for second-degree relatives (grandparents, aunts, and uncles) of patients with anxiety neurosis (panic disorder) was 9.5% but only 1.4% for the second-degree relatives of controls.

In the black family studied in this paper, 33% of the probands' second-degree relatives with sleep paralysis also had panic attacks (5 of 15). This raises the question, in addition to that of sleep paralysis and panic disorder being different clinical manifestations of the same disorder, of whether the inheritability of sleep paralysis is the same as panic disorder. Certainly, the black family studied here has a prevalence of panic disorder similar to the pattern of prevalence in families in which panic disorders seem to run. Since 20 years is the risk age for the development of panic disorders, the prevalence of panic disorders in the black family studied may be underestimated; eleven of them were younger than 20 years (five with sleep paralysis and six without). More family studies need to be done to verify this hypothesis.

Sleep paralysis is traditionally thought of as a component of the narcolepsy tetrad of sleep attacks (cataplexy, sleep paralysis, and hypnogenic hallucinations). However, sleep paralysis may occur as an isolated entity and not in association with narcolepsy or cataplexy. A more thorough review of the literature on isolated sleep paralysis and its relationship to narcolepsy has been presented elsewhere and will not be presented here. New information pertinent to the discussion of isolated sleep paralysis in blacks will, however, be presented. First, it has been noted by sleep disorder researchers that blacks are more predisposed than whites to developing narcolepsy. Narcolepsy is thought to be a hereditary affection transferred in an autosomally dominant manner, and it may be that isolated sleep paralysis and narcolepsy are manifestations of varying penetrance of the same hereditary disorder. In view of the previous discussion suggesting that sleep paralysis and panic disorder may be different clinical manifestations of the same disorder, another new interesting finding is that electroencephalographic patterns are similar in patients with panic disorder and narcolepsy, suggesting a common electrocortical etiology.[21] These findings do not lend support to the Roth et al.[9] hypothesis that sleep paralysis is an independent nosologic and genetic entity that is separate from narcolepsy.

Roth et al.[9] reported that in the two white families they studied, the malady of sleep paralysis was invariably transmitted to the children by mother. Mothers in that study transferred the disease to 56.2% of their daughters and 43.8% of their sons. They did not find a single case in which the affliction had been transmitted by a man. They assert this pattern fits the mode of genetic transmission when the pathologic gene is dominant and on the X chromosome (i.e., half the children—both male and female—of the affected mothers would be affected, and the affected men would transmit the disease to all of their daughters but to none of their sons). The results of the black family study for sleep paralysis were not definite enough to assert whether the genetic predisposition for the development of sleep paralysis was autosomal dominant with mixed penetrance (as in narcolepsy), or X-linked dominant (as suggested by Roth et al.[9]), because the afflicted men in the study had a small number of offspring, who were unavailable to be interviewed. It is clear that there is a dominant pathologic gene involved. More black family studies will need to be done to assert whether the gene is on an autosomal or X-linked chromosome. Despite the likelihood of sleep paralysis being transmitted by a dominant gene, two thirds of the callers did not think sleep paralysis ran in their families. Such a mode of genetic transmission implies that the callers' family members may have had sleep paralysis but never discussed the problem, possibly due to a general tendency in blacks to avoid any discussion of any problems that might indicate a nervous condition. In fact, many subjects with sleep paralysis remarked they never discussed their experiences with others for fear they would be viewed as "crazy."

Ettedgui and Bridges[22] note that a significant percentage of patients with post-traumatic stress disorder experience panic attacks. Burstein[23] and Falcon et al.[24] make a similar observation and go on to point out that antidepressant medication is useful in alleviating post-traumatic stress disorder symptoms. Burstein[23] hypothesized that the arousal-prevention action of the antidepressant medication relieved the post-traumatic stress syndrome patients of their dream disturbances, which were of a REM anxiety nature. Also, Falcon et al.[24] hypothesized that post-traumatic stress disorder may be a term for "heterogeneous group of patients suffering from various other tricyclic-responsive syndromes, especially panic disorder or major depressive disorder."[24] The following all point to a possible connection between sleep paralysis and post-traumatic stress disorders: the proposed relationships between post-traumatic stress disorder and panic disorders; the finding that the only social phenomenon associated with sleep paralysis was "combat fatigue;"[8] the use of tricyclics to treat sleep paralysis[25-28] and post-traumatic stress disorder; the finding that the subjects (callers and family members) with sleep paralysis and panic attacks were more likely than subjects with sleep paralysis and no panic attacks to that report stress caused sleep paralysis. These factors, plus the similar proposed etiologies of an abnormal hypersensitivity of the central adrenergic nervous system in both post-traumatic stress disorder[29] and sleep paralysis, indicate the need to investigate the prevalence of isolated sleep paralysis in patients with post-traumatic stress disorder.

CONCLUSIONS

Isolated sleep paralysis is more common in black subjects, and black subjects with sleep paralysis are more predisposed to having the least common pattern of reoccurrence—one or more episodes per month over a period of years. Because isolated sleep paralysis is a tricyclic-responsive syndrome and has features similar to panic disorder, it is strongly suspected that the two syndromes are different clinical manifestations of the same disorder. In addition, as with panic disorder, isolated sleep paralysis can be shown to have a genetic component to its etiology. The genetic locus for the two syndromes may be the same as well. This also implies different manifestations of the same disorder.

The syndrome of isolated sleep paralysis in blacks appears to be due to genetic factors with varying penetrance and due to environmental factors of stress. It remains to be seen whether isolated sleep paralysis can conclusively be shown to be due to an overaroused central adrenergic system (that was at risk because of a genetic and stressful-environmental predisposition) that is also related to the common and more severe disease of hypertension in blacks. Genuine, ethical research on blacks regarding these issues may well answer some long unanswered questions about stress, anxiety, and psychophysiologic disorders for mankind in general. It may also provide grounds for scientific discourse with black Africa.

COMMENTARY

The CMHC research team refined our research in this second article on isolated sleep paralysis and learned more about this problem within the black community. Based on the preliminary findings from the first study on states of consciousness, this time we looked for a relationship between stress and isolated sleep paralysis. Since the termination of an isolated sleep paralysis attack often occurred with a panic episode, we looked at the relationship between the stress disorder of panic disorder and isolated sleep paralysis and again struck gold. There was a significant correlation between the subjects who had a high frequency of isolated sleep paralysis and panic disorder. We looked at the issue of genetics and isolated sleep paralysis but did not have enough evidence to show the specific genetic patterns for this problem.

I realized the impact of our work when I was looking through the bible of sleep textbooks, *Principles and Practice of Sleep Medicine*, 2nd ed. (W. B. Saunders Company; 1994). In the book, Thomas Uhde's chapter, "The Anxiety Disorders," highlighted CMHCs research on the relationship between isolated sleep paralysis and panic disorder and given a quarter of a page of space! This acknowledgement is even more considerable knowing that one of the book's three editors, Dr. W. C. Dement, had poo-pooed my work years before. Needless to say, I was glad I had not listened to Dr. Dement's negative comments and was overjoyed that I had continued to feel the CMHC research team work is important.

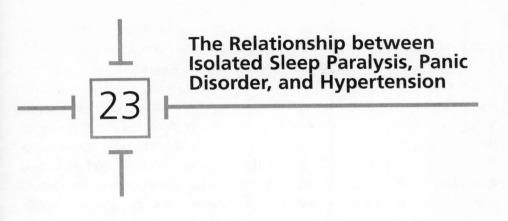

The Relationship between Isolated Sleep Paralysis, Panic Disorder, and Hypertension

23

A hypothesis is proposed that there exists a subgroup of African-American, hypertensive patients whose hypertension could have been prevented by the early detection and treatment of easily recognizable symptoms that signal the initiation of the pathophysiologic processes that lead to essential hypertension.

A pilot study of 31 patients with elevated blood pressure revealed that 41.9% had isolated sleep paralysis, 35.5% had panic attacks, and 9.7% had panic disorder. These proposed hyperadrenergic phenomena might be related to the development of hypertension in certain individuals.

INTRODUCTION

Previous studies have revealed that isolated sleep paralysis is common in African Americans[1,2] and that this altered state of consciousness[3] may indicate greater vulnerability to stress and may serve as a predisposition to developing panic disorder. After an episode of isolated sleep paralysis, an individual experiences symptoms that are produced by adrenergic stimulation (e.g., tachycardia, tremulousness, sweating, panic). The iso-

Originally printed as Bell Carl C, Hildreth Carolyn J, Jenkins Esther J, Carter Cynthia. The relationship between isolated sleep paralysis and panic disorder to hypertension. *J Natl Med Assoc.* 1988;80:289–294. Presented at the 92nd Annual Convention of the NMA, New Orleans, LA, August 1, 1987.

lated sleep paralysis appears to be caused by a dysrhythmia of the sleep/awake cycle, controlled in part by adrenergic mechanisms. This evidence suggests that adrenergic dysfunction is involved in isolated sleep paralysis.

Similarly, adrenergic dysfunction appears to be involved in the symptoms of panic disorder.[4] This hypothesis is derived from the following observations: individuals who experience panic disorder have symptoms produced by adrenergic stimulation;[5-7] pharmacologic agents such as a-adrenergic agonists, tricyclic antidepressants, and benzodiazepines, which decrease adrenergic activity in the locus ceruleus, decrease symptoms of panic;[8-10] patients with panic anxiety have increased plasma levels of 3-methoxy-4-hydroxyphenylethylene, implying increased adrenergic activity.[11]

Although the lateral tegmentum nuclei appear to be the central nervous system's adrenergic center that is specifically related to blood pressure regulation, there is evidence that the locus ceruleus complex plays a role in cardiovascular regulatory mechanisms, including activation of arterial-pressure elevating systems.[12] Further evidence indicates that blood pressure is elevated during panic attacks[5-7] and that adrenergic mechanisms may play a role in the production of both anxiety and high blood pressure. The relationship between anxiety and high blood pressure is also indicated because anti-hypertensive therapy (such as clonidine) appears to reduce blood pressure through a central nervous system mechanism and has been shown to reduce panic anxiety as well.[5,8,10,11]

Other evidence supporting the relationship between adrenergic overactivity, anxiety, and high blood pressure is seen in the example of delirium tremens. This withdrawal syndrome is produced by overactivity of the locus ceruleus, is characterized by increased blood pressure and symptoms of anxiety, and can also be treated with clonidine.[13] Thus, evidence continues to mount indicating that hypertension is indeed a psycho-physiologic disorder and that stress, anxiety, anger, and high blood pressure are related intimately.[14]

Understanding that African Americans have a disproportionate prevalence of hypertension and a disproportionate prevalence of stress[15] and that a relationship exists between these two phenomena, the authors decided to look for the presence of "stress syndromes" (specifically, isolated sleep paralysis, panic attacks, and panic disorder) in a small sample of African-American, hypertensive patients.

A review of the literature indicated that this may have been a good line of reasoning, based on a number of existing studies that make a connection between stress, isolated sleep paralysis and panic disorder;[1,2] stress and panic disorder;[16-18] and panic disorder and cardiovascular problems.[19-23] This latter group of studies is particularly instructive. For example, one study involved a six-year follow-up of 112 subjects with anxiety neurosis (panic disorder) and of 110 controls; it was demonstrated that 17% of the patients with anxiety neurosis developed hypertension, compared with 7% of the controls (significant at the $p < 0.05$ level).[22] In the same study, 19 of the 22 patients with anxiety neurosis, who later developed hypertension, developed their hypertension within two years of initiation of their anxiety symptoms.[20] Another retrospective study found that in 55 cases of panic disorder, 15% of the patients were hypertensive, compared with 9% in the adult primary care population that served as controls (significant at the $p < 0.05$ level).[21]

It appears that there may be a subset of hypertensive patients whose hypertension is heralded by the onset of panic disorder. In the previous work of Bell et al.,[1,2] subjects with isolated sleep paralysis were at risk for developing panic disorder, and it seems that blacks have a greater prevalence of isolated sleep paralysis than whites. Blacks may also have a greater prevalence of anxiety disorders than whites[24]; certainly, blacks are more often exposed to the types of stressors that would produce anxiety disorders.

Based on all these pieces of evidence, the authors decided to investigate the relationship between isolated sleep paralysis (also known as "the witch is riding you"), panic disorder, and hypertension. The hypothesis was that there exists a subset of African Americans whose hypertension began from excessive adrenergic reactivity (identifiable by the presence of isolated sleep paralysis) and who were subjected to excessive stress (resulting in the development of panic disorder) that initiated pathophysiologic cardiovascular processes that developed into essential hypertension. Further, the treatment of these readily identifiable precursors of hypertension in this subset of hypertensive patients will be discussed as a means of prevention.

METHODS

Black adult patients with known or apparent episodic hypertension were interviewed using the questionnaire developed by Bell et al.[1,2] This questionnaire defines isolated sleep paralysis for the patient and requests that patients who have experienced isolated sleep paralysis describe a typical episode to determine the validity of their report. Information was obtained about events, if any, that were perceived to precipitate an episode or prevent episodes. Information was also gathered on the duration and frequency of sleep paralysis attacks, family history of sleep paralysis, and whether family members also had a history of hypertension. Patients were then asked for a history of symptoms related to their panic attacks. *The Diagnostic and Statistical Manual of Mental Disorders*, 3rd ed. (DSM-III)[25] criteria were used.

Patients having isolated sleep paralysis and panic attacks or panic disorder as well as patients having panic attacks or panic disorder alone were felt to have readily identifiable symptoms of anxiety. These patients were informed of the authors' hypothesis that such symptoms of anxiety may be indicative of adrenergic dysfunction, which could be a cause of their hypertension. Patients were also informed that the treatment of their anxiety might, in addition to reducing their discomfort, influence the course of their hypertension.

After a discussion of the possible major side effects of treatment,[26] the patients were started on desipramine: 50 mg at bedtime, with doses increased by 50 mg at 30-day intervals until a ceiling dose of 150 mg was attained. Baseline electrocardiograms (if not present on the chart) were performed and were repeated after each increment of tricyclic antidepressant dose. Patients were interviewed about their symptoms of anxiety, and blood pressure was monitored approximately every two weeks by one of the authors, an internist.

RESULTS

Thirty-one patients were interviewed. Twenty-nine had hypertension and two had apparent episodically elevated blood pressure. Seventy-seven percent of the patients were female and 23% were male. The mean age of the patient population was 52 years old. The mean personal or family income was $6,357 per year, and the mean educational attainment was 9.7 years. Of the patients, 41.9% reported at least one episode of isolated sleep paralysis and 30.8% reported having sleep paralysis disorder, i.e., at least one episode of sleep paralysis per month. A vast majority of the patients were unable to report whether isolated sleep paralysis ran in their family; however, 64.5% reported a family history of hypertension. Of the patients reporting, 30.5% met the DSM-III criteria for panic attacks and two additional patients bordered on meeting the criteria. Three patients met the DSM-III criteria for panic disorder (i.e., at least four attacks within a four-week period), and two other patients fell slightly short of having panic attacks frequently enough to be considered panic disorder. It was found that 9.7% of the study subjects had definite criteria for panic disorder, and considering the two borderline cases, this percentage may be as high as 16.1%. Of the 13 patients with isolated sleep paralysis, three had panic disorder, one bordered on having panic disorder, two had panic attacks, and two bordered on having panic attacks. Five of the 13 denied ever having panic attacks. Of the 18 patients who denied having isolated sleep paralysis, 13 also denied having any episodes of panic attacks, four reported having panic attacks, and one almost met the criteria for having panic disorder (see Table 1).

Eight patients (25.8%) were started on desipramine. One patient dropped out early and was lost for follow-up. Another dropped out after four days of being on the medication due to intolerable side effects. Of the six others, only four were consistent with scheduled appointments for follow-up.

All of the patients reported improvement in overall wellbeing and felt that their ability to cope with stress was improved. They all noted a decreased frequency and severity of their panic attacks over the course of treatment.

One of the two patients with episodically elevated blood pressure dropped out early but showed persistent normalization of blood pressure while on desipramine. This same patient presented with a blood pressure recording of 178/90 mm Hg while having a panic attack. When the patient was started on desipramine, her blood pressure was recorded at 136/80 mm Hg. After taking 50 mg desipramine for two weeks, the next blood pressure reading was 114/76 mm Hg. Two weeks later, while still on desipramine (50 mg at bedtime), the patient was seen during another anxiety reaction, albeit less severe than the one during her first visit, and her blood pressure was recorded at 148/100 mm Hg. During this visit, the patient was started on 100 mg desipramine at bedtime, and her blood pressure was recorded at 142/72 mm Hg during her final visit two weeks later.

TABLE 23.1. Tabulation of Patients with Hypertension, Isolated Sleep Paralysis, Panic Attacks, and Panic Disorder

Patient No.	CONDITION			
	Hypertension	Sleep Paralysis	Panic Attacks	Panic Disorder
1	+	—	—	—
2	+	—	—	—
3	+	—	—	—
4	+	—	—	—
5	+	—	—	—
6	+	—	—	—
7	+	—	—	—
8	+	—	—	—
9	+	—	—	—
10	+	—	—	—
11	+	—	—	—
12	+	—	—	—
13	+	—	—	—
14	episodic	+	+	+
15	+	+	+	—
16	+	+	border	—
17	+	+	+	+
18	+	—	+	—
19	+	—	+	—
20	episodic	—	+	border
21	+	+	border	—
22	+	+	—	—
23	+	+	—	—
24	+	—	+	—
25	+	—	+	—
26	+	+	+	—
27	+	+	—	—
28	+	+	—	—
29	+	+	—	—
30	+	+	+	+
31	+	+	+	border
Total number of patients				
31	100% (N=31)	41.9% (N=13)	35.5% (N=11)	9.7% (N=3)

The other patient with episodically elevated blood pressure showed consistent normalization of her blood pressure while on tricyclic antidepressant medication treatment. Her previous blood pressure recordings were 140/90 mm Hg to 144/90 mm Hg, but during treatment of her anxiety symptoms (isolated sleep paralysis and panic disorder), she had stable normalization of her blood pressure, with a mean reading of 125/81 mm Hg. Neither of these two patients with episodically elevated blood pressure were on anti-hypertensive medications. Although symptoms of anxiety were greatly reduced for the four other patients, no pattern of improved hypertension control could be shown; their blood pressure did not vary from the level of control already obtained from their usual anti-hypertensive regimens.

DISCUSSION

The finding that 41.9% of 31 patients with hypertension had isolated sleep paralysis can be compared with previous findings that 41% of 108 randomly sampled, healthy, anxious, and post-psychotic subjects had sleep paralysis[1] and that 51.6% of 64 family members had isolated sleep paralysis.[2] Both the current study and the previous two studies report a significantly higher prevalence of isolated sleep paralysis than a recent study performed in Nigeria, in which 164 medical students were reported to have a prevalence of 26.1%.[27]

The reasons for this discrepancy are several. First, the demographics of the four groups differed significantly; the ages and socioeconomic status of the Nigerian and African-American subjects studied were not similar. Secondly, the previous studies on African-American subjects indicated that isolated sleep paralysis might be related to stress.[1,2] Perhaps living in an all-black context such as in Nigeria is less stress-provoking than living in a racist, predominantly white society. Thirdly, while the prevalence of isolated sleep paralysis in the control subjects did not significantly differ from that in the anxious and post-psychotic subjects in the random survey, that population was still weighted heavily with psychiatric subjects. This may account for the greater prevalence of isolated sleep paralysis when compared with the Nigerian sample. Similarly, because isolated sleep paralysis does seem to run in families, the family members studied may have been more predisposed to developing isolated sleep paralysis than the Nigerian population. Finally, the Nigerian population may be less prone to adrenergic dysfunction than the African-American populations. Evidence for this may be gleaned from the considerable difference in the reports of a family history of hypertension. The hypertensive patients reported that 64.6% of their family members also had hypertension, and the family studied had a history of hypertension; only 19% of the Nigerian medical students reported a family history of hypertension.[27] In an earlier study using telephone interviews, 84% of the subjects with isolated sleep paralysis reported a family history of hypertension.[2]

The current study was similar to the family and telephone interview study[2] in that it also found a significant relationship between the presence of isolated sleep paralysis and the presence of panic attacks (x^2 [1] = 4.91, p < 0.05). In addition, all of the hypertensive patients in the current study who had panic disorder also had isolated sleep paralysis. This is comparable to the family study, in which all of the patients with panic disorder also had isolated sleep paralysis.[2] Only one hypertensive patient who denied having isolated sleep paralysis came close to having panic attacks frequently enough to qualify for a diagnosis of panic disorder. This was also similar to the finding that of the family members who denied having isolated sleep paralysis, none had panic disorder.[2] In comparing the hypertensive patients with isolated sleep paralysis patients and other subjects with sleep paralysis,[2] it was found that the frequency of having isolated sleep paralysis disorder (i.e., one or more episode of isolated sleep paralysis per month) was not significantly different (see Table 2).

The two patients having episodic hypertension and panic attacks (one with panic disorder and the other borderline on meeting the criteria of panic disorder) may be future members of the proposed subset of African-American patients who developed fixed essential hypertension secondary to the development of panic disorder. Of interest is that desipramine seemed to normalize their episodic hypertension. It may be that through early intervention, these patients with panic symptoms can be prevented from developing permanent essential hypertension. The four patients who had histories of long-standing, essential hypertension did not have any better control of their hypertension with the addition of desipramine to their anti-hypertensive regimen. This supports the hypothesis that once the pathophysiology of essential hypertension is permanently set in place by the adrenergic mechanisms responsible for the panic symptoms, the damage has been done; the condition can no longer be prevented but only controlled.

TABLE 23.2. Comparison of Previous Studies on Isolated Sleep Paralysis

Studies	Sleep Paral. % (No./Tot.)	Fam. Hist. Hyptens. % (No./Tot.)	Sleep Paral. Dis. * % (No./Tot.)	Panic Dis.* % (No./Tot.)	Hyptens.* % (No./Tot.)
States of consciousness study[1] (N=108)	41.0 (44/108)	?	27.3 (12/44)	?	?
Telephone interview study[2] (N=25)	100 (25/25)	84.0 (21/25)	48.0 (12/25)	16.0 (4/25)	32.0 (21/25)
Family study[2] (N=64)	51.6 (33/64)	100 (64/64)	27.3 (9/33)	15.2 (5/33)	24.2 (8/33)
Nigerian study[27] (N=164)	26.1 (43/164)	18.9 (31/164)	?	?	2.3 (1/43)
Hypertensive patient study (N=31)	41/9 (13/31)	64.6 (20/31)	30.8 (4/13) 38.5 (5/13)**	23.1 (3/13)	100 (13/13)

*These percentages, numbers, and totals refer only to those subjects who had isolated sleep paralysis in the study.
**This percentage and number includes those two patients who bordered on meeting the criteria for panic disorder.

Whether the relationships between isolated sleep paralysis, panic attacks, panic disorder, and hypertension are causal, associational, or simply accidental, is too complex to determine from this pilot study. Perhaps the hypertensive patient sample rather than the general population has a greater prevalence of isolated sleep paralysis and panic disorder because the somatic symptoms associated with these phenomena would lead hypertensive patients to a primary care physician's office.[28,29] There may also be, however, a subset of hypertensive patients whose hypertension's etiology is a previously existing adrenergic dysfunction that produces isolated sleep paralysis, panic attacks, and panic disorder. Only larger, well controlled, and better-designed studies will tell.

CONCLUSIONS

Isolated sleep paralysis, panic attacks, and panic disorders are prevalent in African-American, hypertensive patients. Hypertensive patients with isolated sleep paralysis were more likely to have panic attacks than were hypertensive patients without isolated sleep paralysis. These findings matched previous studies on isolated sleep paralysis in African Americans.

Perhaps a role exists for the evaluation and treatment of patients with tricyclic antidepressants (such as desipramine) who have marked elevations of blood pressure in response to anxiety manifested by frequent episodes of isolated sleep paralysis and panic attacks. Such treatment might prevent the future development of sustained high blood pressure. Would it be productive to screen hypertensive patients for stress indicators like those explored in this study? Should a physician choose a centrally acting anti-hypertensive agent to treat such patients? The presence of stress factors might imply a central adrenergic dysfunction that may also be of etiologic significance in the patients' hypertension.

COMMENTARY

Because stress and hypertension have been closely associated within the African-American community, we decided to explore the connection between isolated sleep paralysis and hypertension in our third study. We received a great deal of help from an African-American internist, Dr. Carolyn Hildreth, who collaborated with the CMHC research team on the project. Unfortunately, we didn't get enough specific information to draw a solid conclusion about whether there was a strong relationship. This issue still needs further exploration.

CMHC's research has been replicated by a group of independent researchers in New York (Friedman S, Paradis CM, Hatch M. Characteristics of African-American and white patients with panic disorder and agoraphobia. *Hosp and Community Psychiatry*. 1994;45:798–803). Their results are essentially the same as those found by CMHC's research team: "although

African-American and white patients show similar symptoms of panic disorder, African-American patients had more unnecessary psychiatric hospitalizations, a higher rate of medical emergency room visits, *a higher incidence of isolated sleep paralysis* [italics added], greater likelihood of childhood trauma, and a greater number of life stressors." This same research group published another article on the prevalence of isolated sleep paralysis in African Americans with panic disorder that supported our original work (Paradis CM, Friedman S, Hatch MJ. Isolated sleep paralysis in African-Americans with panic disorder. *J Cultural Diversity and Mental Health*. 1995;3:69–76). Dr. Angela Neal and some of her colleagues have further investigated the relationship between panic disorder and hypertension in African Americans (Neal AM, Rich LN, Smucker WD. The presence of panic disorder among African-American hypertensives: a pilot study. *J Black Psychology*. 1994;20:29–35). They have found support for a relationship between the two phenomena, which strengthens the proof that stress is related to hypertension in African Americans. I came across an article that supported CMHC's observation that hypertension and panic attacks were related (Davies SJC, Ghahramani P, Jackson PR, Noble TW, Hardy PG, Hippisley-Cox J, Yeo WW, Ramsay LE. Association of panic disorder and panic attacks with hypertension. *Am J Med*. 1999;107:310–316). The study found that panic attacks were significantly greater in primary care patients with hypertension (17%, $p < 0.05$) and in hospital-based hypertensive patients (19%, $p < 0.01$) than in normotensive patients (11%).

When I was appointed to the Planning Boards for Dr. David Satcher's *Surgeon General's Report on Mental Health: Culture, Race, and Ethnicity* (published 2001, see www.surgeongeneral.gov), I had to work really hard to get isolated sleep paralysis into the report. In my mind, our work on isolated sleep paralysis met the criteria of being evidence-based—a criteria to be included in any Surgeon General's reports, as our findings had been replicated by two independent researchers. Even though the states of consciousness approach developed by our African-American research team had yielded some important fruit for the black community, our work wasn't as well known since we'd published it in the JNMA. I recently discovered that a European-American sleep researcher has received funding to study isolated sleep paralysis in African Americans, and I'm very interested in what his research findings will be.

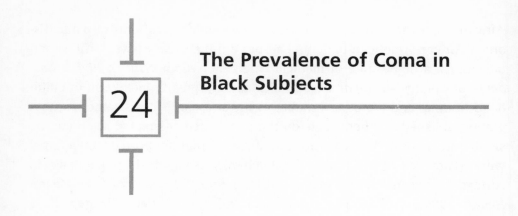

The Prevalence of Coma in Black Subjects

24

Coma, commonly known as "being unconscious" or "out cold," is a state of consciousness characterized by a total inability to perceive incoming stimuli. A retrospective phenomenologic study found that 10 of 36 control, 19 of 36 pre-care, and 20 of 36 after-care subjects (49 of 108, or 45.4%) had experienced coma at least once during their lives. The implications of these findings are discussed.

INTRODUCTION

Coma, or loss of consciousness, is considered one of 18 states of consciousness (the others being dreaming, deep sleep, sleep paralysis, daydreaming, repressed memory, trance, meditation, internal scanning, regression, fragmentation, lethargy, hyperalertness, frenzy, rapture, intoxication, expanded consciousness, and normal waking state)[1] that signal the possibility of a serious neurologic event that may result in neuropsychological impairment. The etiology of coma may be alcohol, epilepsy, infection, opium and other drugs, uremia, trauma, insulin (too much or too little),

Originally printed as Bell Carl C, Thompson Belinda, Shorter-Gooden Kumea, Shakoor Bambade, Dew Donald, Hughley Eugene, Mays Raymond. Prevalence of episodes of coma in black subjects. *J Natl Med Assoc.* 1985;77:391–395.

poison, or shock. These etiologies may be remembered with the help of the mnemonic AEIOU TIPS.

In response to the lack of basic psychiatric knowledge on black populations, the CMHC in Chicago began a research project to qualify and quantify the states of consciousness as experienced by blacks. Three groups were chosen for study: control subjects who had never suffered mental illness, pre-care subjects who had been treated for mental illness only as outpatients, aftercare subjects who had received both outpatient and inpatient treatment for mental illness. This paper focuses on the subjects' reports of their experience with coma.

METHODS

Thirty-six patients from each of CMHC's pre-care and aftercare programs were selected at random to participate in the project. Thirty-six control subjects were selected from the research team's nominations of individuals known to them personally. A structured interview was designed in which a trained interviewer read the definition of coma and gave examples to the 108 total research subjects. The subjects were asked to decide whether they had experienced this state of consciousness and if so, to tell the interviewer about it. Subjects who had not experienced coma were asked whether they had ever heard of it or knew someone who had experienced it. This part of the questionnaire was designed to ensure that the subjects understood the nature of coma and that their reported experience matched the definition given. Once it was established that the subject had experienced the defined state, a standard series of questions was asked to determine whether the state of coma could be self-induced or self-terminated, whether it could be induced or terminated by others, and whether the subject had any control over it. Subjects were asked if they wanted to experience the state more often and to explain why or why not. They were asked how often coma occurred and how long it lasted. They were asked whether coma made them comfortable or uncomfortable, and how; whether it ever got them into trouble or difficulty, and how; and whether it ever helped them to cope, and how. Subjects were asked if their experience with coma had changed with age and if so, how. They were also asked about their experience with other states of consciousness. The interviews were audio taped and reviewed by the principal investigator to check for interviewing technique consistency and for validity of the subjects' reports.

Subjects were also given objective written tests: Holmes-Rahe Social Readjustment Scale, Saafir Stress-Anxiety Diagnostic Scale, Millon Clinical Multiaxial Inventory. Demographic data were collected.

RESULTS

Of the 108 subjects, 49 (45.4%) reported having experienced at least one state of coma. Of these 49, there were 10 controls, 19 pre-care subjects, and 20 aftercare subjects (27.8%, 52.8%, and 55.6%, respectively). Trauma accounted for 37 of the 49 reported episodes. Accounting for the remaining twelve episodes were six reports of infection; three reports of drug overdose; and one report each of nearly drowning, diabetic coma, and pain from sickle cell crisis (see Table 1). Unconsciousness resulting from surgery was excluded when examining the causes of coma. Sixteen subjects had lost consciousness because of non-surgical coma more than once; however, the findings in Table 1 indicate only the most severe episode of coma experienced by each subject. One of the control subjects had an episode of trauma that resulted in a mild coma in childhood. Ten of the pre-care subjects experienced their coma in childhood: five episodes were mild, lasting less than 30 minutes; four were moderate, lasting more than 30 minutes but less than 24 hours; one was of unknown duration. Eight of the aftercare subjects had had a state of coma during childhood: three episodes were mild, three were moderate, and two were severe, lasting more than 24 hours.

Eighteen of the 49 subjects (36.7%) reported having had a mild coma (lasting less than 30 minutes). Eighteen of the 49 subjects (36.7%) reported having had a coma of moderate severity (lasting more than 30 minutes but less than 24 hours). Seven of the 49 subjects (14.3%) reported having had a severe coma (lasting more than 24 hours). Six subjects (12.2%) did not know the duration of their loss of consciousness.

Of the 59 subjects who had never experienced "non-surgical coma," 19 had experienced surgical events in which anesthesia induced the coma. If anesthesia-induced unconsciousness were considered a form of coma, it would bring the total number of subjects that experienced at least one episode of coma to 68, or 73%. In all, 32 of the 108 total subjects had experienced surgery that called for the induction of a "controlled coma."

Of the total test subjects, 52 were men and 56 were women. The average age was 31.3 years and the average educational level was 13.8

TABLE 24.1. Causes of Subjects' Longest Episode of "Nonsurgical Coma"

Type of Coma	Control (N=10) No.	Pre-care (N=19) No.	Aftercare (N=20) No.
Mild (<30 min.)			
Trauma	—	—	2
Interpersonal trauma	1	1	1
Sports trauma	2	1	—
Childhood trauma	1	4	2
Interpersonal childhood trauma	—	1	—
Drugs	—	1	—
Childhood diabetes	—	—	1
Moderate (30 min.–24 hrs.)			
Trauma	—	1	2
Interpersonal trauma	1	1	—
Sports trauma	1	—	—
Childhood trauma	—	2	3
Interpersonal childhood trauma	—	1	—
Near drowning	1	—	—
Pain	1	—	—
Infection	—	—	2
Childhood infection	—	1	—
Drugs	—	—	1
Severe (>24 hr)			
Trauma	—	1	1
Childhood trauma	—	—	1
Interpersonal childhood trauma	—	—	1
Infection	1	2	—
Duration unknown			
Trauma	—	—	2
Interpersonal trauma	1	—	1
Childhood trauma	—	1	—
Drugs	—	1	—

years. Twenty-three subjects were living with spouses (21.3%). There were 23 male (64%) control subjects, 14 male (39%) pre-care subjects, and 15 male (42%) aftercare subjects. The average age in all three groups was early 30s. For average number of years of formal education, the controls had 15.4, the pre-care subjects had 13.6, and the aftercare subjects had 12.5. Of the control subjects, 41.7% were living with a spouse, compared with 5.6% of the pre-care sample and 11.1% of the aftercare sample. Of the subjects who had experienced coma, nine of the ten controls were male, 10 of the 19 pre-care subjects were male, and 10 of the 20 aftercare subjects were male.

The findings of the objective tests are reported in an earlier article on sleep paralysis[2] (see Chapter 21). Additional reports will be forthcoming on the other states of consciousness; a more detailed analysis of the objective tests and their relationship to the states of consciousness; and the use of altering states of consciousness to master stress.[3]

DISCUSSION

States of coma occurred in this cohort at a rate of 45.4%—an extremely high rate of exposure to a potentially serious neurologic event that can have serious implications for neuropsychological impairment. Thirty-seven of the comas (75.5%) were due to trauma or concussion, i.e., head injury severe enough to cause a loss of consciousness. Concussion has been known to cause post-concussion syndrome (objectively identifiable on electroencephalogram with somnographic patterns in nocturnal sleep[4]), which may consist of various somatic sequelae such as headache, dizziness, nausea, and vasomotor instability causing hyperhidrosis.[5] It has been stated, however, that "the most consistent consequence of a head injury is some disorder of mental functioning, either temporary or permanent."[6] After a concussion of moderate severity, there is measurable impairment of cognitive functioning attributed to fatigue, inattention, and defects in rapid information processing.[7] Patients may complain of memory and concentration difficulties. Psychological symptoms of anxiety, fear, insomnia, restlessness, fatigue, nervousness, and depression have also been described.[8] Clinicians have noted the following: personality changes like reduced drive, or apathy; affective changes of euphoria, irritability, lability, or blunted affect; a decrease in the ability to adapt and cope with new environmental stress; a decrease in social restraint and judgment; and exaggeration or reversal of personality traits. After a more severe injury, associated with coma of some hours' duration, the patient may be in a state of fragmentation (disordered consciousness or psychosis) for many hours or days. As 16 of the 49 subjects reported having had at least one moderate or severe concussion, this neurologic event may have altered their lives. One study found that severe behavioral and aggressive disorders in children and adolescents were related to serious craniofacial trauma.[9] The episodes of childhood coma in the present study's sample was 17.6% (1% in the control subjects and 16.6% in the psychiatric pre-care and after-care subjects). Coma in childhood may have etiologic significance for the development of psychiatric disorders in later life, or it may have an associational rather than causal correlation.

Ten of the 49 subjects had been the victims of interpersonal violence that resulted in coma. Of 702 patients admitted for head injuries over a one-year period to Cook County Hospital, Chicago, interpersonal injuries accounted for the majority of the injuries to adults (55.7%).[10] Of this sample, 77.6% were black, 80% were male, and 70% had an annual income below $6,000. Fatal injuries were reported for 2.4% of the sample.[10] Severe spouse beatings occur in about 5% of US households and may have greater incidence in black households.[11]

There is some evidence that cerebral insult resulting in unconsciousness or neuropsychological impairment may be partly responsible for interpersonal violence. A study of 130 violent patients found that 55.4% had been unconscious because of injury or illness.[12] Researchers hypothesized that some of the difficulties of many of the patients were the result of minimal brain damage.[12] This hypothesis is supported by the findings of Dr. R. Langevin, who reported to the Canadian Psychiatric Association that one fourth to one third of violent offenders had neuropsychological impairment, compared with nonviolent offenders who had none. The finding that 45.4% of this population had experienced at least one state of coma during their lives and the association of states of coma with violent individuals may better help to understand the high incidence of black-on-black violence.

The relation between coma and violence may be of considerable importance in understanding murders, a vast majority of which are "crimes of rage" or "crimes of passion," involving acquaintances or relatives. These crimes, classified as primary homicides, were responsible for 75% of all murders in the US from 1976 to 1979.[13] These homicides were overwhelmingly intraracial, specifically, between blacks. Currently, homicide is the leading cause of death of black men aged 15–44 and may account for up to one third of all the deaths of black men in this age range. Clearly, an environment that produces a high occurrence of coma resulting from traumatic incidents and other factors must be changed, since these incidents may result from violence and neglect, which cause more violence and neglect. Rather than collect FBI and police "body count" statistics on the number of black-on-black murders, there must be a positive intervention in this vicious cycle. Various governmental agencies must be mandated to observe patients with head injury and provide them with adequate follow-up services to prevent their being continued victims of head injury. Rose[14] demonstrated that there were 80% of black homicide offenders compared to 47% of victims with histories of episodic fighting. Dennis et al.[15] demonstrated in a study of black homicide that offenders and assault victims (proxies for homicide victims) engaged in fighting at a much higher rate than the controls of their population. The authors of this paper hypothesize that the early identification of black individuals presenting to emergency rooms with concussion from black interpersonal violence could help individuals benefit from prevention services designed to combat black-on-black murder. For example, a black woman presenting to the emergency room with a concussion from spousal abuse could engage in family counseling for her family. Such therapeutic counseling might curb future spousal abuse that could have resulted in black-on-black murder.

Twenty-nine of the 49 subjects were male (59.2%) and 20 were female (40.8%). Control males experienced at least one episode of coma at a rate of 39.1%, whereas pre-care males and aftercare males experienced coma at a rate of 71.4% and 66.7%, respectively. Control females had states of coma at a rate of 7.7%, compared with pre-care females who had it at a rate of 45.5% and aftercare females at a rate of 47.6%. Twice as many men as women may present to emergency rooms for treatment of head injuries[6]; it is suspected, therefore, that the variance in number between men and women in the study groups is caused by lifestyle differences related to sex. Psychiatric male subjects (pre-care and aftercare) had experienced coma (51.3%) at a greater rate than the non-psychiatric male subjects (39.1%). More than five times the female psychiatric subjects

(44.2%) than non-psychiatric women (7.7%) had experienced coma. These findings may be caused by a number of variables, such as the small size of the population, causing skewing of the results; educational differences between the groups; or the significance that episodes of coma may have in the etiology of psychiatric disorders. More investigation on larger populations controlled for age, sex, education, and socioeconomic status is warranted to further delineate the problem.

It may well be that, depending on the circumstances, a coma will seriously influence the development of an individual's narcissistic personality components, because unconsciousness challenges feelings of grandiosity and omnipotence; an extreme sense of vulnerability also remains and may be handled in a constructive or destructive manner.[16,17] The psychological response of the black individual and the black community regarding the high frequency of coma in black subjects, psychiatric and non-psychiatric, must be considered. The response has primarily been fear or denial. The time has come for the black community to honestly face the problem and hold itself and society accountable for finding the solution.

CONCLUSIONS

The finding that 27.8% of the control, 52.8% of the pre-care, and 55.6% of the aftercare subjects (45.4% of the total study population of 108) experienced at least one state of coma is an indication that coma may be a common occurrence in the black population, both psychiatric and non-psychiatric. Furthermore, 75.7% of the reported comas were caused by trauma or concussion, and 20.4% had been caused by interpersonal injury. This data is consistent with the findings from two inner-city studies describing clinical head injuries, for which interpersonal violence was often responsible (49.7% in one study[10] and 37% in the other[18]). This information, along with the finding that explosive rage may appear in a previously normal subject after head trauma or other cerebral insults,[19] demands further investigation in the etiology of black-on-black violence, a national public health problem.

The finding that the two types of psychiatric patients, pre-care, and aftercare, had experienced nearly twice as many states of coma as controls leads to questions about the role of coma in the etiology of psychiatric states in blacks. Follow-up of patients who have received immediate medical attention for states of coma is essential; it may aid in the prevention of black-on-black violence and reduce the morbidity of post-concussion syndrome.

The high number of "nonsurgical coma," childhood coma, and surgical events necessitating anesthetics to induce a "controlled coma" are indications of the large amount of violence, trauma, and illness in the black population examined. The facts suggest a sad statement about the quality of life of some black populations, psychiatric and non-psychiatric. More must be done to aid these populations.

COMMENTARY

Our states of consciousness research yielded interesting findings about isolated sleep paralysis in African Americans, but we also learned something intriguing about states of coma in our population. To our surprise, we found that many of our subjects reported physical trauma that caused them a loss of consciousness. We were surprised at the amount of surgery our population had undergone as well. Our observations of our African-American population revealed a great deal of exposure to incidents—frequently head injury—that could compromise neurologic functioning. I became interested in coma while examining the relationship between head injury and personality changes. In addition, because of my earlier interest in violence (see Chapter 10), and because of the possibility of head injury being a factor in causing violence, I became even more interested in the topic. This interest led me to review the literature and publish parts one and two of "Coma and the Etiology of Violence" (see Chapters 11 and 12). I also published a guest editorial entitled "Neuropsychiatry and Gun Safety" (*J Neuropsychiatry*. May 1990).

With the help of Dr. Ihsan Salloum, a psychiatric resident from the Chicago Medical School, the CMHC research team continued our investigations of head injury in an African-American psychiatric population. While doing his outpatient psychiatric training at the CMHC, Dr. Salloum constituted a research team to explore how a head injury influenced the treatment of psychiatric patients (Treatment compliance and hostility levels of head-injured psychiatric outpatients. *J Natl Med Assoc.* August 1990). Head-injured patients were more likely to experience difficulties in their interpersonal relationship with their therapists compared to non-head-injured patients. The head-injured group had higher hostility scores, although the difference did not reach significance.

Considering the levels of violence within some African-American communities, there is still a great deal to be discovered in this investigation. Our work in this area wasn't very sophisticated; yet, it uncovered a significant problem that needs more study. My only hope is that someone reading this book will pick up the gauntlet and do this area of research more justice than we were able with our limited resources.

Section Five

CULTURAL SENSITIVITY

AND

RACISM

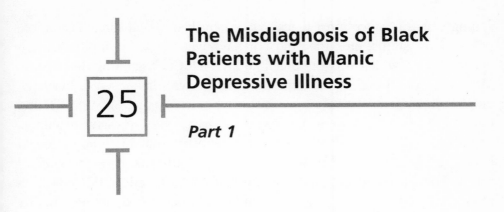

The Misdiagnosis of Black Patients with Manic Depressive Illness

Part 1

It has been shown repeatedly that, contrary to earlier beliefs, blacks may well demonstrate similar prevalence rates for manic depressive illness as whites. Yet, the authors believe that black manic depressive patients are frequently misdiagnosed as being chronic undifferentiated schizophrenics and are treated with major tranquilizers, when lithium is the drug of choice. This contention is supported by three case histories and some institutional dynamics that cause this form of iatrogenic morbidity to continue preying upon black psychiatric patients.

INTRODUCTION

It has been repeatedly reported that blacks have lower rates of affective disorders when compared with whites. According to Thomas and Sillen, earlier reports by those such as Babcock (1895), O'Malley (1914), Green (1914), and Bevis (1921), attributed this finding to blacks' state of primitive mentality.[1] In the 1960s, several studies also reported racial differences, with respect to the incidence of affective illness; the etiology of these differences was then attributed to psychodynamic theory. The rea-

Originally printed as Bell Carl C, Mehta Harshad. The misdiagnosis of black patients with manic depressive illness. *J Natl Med Assoc.* 1980;72:141–145.

soning was that since most blacks were deprived of self-esteem, material possessions, status, etc., they did not have what was required to experience a "loss," which was the precipitating factor to triggering depression. Malzberg[2] found that manic depressive illness was diagnosed in blacks at one-fourth the rate it was diagnosed in whites. Prange and Vitols found that only 1% of blacks were diagnosed with psychotic depressive reactions, compared with 4.3% of whites.[3] Jaco reported that his study showed blacks having affective disorders at one-seventh the rate of whites.[4] Johnson et al. could not find one case of a black patient diagnosed as manic depressive during three years of admissions at Bellevue Psychiatric Hospital.[5]

In diagnosing schizophrenia, there again appears to be racial differences, with blacks exhibiting a higher rate. Favis and Dunham report a 25% higher rate among blacks.[6] Frumkin[7] and Malzberg[2] both reported that black patients received a diagnosis of schizophrenia on first admission over two times more than white patients. Taube,[8] at the National Institute of Mental Health (NIMH), found that blacks have over a 65% higher rate than whites.

While there have been several attempts to demonstrate that these diagnostic differences tend to reflect a subtle form of institutionalized racism, the lack of recognition that blacks seem to have as high a rate of affective illness as whites continues. Simon et al. pointed out, "This hesitancy to diagnose blacks as affectively ill is more than compensated for by a strong tendency to diagnose blacks as schizophrenic more frequently than whites."[9] This study demonstrated that the hospital diagnosis strongly correlated with race; a diagnosis of schizophrenia rather than affective illness was given more frequently to blacks than to whites. When the project's personnel made independent diagnoses, however, race and diagnosis were not found to be related. This is consistent with Helzer's finding that the clinical and familial expression of bipolar affective illness is similar in both white and black men (with the exception of a greater degree of alcoholism in paternal relatives of black men).[10] In 1976, Cannon and Locke[11] of NIMH reported that the tendency toward diagnostic confusion in the treatment of black patients continues at an alarming rate.

The purpose of this paper is to demonstrate that black manic depressive patients are still frequently misdiagnosed in 1979. This paper will also outline some of the institutional forces that cause this harmful carelessness to continue. While statistical data are presently incomplete, the use of individual cases adequately indicates the alarming degree of iatrogenic morbidity caused by diagnostic haphazardness.

BACKGROUND

The mental health system in Illinois is a fairly standard system in that the state is regionalized, i.e., set up into specific target areas to be serviced by specific state institutions. Region 2 is one such region, composed of Chicago and several surrounding counties. Region 2 is divided into 53 planning areas with one or more making up eight sub-regions. Sub-region 12, on the Southside of Chicago, has a target population of 700,000 and is composed of six planning areas consisting of South Shore, Chatham Avalon, Roseland, Southwest, Southeast, and Beverly Morgan. The first four areas are primarily inhabited by black residents, with 25% of the population on welfare in each area. Patients of Sub-region 12 are served by Tinley Park Hospital, which has a total of 220 total adult psychiatric beds. Tinley Park also serves two other sub-regions and as a result, 220 psychiatric beds serve a target population of three million. The beds utilized by patients of Sub-region 12 range between 110 and 140 of the 220 "first come-first served" state hospital beds. Sub-region 12 has six outpatient psychiatric clinics whose target population lives in the six planning areas comprising Sub-region 12. Five clinics are operated by Chicago's Department of Mental Health and one by Jackson Park Hospital, a general medical hospital. The state aids Jackson Park in maintaining an additional 14–21-day-stay unit with 14 beds.[12]

Patients who develop psychotic illness in Sub-region 12 either enter the state hospital system via the intake center at Tinley Park or are serviced at Jackson Park's 24-hour Psychiatric Emergency Service, where patients are hospitalized in a private facility, referred for hospitalization at Tinley Park, or treated in the crisis intervention program. The average stay at Tinley Park is two to three weeks, which is about the same at Jackson Park. On discharge, patients are referred for aftercare treatment at one of the six outpatient clinics. The focus of treatment at both Jackson Park and Tinley Park tends to be the medical management of acute psychotic episodes. This continues on an outpatient basis at the various outpatient clinics with additional work on the patients' social and interpersonal environment. As a result of the focus on medical management, a clear differentiation between manic depressive illness and schizophrenia is essential. Unfortunately, as already noted, blacks tend to receive more than their share of schizophrenic diagnoses.

Tinley Park has statistics only regarding whether patients are diagnosed as mentally ill or developmentally disabled. As a result, it is quite difficult to demonstrate hard data on the percentage of patients diagnosed as manic depressive or schizophrenic. However, the authors have been struck by the many black patients with manic depressive illness being misdiagnosed as being chronic undifferentiated schizophrenics. Because this could not be supported by State of Illinois diagnostic statistics, the authors decided to examine case histories of Jackson Park's outpatient clinic patients who had been diagnosed and treated as manic depressives.

CASE HISTORIES

Case 1

Mrs. A, a 70-year-old black female, was first hospitalized in 1970 at Tinley Park Mental Health Center (TPMHC) with clinical findings of flight of ideas, hyperactivity, confusion, excessive talking, and paranoia. She was diagnosed with manic depressive illness and was discharged on chlorpromazine 200 mg twice a day. She functioned optimally until about six months later, when she was re-hospitalized at TPMHC with a history of combativeness, hyperactivity, confusion, paranoid thinking, irritability, accelerated rate of speech, and grandiose ideations. At this time, a diagnosis of schizophrenia, schizoaffective type, was made and the patient was treated with amitriptyline 25 mg three times a day. Twelve days later with remission of symptomatology, Mrs. A was discharged to a community mental health clinic for follow-up. Remission continued for four months.

During October 1971, she was re-hospitalized for nine days at TPMHC with confusion, hallucinations, delusions, verbosity, incoherence, and circumstantiality. A diagnosis of schizophrenia, chronic undifferentiated type, was made and the patient was discharged to a community mental health clinic on chlorpromazine 300 mg three times a day and trifluoperazine 15 mg twice a day. The fourth hospitalization occurred eleven months later due to a history of paranoid implications, hostility, loose associations, and fragmented thought processes. At this time, a diagnosis of anxiety neurosis was made and the patient was treated with amitriptyline 25 mg three times a day. A year later, she was re-hospitalized the fifth time for follow-up. Remission continued for 22 days with a diagnosis of alcoholism and cerebral atherosclerosis. Clinical findings at this time were arrest for misdemeanor charges, irritability, grandiosity, and hyperactivity. Again, she was discharged to a local clinic for follow-up while on chlorpromazine 50 mg twice a day and trihexyphenidyl 2 mg daily. Ten weeks later, she was re-hospitalized for four weeks with a diagnosis of acute psychotic episode associated with alcoholism and with clinical findings of bizarre behavior, making phone calls at all hours day and night, hostility, and uncooperativeness. She was treated with fluphenazine enanthate 25 mg intramuscularly and benztropine mesylate 2 mg daily.

The seventh hospitalization occurred four months later during May 1974 due to agitation, elation, disturbing behavior, and flighty speech. The diagnosis of manic depressive illness was made and she was treated with fluphenazine decanoate 25 mg intramuscularly every two weeks. This time, the remission of her illness continued for two years later, when she was re-hospitalized in April 1976 with a history of shoplifting, hyperactivity, confusion, talkativeness, flight of ideas, delusions, and hallucinations. She was discharged after 23 days on no medication, with a diagnosis of schizophrenia, chronic undifferentiated type. A year later, she was re-hospitalized for one week, with disorderly conduct, agitation, hyperactivity, confusion, disorganized verbal output, and irritability. The diagnosis of manic depressive illness was made, and she was treated with lithium carbonate 300 mg three times a day (her first treatment with lithium) and haloperidol 5 mg three times a day.

Currently, the patient has been followed at Jackson Park's outpatient clinic for over two years while on lithium carbonate and supportive psychotherapy. Although there have been a few episodes of hypomania and depression, she has been successfully maintained on lithium and has been able to avoid further hospitalizations. Currently, Mrs. A enjoys complete remission of symptomatology, has stable interpersonal relationships, and is living independently.

Case 2

Mrs. B is a 30-year-old black female who was first hospitalized at TPMHC at the age of 21 in 1970 with a history of agitation, excitability, disrobing herself, pressured speech, talkativeness, ideas of reference, and uncooperativeness. She was diagnosed as schizophrenic, chronic undifferentiated type, and was discharged after four weeks on chlorpromazine 100 mg four times a day, trifluoperazine 5 mg twice a day, and benztropine mesylate 2 mg twice a day. In 1973, she was re-hospitalized with a diagnosis of schizophrenia, chronic undifferentiated type. At this time, she had religious preoccupation, ran from house to house, was agitated, irritable, and delusional. She was treated with thiothixene 5 mg and trifluoperazine 5 mg, both three times a day, and trihexyphenidyl 2 mg twice a day.

The third hospitalization occurred two years later in 1975 when she was hospitalized for seven days with a diagnosis of schizophrenia, paranoid type. This time she had religious preoccupation (stating "I have the Holy Spirit in me"), grandiosity, agitation, insomnia, psychomotor excitation, irritability, euphoria, and talkativeness. She was discharged on fluphenazine decanoate 25 mg intramuscularly every ten days and thioridazine 200 mg twice a day. The fourth hospitalization occurred two years later in 1977, with a diagnosis of schizophrenia, paranoid type. The patient had pressured speech, irritability, religious preoccupation, elated mood, delusions, and paranoid ideation. She was discharged on haloperidol 5 mg three times a day. Nine months later, she was re-hospitalized for a fifth time with a diagnosis of schizophrenia, chronic undifferentiated type. Clinical findings included wandering in the street, laughing and talking constantly, sexual preoccupation, insomnia, pressured speech, hallucinations, and delusions.

The sixth hospitalization occurred six months later, and the patient was diagnosed as having schizoaffective illness because she displayed delusions, agitation, and restlessness. She was treated with haloperidol 10 mg three times a day and discharged nine days later with complete remission of symptoms. Since her fifth hospitalization, the patient had been followed regularly at Jackson Park's outpatient clinic on lithium carbonate four times a day and supportive psychotherapy. She had done so well that she dropped out of treatment, resulting in the sixth hospitalization. Since that hospitalization, she has remained symptom free, exhibited good interpersonal relationships, and failed to exhibit deterioration in personality. She is quite pleased with the lithium because it calms her down and keeps her from getting too excited and yet does not sedate like the major tranquilizers she had been given in the past.

Case 3

Mrs. C is a 28-year-old black female who was first hospitalized at TPMHC during December 1972 at the age of 20 with a diagnosis of schizophrenia, schizoaffective type, depressed. At that time the clinical findings were irrelevant speech, disorganized thought processes, and cooperative. She was discharged on thioridazine 100 mg twice a day, imipramine hydrochloride 50 mg three times a day. The next hospitalization took place in August 1975 for seven weeks, when she was diagnosed as having schizophrenic reaction. She was treated with fluphenazine decanoate 25 mg intramuscularly every two weeks, chlorpromazine 200 mg three times a day, trifluoperazine 5 mg twice a day, trihexyphenidyl 2 mg twice a day. Her clinical picture at this time was described as including psychomotor agitation, auditory hallucinations, and visual hallucinations. Ten months later, she was hospitalized for a third time with a history of depressed mood, slow responses, auditory hallucinations, and confused thinking, with a diagnosis of schizophrenia, chronic undifferentiated type being made. She was discharged after seven days on fluphenazine decanoate 25 mg intramuscularly, and thioridazine 50 mg in the morning and 100 mg at bedtime.

The fourth hospitalization took place eight months later in February 1977, when she was given a diagnosis of schizophrenia, chronic undifferentiated type. She was hospitalized this time for calling the police, neglecting her children, and agitation. She was treated with chlorpromazine 100 mg twice a day. Following her last hospitalization, Mrs. C came to the Jackson Park clinic with irritability, flight of ideas, insomnia, distractibility, and pressured speech. At this time, a diagnosis of manic depressive illness was made, and the patient was placed on lithium carbonate 300 mg four times a day. The patient has managed to avoid hospitalization for two and a half years and has been asymptomatic. She has exhibited good interpersonal relatedness and a good range of affect. Like patient B, Mrs. C is glad she no longer has to feel "drugged" by major tranquilizers in order to carry out her daily activities.

DISCUSSION

From the above case histories, which clearly manifest manic phenomenology, one wonders how it is that such symptomatology was misdiagnosed as schizophrenia, especially chronic undifferentiated type. Admittedly, the problem is quite complex; yet, we would like to present a few possible explanations.

The problem clearly has its root in how these patients are treated. The patients with psychosis are hospitalized on short-stay hospital units (two to three weeks). Since the patients are hospitalized in a fragmented state, little history is obtained from them. Because of cognitive disorganization, the patients cannot fully verbalize their thought processes. Thus, it is difficult for the inpatient psychiatrist to establish a firm diagnosis. As Taylor and Abrams point out, "…over diagnosis of schizophrenia results from failure to recognize mania and from the belief that certain psychopathological phenomena (e.g., persecutory delusions, auditory hallucinations, catatonia, first-rank symptoms) occur only in patients with schizophrenia."[13] In addition, the language barrier between the patient and physician (many of whom are foreign medical graduates and unfamiliar with cultural aspects of black patients' language and behavior) makes for further difficulties leading to difficulties in interpretation and consequently, leads to misdiagnosis.

Often, the fragmented speech of a manic patient with pressured speech appears the same as the fragmented speech of the schizophrenic patient with cognitive slippage. By the time the psychosis is somewhat under control with neuroleptic therapy, the patient is discharged to aftercare facilities for follow-up. Once on outpatient status, the patient is likely to be treated for the diagnosis for which they were discharged. This is likely due to several factors: time constraints that outpatient clinics must function within in order to service their patient load; the difficulty with which lithium blood levels are obtained; language and cultural barriers; and the schizophreniform appearance of manic depressive illness. When hospitalized again, the prior diagnosis plays a heavy role in arriving at the current diagnosis, thus repeating the vicious cycle of misdiagnosis, improper management, and increase in iatrogenic morbidity. If correct evaluations fail to occur and the patient does not get prophylactic benefit of lithium carbonate therapy, the patient will have further psychotic breaks, increased recidivism, and unwanted neurological and other adverse effects of long-term neuroleptic therapy.

In addition to the management dynamics of patient care, there are obviously other factors leading to the misdiagnosis of black manic depressive patients. For one, it is a common belief that manic depressive illness is clustered in higher socioeconomic patients.[14] This belief tends to support the notion that black patients (frequently at the bottom of the socioeconomic totem pole) do not get affective illnesses. The authors believe that such myths significantly contribute to the misdiagnosis of a patient exhibiting euphoria, pressured speech, poor interpersonal relatedness, hyperactivity, and a lack of personality deterioration as having schizophrenia, chronic undifferentiated type. It is felt that these myths are rooted in a pervasive, covert form of racism that has been institutionalized in psychiatry to the point that low prevalence and incidence of manic depressive illness in blacks is given. The schizophreniform nature of manic depressive illness might understandably lead to a misdiagnosis of paranoid schizophrenia or catatonic schizophrenia.[13] However, a repeated diagnosis of schizophrenia, chronic undifferentiated type, in a patient with manic symptoms is almost inconceivable because the two clinical pictures of mania and schizophrenia are so different. Patients are given the schizophrenic diagnosis because they are of a lower socioeconomic class and nonwhite, especially if it is the first acute psychotic episode (as with Mrs. B), whether it is due to manic depressive illness, schizophrenia, acute type, drug abuse, borderline syndrome, hysterical psychosis, etc.

CONCLUSIONS

While hard statistical data are not presently available, a clear trend regarding the misdiagnosis of manic black psychiatric patients has been uncovered. Specifically, the patients who demonstrate obvious manic symptomatology in their case histories and who do quite well on lithium carbonate therapy are frequently diagnosed as schizophrenics, chronic undifferentiated type. This diagnosis carries poor prognostic implications and tends to lead to treatment with neuroleptic medication, which results in an iatrogenic morbidity from poor medication compliance, relegation to low-intensity supportive therapy, neurologic complications from long-term neuroleptic treatment, high re-hospitalization rates, and discomfort from neuroleptic therapy side effects. It is felt that this misdiagnosis is rooted in the lack of recognition that black patients suffer from manic depressive illness and in the patient management dynamics in a community with less-than-adequate resources for patient care. Physicians must keep dispelling myths that blacks are an unsophisticated people with a limited number of diagnostic categories, which result in blacks receiving unsophisticated medical care.

COMMENTARY

While I was a psychiatric resident at the Illinois State Psychiatric Institute, a white colleague turned me on to an invaluable book, *Racism and Psychiatry*, written by Alexander Thomas and Samuel Sillen, which provided a fascinating outline of the history of racism in the field of psychiatry. Several racist myths about African-American mental health were exposed. For example, "drapetomania" was the diagnosis given to slaves who tried to run away, and whipping was the treatment prescribed. "Dysesthesia Aethopica" was a disorder that was said to cause slaves to be troublesome, and treatment for this problem was hard work in the open air and sunshine.

Thomas and Sillen also did an outstanding job of documenting how African Americans supposedly had lower rates of affective disorders compared to whites. According to their research, which still holds true today, many African Americans receive their mental health care from poorly funded public mental health systems. Such systems generally do not offer patients a comprehensive, careful assessment of their psychiatric problems. Since the correct diagnosis is critical to receiving proper treatment, it is not hard to conclude that many African-American patients were and are misdiagnosed. Thus, they were not receiving appropriate treatment for their problems.

Because of the information presented in *Racism and Psychiatry* and my own observations, I did a point prevalence study of African-American patients with manic depressive illness. I identified every patient in Jackson Park Hospital's Psychiatric Outpatient Clinic who had been diagnosed as having manic depressive illness and reviewed each patient's past histories for other diagnoses. The results were alarming. Most of the patients had been misdiagnosed as having schizophrenia and had been given inappropriate treatments for years.

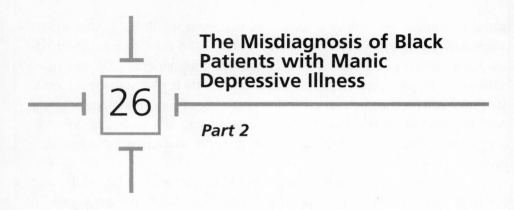

The Misdiagnosis of Black Patients with Manic Depressive Illness

Part 2

In a previous article (J Natl Med Assoc. 1980;72:141), the authors proposed that despite several attempts to disprove the myth that blacks do not demonstrate similar prevalence rates of manic depressive illness as whites, many black patients with manic depressive illness are frequently misdiagnosed. In a survey of the outpatient psychiatric clinic at Jackson Park Hospital, it was found that black patients in this clinic have similar prevalence rates of manic depressive illness when compared to surveys of white patient populations. In addition, it was found that the demographic characteristics of this subgroup of manic depressive patients were very similar to those found in white manic depressive patients. Yet, when the past histories of these black manic depressive patients were reviewed, there were large numbers of patients who received a diagnosis of schizophrenia and thus were not considered for treatment with lithium.

INTRODUCTION

Earlier studies[1-5] have reported that black patients are diagnosed with affective illness at a rate one-fourth that of whites, while estimates of

---

Originally printed as Bell Carl C, Mehta Harshad. The misdiagnosis of black patients with manic depressive illness: second in a series. *J Natl Med Assoc.* 1981;73:101–107. Presented at the 133rd Annual Meeting of the APA, San Francisco, CA, May 8, 1980.

the rate of schizophrenia in blacks has been twice that of whites.[4-7] Attempts have been made to show that these differences were due not to the actual incidence of manic depressive illness in blacks, as reflected by an accurate diagnostic assessment, but rather due to institutional racism.[4-10] Nevertheless, it has been the authors' contention that the misdiagnosis of black manic depressive patients continues at an alarming rate.

In an earlier article on the misdiagnosis of black manic depressive patients, the authors pointed out some of the institutional dynamics that cause this form of iatrogenic morbidity to persist.[11] Briefly, the patient who becomes acutely psychotic tends to be medically managed through brief hospitalization and crisis intervention.[12] This form of management relies heavily on controlling psychotic symptoms with medication and allows for a speedy referral to outpatient clinics, where medical management continues with brief monthly medication evaluations. As a patient's niche (housing, social support system, economic support system, etc.) in a lower socioeconomic community is extremely difficult to reestablish once lost, this treatment modality is a necessary and useful one. However, this form of treatment also means that once an acutely psychotic patient reaches a coherent state (which would allow the gathering of information necessary to differentiate the fragmented state of mania from schizophrenia), he or she is quickly referred. Unfortunately, the patient is often referred with a diagnosis of schizophrenia, a diagnosis that is maintained when the patient reaches a clinic. This catchall diagnosis, along with factors like lack of recognition that blacks may have affective illness, the general lack of recognition of manic symptoms, language barriers between doctors and patients, and the poor availability of lithium blood-level testing in an inner-city black population, tends to preclude a therapeutic trial of lithium in a black patient who clearly has a history of manic symptoms and who demonstrates manic signs in the clinical interview.

The authors reviewed three cases of manic depressive illness that were being successfully treated with lithium.[11] While there were numerous references to these patients' hyperactivity, pressured speech, elated mood, interpersonal relatedness, distractibility, flight of ideas, grandiose delusions, and excitability, a large percentage of these patients' final diagnoses was schizophrenia and chronic undifferentiated schizophrenia. These patients reported that major tranquilizers made them feel drugged and unable to perform the activities of daily living; yet, they were often placed on major tranquilizers despite the fact that none exhibited the flat affect, avoidant interpersonal style, and unmotivated picture of the schizophrenic patient. While it was felt that these cases identified a significant trend, more documentation was needed to better establish scientific validity of the contention that the trend of misdiagnosing black manic depressive patients did in fact exist. This paper provides additional documentation.

PROCEDURE

As the State of Illinois did not have diagnostic statistics on its patient population, charts of current cases at Jackson Park Hospital's outpatient clinic were reviewed. Patients with a diagnosis of manic depressive illness were selected for the study. Their history of illness was reviewed and information (admission note, psychiatric evaluation, and discharge summary) about each hospitalization was requested. This information was reviewed for consistency of descriptive data with the diagnostic category and treatment, which was then tabulated in order to present demographic data.

FINDINGS

Of the 272 outpatients at Jackson Park Hospital's outpatient clinic, the authors identified 22 who had had a diagnosis of manic depressive illness. Table 1 presents these patients' demographic data. The typical manic depressive patient found in the clinic was likely to be in the aftercare program, female, black, 40 years old, working, taking lithium only, and was likely to have slightly more than 12 years of education (see Table 2). It is also noted that such patients account for about 8% of a predominately black outpatient population.

Two of the 22 patients were never hospitalized, and six patients had incomplete record status regarding information from past hospitalizations (see Table 3).

The average age of first hospitalization was 33.2 years (the youngest was 20; the oldest, 63). The average number of hospitalizations

TABLE 26.1. Demographic Data on Manic Depressive Patients at Jackson Park Hospital Outpatient Clinic

Pat./ Age	Sex	Race	Yrs. of Educ.	Prog.	Record Status	Employment Status	Current Medication
A/72	F	B	18	Senior	Complete	Retired	Lithium 300 mg TID
B/32	F	B	11	Aftercare	Complete	Unempl.	Lithium 300 mg TID
C/28	F	B	9	Aftercare	Complete	Unempl.	Lithium 300 mg TID Chloroprom. 200 mg HS
D/41	F	B	6	Aftercare	Complete	Babysitter	Lithium 300 mg TID
E/36	F	W	10	Aftercare	Complete	Housewife	Lithium 300 mg TID Fluphenazine D 20 mg IM q 4 wks Trihexyphenidyl 2 mg daily
F/36	F	B	15	Aftercare	Complete	Employed	Lithium 300 mg TID
G/27	M	B	13	Aftercare	Complete	On & off	Lithium 300 mg QID Chloroprom. 500 mg HS
H/67	F	B	10	Senior	Complete	Babysitter	Lithium 300 mg TID
I/36	F	B	12	Aftercare	Complete	Unempl.	Haloperidol 2 mg HS PRN
J/30	F	B	12	Aftercare	Complete	Employed	Fluphenazine D 25 mg IM q 4 wks Thioridazine 50 mg HS Trihexyphenidyl 2 mg HS
K/48	F	B	12	Aftercare	Complete	Unempl.	Loxapine 10 mg one or two HS
L/32	F	B	11	Aftercare	Complete	Employed	Trifluoperazine 2 mg BID Imipramine 25 mg BID
M/48	F	B	18	Aftercare	Complete	Employed	Lithium 300 mg QID Chloroprom. 100 mg HS Chloroprom. 25 mg BID
N/25	M	B	12	Aftercare	Complete	Employed	Fluphenazine 10 mg BID
O/47	F	B	18	Pre-care	None	Employed	Lithium 300 mg TID
P/36	F	B	7	Pre-care	None	Unempl.	Lithium 300 mg TID
Q/63	F	B	8	Senior	Incompl.	Unempl.	Lithium 300 mg TID Thioridazine 50 mg HS
R/21	F	B	15	Aftercare	Incompl.	Student	Lithium 300 mg TID
S/29	F	B	12	Aftercare	Incompl.	Employed	Lithium 300 mg TID
T/42	F	B	14	Aftercare	Incompl.	Employed	Lithium 300 mg TID
U/48	F	B	12	Aftercare	Incompl.	Unempl.	Lithium 300 mg TID
V/38	F	B	16	Aftercare	Incompl.	Employed	Trifluoperazine 5 mg HS Benztropine 1 mg HS

TABLE 26.2. Demographic Data on Manic Depressive Patients at Jackson Park Hospital Outpatient Clinic

Patients by Program			
	No. Total	No. Manic Depressive	%
Pre-care patients	70	2	2.9
Aftercare patients	181	17	9.4
Senior-age patients	21	3	14.3
Total no. of clinic patients	**272**		**100**
Total no. of manic depressive patients* **		**22**	**8.1**

Manic Depressive Patients by Gender, Race, Employment Status, and Treatment		
	No.	%
Female	20	90.9
Male	2	9.1
Black	21	95.5
White	1	4.5
Working	14	63.6
Treated with lithium alone	11	50
Treated with low doses of major tranquilizers only	6	27.3
Treated with lithium and low doses of major tranquilizers	5	22.7

*The average number of years of education of manic depressive patients was 12.3; 8 patients (36.4% of sample) had some college education.
**The average age of all manic depressive patients at the clinic was 40 (the youngest was 21; the oldest, 72).

TABLE 26.3. Case History Demographic Data on Manic Depressive Patients

	No.	%
Manic depressive patients never hospitalized	2	9.1
Manic depressive patients with incomplete records	6	27.3
Manic depressive patients with complete records	14	63.6

Note: The average age of first hospitalization was 33.2 years (the youngest was 20; the oldest, 63).
The average number of hospitalizations was 6.8.
The average length of hospital stay was 21.8 days (shortest stay 1 day, longest stay 352 days; 46.2% with a stay of 14 days or less).

was 6.8. The average length of hospital stay was 21.8 days (shortest stay 1 day, longest stay, 352 days; 46.2% with a stay of 14 days or less). When data for the 14 patients with complete inpatient hospitalization records was tabulated, it was found that the average age at their first hospitalization was 33, the average number of hospitalizations was approximately 7, and the average length of hospital stay was approximately 22 days. All together, these 14 patients had been hospitalized 83 times. Table 4 presents a breakdown of their diagnostic events with regard to diagnosis and whether the patient was hospitalized in a state or private hospital.

TABLE 26.4. Breakdown of Diagnostic Events at Jackson Park Hospital Outpatient Clinic

| | Total | PRIVATE HOSPITAL | | | | PUBLIC HOSPITAL | | | |
| | Diag. | Tot. | | Manic | | Tot. | | Manic | |
Pat.	Evnts	No.	Schizo.	Depr.	Other	No.	Schizo.	Depr.	Other
A	12	3	0	3	0	9	2	3	4
B	5	0	0	0	0	5	4	0	1
C	4	0	0	0	0	4	3	0	1
D	6	2	1	0	1	4	2	0	2
E	5	5	3	0	2	0	0	0	0
F	4	4	0	3	1	0	0	0	0
G	25	3	1	1	1	22	4	14	4
H	1	1	0	0	1	0	0	0	0
I	2	0	0	0	0	2	2	0	0
J	5	0	0	0	0	5	4	0	1
K	4	0	0	0	0	4	4	0	0
L	1	1	1	0	0	0	0	0	0
M	4	4	0	4	0	0	0	0	0
N	5	0	0	0	0	5	4	0	1
Totals									
14	83	23	6	11	6	60	29	17	14

Note: Other diagnoses included the following: schizoaffective disorder, anxiety neurosis, psychosis with atherosclerosis, psychosis with drug intoxication, acute psychotic episode with alcohol addiction, alcoholism, depressive neurosis, psychotic depression, affective disorder, personality disorder (antisocial type).

Clearly, the figures show a substantial difference in diagnostic trends at private and state hospitals in which the black manic depressive patients were hospitalized. If hospitalized in a private hospital, there was a 47.8% likelihood of these patients receiving a diagnosis of manic depressive; if hospitalized in a public hospital, the likelihood of their receiving this diagnosis was only 28.3%. On the other hand, if hospitalized in a public hospital, these patients were apt to be diagnosed as schizophrenic 48.3% of the time; if hospitalized in a private hospital, their chance of diagnosis with schizophrenia was only 26.1%. Furthermore, 19 (62.1%) of the 29 public hospital diagnostic events which found these patients schizophrenic classified them as having the chronic undifferentiated type.

Table 5 demonstrates the public hospital's preferential use of major tranquilizers for the treatment of these black manic depressive patients, compared to the use of lithium (either in combination or alone) in the private hospital setting.

TABLE 26.5. Breakdown of Treatment Events

Total Rx		PRIVATE HOSPITAL					PUBLIC HOSPITAL			
Pat. Evnts	Tot.	Anti-psych.	Anti-depr.	LiCO$_3$	LiCO$_3$ & Other	Tot.	Anti-psych.	Anti-depr.	LiCO$_3$	LiCO$_3$ & Other
A 12	3	0	0	2	1	9*	6	1	0	1
B 5	0	0	0	0	0	5	5	0	0	0
C 4	0	0	0	0	0	4	4	0	0	0
D 6	2	2	0	0	0	4	4	0	0	0
E 5	5	4	0	1	0	0	0	0	0	0
F 4	4	0	1	0	3	0	0	0	0	0
G 25	3	0	0	0	3	22**	7	0	1	11
H 1	1	0	1	0	0	0	0	0	0	0
I 2	0	0	0	0	0	2	2	0	0	0
J 5	0	0	0	0	0	5+	4	0	0	0
K 4	0	0	0	0	0	4	4	0	0	0
L 1	1	1	0	0	0	0	0	0	0	0
M 4	4	0	0	3	1	0	0	0	0	0
N 5	0	0	0	0	0	5	5	0	0	0
Totals										
14 83	23	7	2	6	8	60	41	1	1	12

*No medication during one hospitalization.
**No medication during three hospitalizations.
+No medication during two hospitalizations.

The use of lithium alone or in combination with other medications occurred for 60.9% of patients hospitalized in a private facility and in only 21.7% of patients hospitalized in a public facility. Major tranquilizers alone were used 30.4% of the time when the patients were in private hospitals and 68.3% of the time while in public hospitals.

Regarding the correlation between diagnosis and medication, it was noted that in both public and private facilities, the use of lithium alone or in combination required a diagnosis of manic depression, while the use of major tranquilizers alone tended to be the treatment for patients diagnosed as being schizophrenic (although a few patients diagnosed as manic depressive received only major tranquilizers upon discharge).

DISCUSSION

The demographic data on this study group demonstrates that black manic depressive patients show the same characteristics as do white manic depressives.[13-16] Yet, why are they misdiagnosed 71.7% of the time in public hospitals and 52.2% of the time in private hospitals? It should be pointed out that the percentage of misdiagnosis in public hospitals would be higher if not for the fact that patients diagnosed as schizophrenic by public facilities were correctly diagnosed with manic depressive illness by a hospitalization event in a private facility. The dynamics of this influence were that once patients had been placed on lithium (usually because of a manic depressive diagnosis arrived at by a private hospital) and had a better treatment outcome than when on major tranquilizers during re-hospitalization in a public hospital, they informed the public hospital staff of their previous diagnosis and treatment, enabling that staff to correctly diagnose them.

One factor contributing to the problem of misdiagnosis is that mania is frequently misdiagnosed as schizophrenia.[17] However, in examining the racial distribution and the subtypes of schizophrenic diagnoses in the patients in misdiagnosis studies,[13,18] it becomes clear that race is a significant factor in whether a patient receives a poor prognosis diagnosis of chronic undifferentiated schizophrenia or a better prognosis diagnosis of paranoid, catatonic, or schizoaffective schizophrenia. Therefore, while the authors admit that there is a general lack of appreciation of the signs and symptoms of mania, this lack does not account for the considerably higher percentage of black manic depressive patients misdiagnosed as chronic undifferentiated schizophrenics.

Another factor in misdiagnosis is whether the hospital is private or public (money is not a factor in this consideration, as the State of Illinois provides an indigent hospitalization grant to cover private hospitalization costs for patients who cannot pay). The physicians in private facilities had a greater recognition of manic depressive symptoms than the physicians in public facilities. It is suspected that this difference lies in the difficulty that state hospitals have in retaining qualified psychiatrists[19] and in the competitive nature of getting appointed to a private hospital staff (e.g., applicants must be board-eligible). It is suspected that the difference is also due to the large number of foreign medical graduates in public facilities, which results in a language barrier between public hospital physicians and black patients. It is not the authors' intent to imply that all state or foreign medical school graduate physicians are inept or inadequately trained; however, the factor of qualified public hospital physicians with a good command of English must remain a consideration in the etiology of misdiagnosing black manic depressive patients with the catchall diagnosis of chronic undifferentiated schizophrenia.

Other factors contributing to this misdiagnosis are time constraints and the availability of serum lithium levels, which have been previously mentioned.[11] Hopefully, all of the factors mentioned will be lessened with the release of the *Diagnostic and Statistical Manual of Mental Disorders*, 3rd ed., published by the American Psychiatric Association. This edition more clearly spells out diagnostic criteria for manic depressive illness and schizophrenia. Regardless if a difference is made, nonetheless, the authors contend that, given scientific validity presented in this study, that the prevalence of manic depressive illness is just as great in blacks as in whites.

Finally, it is of interest that 14.3% of the patients in the senior-age program had diagnoses of manic depressive illness, compared to 9.4% in the aftercare program. While the actual number of these patients is small, it supports a suspicion that "bipolar affective illness may be a relatively common missed diagnosis in the elderly."[20] This should be kept in mind when examining elderly blacks.

CONCLUSIONS

Black manic depressive patients have the same demographic data (i.e., middle aged, female, highly educated, employed, stable pre- and postmorbid personality, etc.) as do white manic depressive patients. Black manic depressive patients are more likely to be diagnosed as schizophrenic, especially chronic undifferentiated schizophrenic, if they are hospitalized in a public hospital. Private hospitals tend to more accurately diagnose black manic depressive patients but a trend to misdiagnose is also evident.

While the factors for being misdiagnosed as schizophrenic are similar for both black and white manic depressive patients, the variable of being black increased the likelihood of misdiagnosis and the likelihood of receiving a subtype diagnostic category of schizophrenia—specifically chronic undifferentiated, which has a poor prognosis. Consequently, these patients do not receive the type of treatment that would allow them maximum recovery from their illness.

RECOMMENDATIONS

It is recommended that all private and public facilities (inpatient or outpatient) serving large populations of black patients perform an audit on their charts in order to ascertain their percentage of black manic depressive patients. If this percentage does not compare to the average (about 8%) found in most general psychiatric facilities that have done a clear study to determine the percentage of manic depressive patients in their population, it is further suggested that the facility take a serious look at patients with other diagnoses who show signs of interpersonal relatedness, have stable post-morbid personalities, are middle-aged or older and became ill during mid-life, are well educated, have a good range of appropriate affect, and show a poor tolerance to major tranquilizers.

COMMENTARY

An abstract of "The Misdiagnosis of Black Patients with Manic Depression" (see Chapter 25) was produced for International Synopses, *Psychiatry Digest*, and was available in four languages by February 1981. Dr. Harshad Mehta and I decided to find out exactly how common the problem was. Consequently, we produced this article.

While we were conducting our research, several other researchers were doing similar research. Dr. Billy E. Jones, a prominent African-

American psychiatrist, and his colleagues in New York were exploring manic depressive illness among poor urban blacks. When they published their results in the *American Journal of Psychiatry* in May 1981, they referenced our work in the area. Because they found results similar to ours, the fact that African Americans with manic depressive illness were being misdiagnosed and consequently harmed could not be denied. Our work received a great deal of attention and was written up in *Clinical Psychiatry News*, a trade newspaper, and in *The SK&F Eskalith Newsletter*, a drug company newsletter. As a result, these articles began a national awareness that African Americans could have psychotic disorders other than just schizophrenia and, I believe, broadened the range of diagnoses applied to them. I still occasionally find these two articles referenced in various other articles on the misdiagnosis of African Americans, on the influence of racial factors on psychiatric diagnosis, and on the topic of African Americans and mental health care. The first was even cited in *Manic-Depressive Illness* by Frederick K. Goodwin and Kay Redfield Jamison (Oxford Press; 1990), which is still considered the "bible" on the disorder. Although these two articles were written more than 20 years ago, they still hold critical information for African Americans obtaining psychiatric services. I cannot emphasize the importance of getting a good assessment before starting any type of treatment.

Four years after I published this article, I became interested in another area of misdiagnosis affecting black patients. As a result, several colleagues and I published the article, "Misdiagnosis of Alcohol-Related Organic Brain Syndrome in Blacks: Implications for Treatment" (In: Brisbane F, Wobble M, eds. *Treatment of Black Alcoholics*. New York: Haworth Press; 1985). This article pointed out that African Americans who had damaged their brains from drinking large amounts of alcohol were frequently misdiagnosed with schizophrenic illness. I presented three cases I had discovered while treating patients at the CMHC and outlined how, because of their misdiagnosis, they were not receiving proper treatment. I outlined as various factors responsible for the misdiagnosis cultural drinking patterns, culturally biased diagnostic criteria, false positive symptoms, as well as other factors listed in the articles on the misdiagnosis of blacks with manic depressive illness. I also pointed out in this article that by giving a patient the wrong diagnosis, the medical treatment a patient received could do more harm than good. Physicians misdiagnosing alcohol-related organic brain damage could inadvertently cause a patient to develop tardive dyskinesia, a neurologic movement disorder caused by anti-psychotic medications. Physicians could cause patients to lose hope and become demoralized if they are told they have schizophrenia, with its attendant poor prognosis. Furthermore, a diagnosis of schizophrenia frequently means poor rehabilitation potential, so alcoholic patients would not be given a fair chance of getting their lives back together.

It turns out that there is evidence that African Americans are at greater risk for developing tardive dyskinesia when put on older anti-psychotic medications. The good news is that in the 21st century, modern medicine has developed newer anti-psychotic medications that do not cause tardive dyskinesia. Unfortunately, research I have been doing with the APA's Psychiatrists Research Network reveals mentally ill African-American patients have been slow to receive newer medications. I suspect this is because newer medications are always so expensive, making their availability limited. In addition, African Americans frequently tell me they are concerned with being "guinea pigs" for modern medicine, and that they are afraid of being involved in research or trying newer treatments. I always remind them of three things. The first is that physicians are scared to death of being sued, so if any physician ever "experiments" on them without their consent, they can sue, sue, sue! Secondly, physicians are scared to death of hurting people; after all, most of us went to medical school to save lives, not harm them. Finally, I ask African Americans to name one time when they have ever gotten the benefit of modern medical care. The answer is next to never; we are the last to receive life-saving treatments such as heart transplants, kidney transplants, bypass surgery, etc. In fact, the only time I can think of was when DNA tests got numerous falsely accused black inmates off death row. The funny thing is that when DNA testing was being proposed, many African Americans were fearful of how it would harm them.

Believe me, European-Americans who mean African Americans harm don't have to do much; they can simply let us wallow in our ignorance and fear of modern medical technology, ultimately making us harm ourselves.

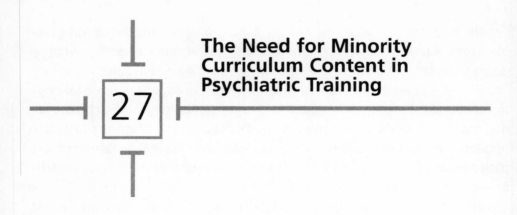

The Need for Minority Curriculum Content in Psychiatric Training

27

It is my pleasure to work in an inner-city general medical hospital with a behavioral medicine component to meet the psychiatric needs of the predominately black population of the area. In addition to myself, an African American, there are two Asians and one Hispanic who function as psychiatrists in the hospital's 24-hour psychiatric emergency service during the day. My responsibility as Director of clinical services has been overseeing the maintenance of the milieu of the psychiatric emergency service, because staff attitudes, values, and behavior greatly influence the behavior patients demonstrate while under acute stress. Since this is a very high-pressure area (both for patients and staff), psychiatric emergency service affords an excellent opportunity to observe how various styles of behavior affect patient care.

While all physicians follow the same procedures, on close inspection, one finds that there is quite a difference in "vibes" in the emergency area, depending on the physician on duty. The type of "vibe" is determined by such things as political power in the general hospital system, treatment orientations, relationship with staff, culture of origin, class of origin, etc.

Originally printed as Bell Carl C. Guest editorial on "The Need for Minority Curriculum Content in Psychiatric Training." *J Natl Med Assoc.* 1980;71:195–196.

While these variables are extremely ethereal, there is something to be said concerning physicians treating patients whose background is very different from their own.

The Hispanic physician maintains a very traditional cultural environment when on duty. He or she is the doctor and as such is responsible for making decisions about patient management. The doctor expects that the patients coming through the service will treat him or her with respect, due to the nature of the position. Being a member of the Catholic faith tends to make this physician a very gentle, soft-spoken person with the opinion that most black people are very mean and cruel to each other. Evidence for this belief is the way blacks freely use of profanity when talking to each other. This physician has frequently stated, "Even the staff talks about one another using such language; they can't like each other." I also pointed out that in Hispanic culture, the type of behavior seen in both black patients and staff is considered vile and sinful. This is the "tradition" philosophy.

Many Asian practitioners maintain a "please, no trouble" milieu. He or she tries very hard to see that everyone is content and that there are no confrontations. They tend to ask the staff's opinion about cases to make sure that the decision is in accord with everyone's feelings about the patient. When making a decision that will be unpopular, they are able to do so after much checking with the staff and patient and after several attempts to persuade all concerned that the plan for treatment is a good one. They talk about how much black people struggle against overwhelming odds and how it is often better to be like the willow in a hurricane and bend, rather than be like the oak and break. This is the "water" philosophy.

Other Asian physicians who have received a great deal of training in an all-black setting tend to have a rather smooth style and a non-threatening yet matter-of-fact approach. They tend to avoid conflict and confrontations but do not check out the plan as much as in the first example for Asians given above. This may be a result of having a better command of English and seemingly having an understanding of African-American subculture phenomena. Thus, they are able to blend their culturally biased expectations with the reality of the black experience. This is the "middle path" philosophy.

My style tends to be "tell it like it is." I speak directly to patients and let them know I realize that they are in a crisis and that I intend to help them if I can. However, I also make it clear that I will not tolerate agitation or violence. I will respect them, and I expect them to respect my staff and me. I am not concerned with tradition or trouble; I will make due with what I have to work with in order to treat the patient. My philosophy is "point-blank."

We see four different styles of handling black psychiatric patients in an emergency service, with each being partially related to the psychiatrist's culture of origin. One sees a similar situation when the white psychiatrist is in a comparable position; his/her style tends to reflect a belief that unlimited resources are available to patients as well as several mythical beliefs about blacks in general, such as the inherent weakness of the black family and the predominance of schizophrenia among blacks. The Hispanic psychiatrist has pointed out to me that my style would bring me ruin in the Hispanic sector of town; Hispanic patients would find it difficult to relate to me since my "point-blank" style is considered rude in their culture.

From my perspective, it seems clear that a large number of black patients is being treated by physicians of other cultures of origin, and that these physicians' ethnocentric attitudes, values, and behaviors have a serious impact on their ability to establish effective physician-patient relations. It is evident that the quality of the rapport between physician and patient determines to a great extent whether or not treatment will be successful.

Fortunately, several attempts have been made to improve the minority curriculum content in training programs. The Black Psychiatrists of America have developed an Academy on Issues on Psychiatry for Black Populations. The Solomon Carter Fuller Institute has researched the problems foreign medical graduates have in treating black psychiatric patients. Howard University is having conference-workshops to examine and deal with the problem. Unfortunately, while the need for minority curriculum content has been recognized, little has been done to implement training in this area. Because this is an extremely important issue, we must see that the recommendations for training programs concerning minority curriculum content have "teeth" in them to insure their implementation. This can be done only by placing political pressure on the various bodies that accredit and fund programs training individuals to care for patients.

For further information, write to Dr. Billy Jones, MD, Black Psychiatrists of America, 56 Hamilton Terrace, New York, NY 10031; Dr. Robert Sharpley, MD, Solomon Fuller Institute, 127 Mt. Auburn Street, Cambridge, MA 02138; Dr. Patricia Dunston, School of Social Work, Howard University, Six and Howard Place, NW, Washington, DC 20059.

COMMENTARY

In 1979, I worked with several other black psychiatrists to develop a chapter on curriculum development and implementation. The goal was to improve psychiatric residents' knowledge and skills necessary for treating African-American patients appropriately. In early 1980, I was a faculty member at the conference, "Training in Mental Health Services for Black Populations," sponsored by the BPA and New York Medical College in Port Chester, New York, where I also addressed the issue. To promote this work, I wrote this guest editorial. Because of my interest in the area, I was asked to speak at the Lafayette Clinic (Detroit), at the New York Hospital's Westchester Division of Cornell Medical Center (New York), and at Adelphi University's Department of Psychology (New York).

My experience advocating for minority curriculum content has shown me that while advocacy is appropriate, the content is lacking. We're in this situation because enough resources haven't been devoted to researching African-American mental health issues. It is my hope that Dr. Satcher's *Culture, Race, and Ethnicity Mental Health* report (see www.surgeongeneral.gov) will help correct this problem. However, I hasten to add that when we were working on this report, we had a major difficulty finding information and research about mental health needs of African-American populations. Much of the work black mental health professionals and I have been has tried to fill some of these information gaps.

Unfortunately, research in the 21st century is so complex that many African-American institutions do not have the administrative, methodological, or statistical infrastructure to do scientifically acceptable research devoid of serious flaws. How, then, will African Americans benefit from some of the very helpful psychiatric research coming down the pike in the near future? My personal solution has been to increase my research training so that my research moves from "bent-nail" to "store-bought, straight nail." This has taken me ten years to accomplish, and I couldn't have done it without the significant support of an extremely dedicated, supportive team of professionals at the CMHC and colleagues at the University of Illinois. Being aware of how things work, we've tried to groom our replacements as well. As a result, the CMHC has established its fourth African-American Mental Health and Wellness Think Tank. This group is composed of nearly twenty African-American physicians, psychiatrists, psychologists, social workers, and nurses who are organizing a research institution that focuses on African-American mental health and wellness issues using 21st-century science. We're trying to build an infrastructure that will mentor younger African-American scientists to fill the information gap about African mental health and wellness, so we can have minority curriculum content in the mental health field. Much of my professional effort has been aiding in filling the content void as well. When I go out and lecture on knowledge and skills needed to treat African-American patients, I have information that is substantive and useful.

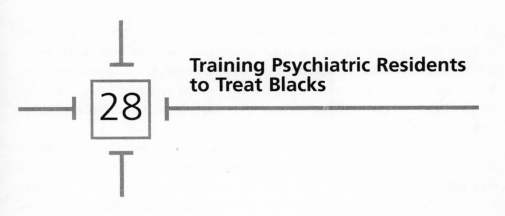

Training Psychiatric Residents to Treat Blacks

28

Since only 600 of the 30,000 psychiatrists in the United States are black, it is apparent that black American psychiatrists cannot meet the needs of all mentally ill blacks in this country. In view of this situation, the authors feel that psychiatric residency training programs should prepare psychiatric residents to treat black patients. This paper describes some of the knowledge base and experience that residents need to treat black psychiatric patients.

INTRODUCTION

Blacks differ from one another in many ways regarding attitudes, values, folkways, mores, ethnic identity, religious beliefs, diet, language, social class, family history, and other distinguishing characteristics. The ethnic aspects of black American lifestyles show a richness and diversity that is quite different from other ethnic groups in America. Examples of how black Americans differ from other American ethnic groups can be found in the system of black folk medicine, diet, music, and language, as well as in a number of vestiges from black African culture and American slavery.

Originally printed as Bell Carl C, Fayen Maurine, Mattox Gail. Training psychiatric residents to treat blacks. *J Natl Med Assoc.* 1988;80:637–641. Presented at the 1985 Annual Meeting of the APA.

Despite these obvious cultural and ethnic differences, the question of what these differences are and how they influence the psychiatric evaluation and treatment of blacks has not been investigated rigorously. The American psychiatric community has also given sparse attention to the "newer" groups of American blacks who have immigrated recently from Africa and the Caribbean.

The knowledge base for the psychiatric assessment and treatment of blacks has gone from blatant pseudoscientific rationalizations (which justified racial segregation and discrimination), to an omission of legitimate differences in assessment and treatment, to the psychiatry's current trend of looking at black psychiatric issues from a truly scientific perspective. It is on this new wave of transcultural/transethnic knowledge that a psychiatric residency training program should base its curriculum content for evaluating minorities.

CURRICULUM CONTENT

A truly sound psychiatric residency should include curriculum content and experiential training that would enable trainees to be knowledgeable and comfortable with transcultural and transethnic issues and situations[1]; after all, America is not a "melting pot" but is rather a cultural and ethnic mosaic that is destined to become even more diverse in the near future. Subjects for didactic courses that would enhance the knowledge and skills necessary to treat black psychiatric patients would include the following:

1. Study of the overt racism in psychiatry prior to the 1970s.[2]

2. Study of the general history of blacks in America, with particular attention to the fact that desegregation in the United States is only 32 years old. This phenomenon is revealing of the historical roots of the social context that affects blacks today.[3]

3. Study of the psychodynamics of stereotyping[4,5] and prejudice[6] and the contemporary myths they generate (blacks are primitive, the black family is a "tangle of pathology," the black family is a matriarchal structure, the black family is in total disarray from the effects of slavery, blacks rarely get depressed or

commit suicide, all blacks are in the lower socioeconomic classes, etc.).[7]

4. Study of the causes of misdiagnosing black patients: (1) different clinical presentations of blacks (e.g., blacks have been reported to have more hallucinatory phenomena than whites), (2) the role of early exposure to alcohol on the development of psychiatric disorders, (3) the use of diagnostic tools that were not standardized on blacks, (4) the consistency with which clinicians apply descriptive diagnostic criteria to blacks, (5) the role of social and cultural distance and racism between the patient and clinician.[8]

5. Study of the consequences of misdiagnosing black patients. Misdiagnosis causes a lifetime of mistreatment with varying degrees of iatrogenic consequences, including poor compliance with treatment, excessive relapses, correctional institutionalization rather than hospitalization, excessive side effects from somatic treatment, decreased recognition of rehabilitation potential, demoralization, and more. Another area deserving attention is how misdiagnosis leads to a lack of an accurate epidemiologic knowledge base for incidence and prevalence assumptions, so as to plan the adequate delivery of mental health services.[9]

6. Study of the ethnic-identity issues with which blacks grapple. This is a necessity for any psychiatrist who attempts psychotherapy with a black patient. Questions of an integration philosophy, a Pan-African stance, a black nationalist stance, or a non-ethnic middle-class stance are bound to be raised in any valid psychotherapeutic treatment of a black patient. Psychiatrists must be familiar with the pros and cons of these ethnic philosophies in order to respond adequately. Similarly, the issue of ethnic isolation, which may bring on suicidal urges and survivor guilt, must be clearly understood to adequately treat the upwardly mobile, middle-class black patient.[10]

7. Study of the psychosocial context of growing up in a milieu where black-on-black murder is the leading cause of death in black men aged 15–44 years. This is essential. An examination of the high rate of head injury, unemployment (two to three times higher than whites'), the ever-present threat of violence from whites, and the widespread availability of liquor in ghetto neighborhoods is also necessary. How this milieu influ-

ences the psychological aspects of narcissism, nihilism, and self-esteem in blacks needs to be understood.[11,12]

These considerations and more should form the base of black minority curriculum content in residency training. The attitudinal milieu in which training also occurs deserves attention. Professional socialization,[13] an appreciation of the cultural pluralism found in the American psychiatric patient population, tolerance, and respect for differences (e.g., an absence of the phenomenon of "hallucinatory whitening"[14]) are all factors that must be attended to by residency training directors in the experiential process of training. Minority role models must be provided for minority trainees, and white residents need to be supervised by minority faculty to better understand interracial and interpersonal dyads.

Unfortunately, the majority of residency training programs do not have a black minority content included in their core curriculums. It is left up to the resident to attend workshops or lectures on black psychiatric issues or elect to take specialized rotations.[1] Such workshops and lectures are offered at the annual meetings of the American Psychiatric Association and the National Medical Association, at the Black Psychiatrists of America's Transcultural Seminar, and during other special efforts initiated by various training programs. Experience with this format has shown that it can be helpful in stimulating interest in transcultural and transethnic issues, but often, the limited nature of this experience only grazes the surface of the knowledge and process base necessary to develop skills needed for treating black patients. On the other hand, the preceptorship format allows for a much more extensive and intimate contact with a black preceptor, and during the course of an elective specialized-curriculum rotation, the resident can be provided with a firm knowledge base on the psychiatric assessment and treatment of black populations. Such a curriculum establishes a well-guided experiential process that shapes attitudes, values, professional socialization, professional identity, and cultural and ethnic pluralism.

In 1985, two psychiatric residents, one from the University of Chicago and one from Northwestern University, elected to take a rotation at the Community Mental Health Council (CMHC) in Chicago. The experience consisted of delivering psychiatric services through a predominately black-staffed community mental health agency to a predominately black patient population on Chicago's Southside. The Council's services included screening and psychiatric assessment, crisis intervention, liaison with an inpatient psychiatric hospital, day treatment, vocational rehabilitation, adult outpatient services, elderly outpatient services, children and adolescent outpatient services, sustaining-care outpatient services, residential services, research on black populations, and community education and development. The residents were exposed to research issues such as the misdiagnosis of blacks with organic brain syndromes associated with alcoholism, the prevalence of coma in blacks, and the prevalence of isolated sleep paralysis in blacks. In addition, the residents witnessed a beginning effort to address black-on-black murder through public education. A synopsis of the residents' experiences follows in an effort to give a first-hand account of the preceptorship model.

RESIDENT EXPERIENCES AT A BLACK COMMUNITY MENTAL HEALTH CENTER

A White Female Psychiatry Resident

I grew up in a suburban community, a moderate-sized mid-western city. At my grade school, the most unique cultural difference was an Irish-Catholic family with less than four children. The biggest cultural change I encountered upon entering high school was meeting and befriending non-Irish Catholics, Poles, and Italians for the first time—mostly middle-class kids from southern California.

I attended medical school in Cleveland. The curriculum included a program for first-year students to follow a pregnant woman through the latter part of her pregnancy, labor, and delivery, and to follow the baby through its first year of pediatric visits. I was assigned to a single, black woman who occasionally lived with her boyfriend. At one time, she had been a professional shoplifter. She decided to take it up again during the ninth month of her pregnancy. She was caught, arrested, and jailed overnight. Two weeks after getting out, the baby was born. When the baby was six months old, my patient "went underground" to avoid federal agents. They were trying to extradite her to Canada so she could testify against her boyfriend on a murder rap.

"Getting to know" my only patient required learning about more than the anatomy, physiology, and psychology of labor and delivery and mothering. It required learning something about "boosting" and jails and required a network of phone calls to the 41 "underground" to get the baby in for his next DPT vaccine. This being my first patient, I was probably a little too strong on idealism and good will; however, the experience sensitized me to issues that would continue to surface throughout my medical training—issues that had to do with racial, cultural, and socioeconomic differences between my patients and me.

My medical school training rotations were through inner-city hospitals, as well as through the Veteran's Association hospital and suburban community hospitals. I needed to learn how to deal with patients and their families from inner-city black, inner-city Appalachian, and suburban Jewish backgrounds. It became increasingly evident to me that I needed to see my patients and their families within a cultural realm if I expected them to take the anti-hypertensive medicine I prescribed, to come to hemodialysis, and to participate in a cancer chemotherapy regimen.

It was from this background that I came to a residency program at the University of Chicago, situated in a racially integrated pocket on the predominantly black Southside of Chicago. The patient population was mixed—university types (faculty and staff), students, people from the middle-class community, and some from the contiguous neighborhoods' housing projects. But the university has no catchment area per se, and for this reason, I wanted some exposure to community psychiatry. I opted, therefore, for an elective rotation with Dr. Carl C. Bell of the CMHC.

It took some time to work out a program. For a while, I simply sat and observed the workings of his office, which included individual patient medication management, medication groups, administrative supervision, and education groups for the day hospital, to name a few. I spent some time with the various subdivisions of the clinic. I made rounds with the psychiatric inpatient liaison worker and discussed caseloads and treatment approaches with the child counselors. I spent a day going to groups, crafts, seminars, and meeting with the administrator to discuss policy. Eventually, I moved to seeing patients under direct supervision regarding the management of their medications. Dr. Bell and I jointly ran the medication groups, and I gave a talk to the education group. My position later evolved to "walk-in physician," where I worked relatively independently, seeing acute cases for diagnosis or for short-term pharmacologic aid to alleviate some of the staff psychiatrists' caseload.

As a white female psychiatry resident, I was working at a center with a predominantly black staff in a black community. The difference between my experiences at the University of Chicago and at the CMHC had little to do with the range of pathology seen or the types of medication and therapy provided. The differences had more to do with focus. The CMHC concerns itself wholeheartedly with the psychological wellbeing of its community and provides psychiatric outpatient and day treatment services. In addition, it provides educational and social programs to the community. Its staff is involved in politics and policy-making at the local, city, and state levels. The CMHC is involved with local businesses and local schools. They have a commitment to, and a concern for, the local population that is evident in all the services provided.

Dr. Bell is interested in areas of research that deal specifically with the idiosyncratic manifestations of psychopathology in the black population. I was exposed to his views and given an adequate bibliography of cross-cultural psychiatry. I was also given the opportunity to read about other minority groups and the individual ethnic differences they bring to psychiatry.

Because I come from a non-pluralistic background, I have concentrated on educating myself in a manner that would show me the heterogeneity of the population to be served by psychiatry. Medical school and psychiatric training do much to educate one about *generic* pathology in the human organism. But especially in psychiatry, if one is to use oneself as an empathic tool, one would do well to be educated pluralistically. In so doing, we learn about a myriad of treatment modalities to deal with the range of psychopathology we encounter. We would do our patients and ourselves a service if we could learn about them within their cultural context.

It would not be impossible to implement the topic of cross-cultural psychiatry into a residency curriculum. A useful way to begin is an example used at the University of Chicago: its incorporated into an emergency psychiatry course taught at the PGY2 level. Residents need to think about patients as persons within a cultural setting early in their training if they are to incorporate pluralistic approaches into their repertoire of skills for dealing with psychiatric patients.

A Black Female Psychiatry Resident

There is a tremendous need to adequately train psychiatry residents to treat minority populations. This need has been emphasized continuously nationwide, yet only a few residency training programs have implemented any change in their core curriculum to include minority content. The majority of psychiatrists today are still trained within a predominately white context with a middle-class orientation. Various methods have been proposed to include minority content in the training process, including workshops, didactic courses, and field experience. Ideally, the best approach would utilize a combination of the above techniques.

I wish to review my own experience with the preceptorship model. As a third-year black psychiatry trainee, I was afforded the opportunity to rotate through the CMHC, located on the Southside of Chicago and serving an inner-city, predominately black population. This rotation was for a six-month period. One day a week was spent on site working with the medical director, Dr. Carl C. Bell. The educational objectives were delineated, and the goals included providing a clinical/administrative/consultative training experience within a black community mental health setting. This was to include the following: (1) orientation to the community mental health systems network of facilities, (2) emergency diagnostic evaluations, (3) brief psychotherapy and medication management, (4) psychiatric consultation with non-medical health staff.

Additionally, it was felt that this experience would result in an enhanced understanding of the complexities of racism and cultural adaptation in terms of how it defines mental health and affects the manifestation of psychopathology.

The rotation began with an orientation phase, which included attending administrative meetings. Following this, the actual clinical experience involved working with the "walk-in" clinic component. This involved providing medication management, diagnostically evaluating patients, and at times, facilitating hospitalization where needed. Children and adolescents were also seen occasionally. Multidisciplinary staffings were attended weekly, and formal supervision also occurred on a weekly basis. Informal supervision was readily available at any time. The clinical experience was supplemented by relevant reading material, which was reviewed and discussed during supervision. The resident was exposed to not only ongoing research projects pertaining to minority mental health issues but to educational projects directed toward the community at large as well.

One valuable component of the experience was working within a "cultural milieu." The predominately black staff was well trained, committed, and adept at functioning efficiently, especially with limited resources. The striking difference between working in a community health setting compared to a major institution was exemplified in such areas as lack of on-site security personnel to assist with agitated patients and the difficult task of arranging for medical and laboratory procedures, such as lithium levels. Thus, the resident had to learn how to maintain a high level of quality care while maneuvering around obstacles.

Because the preceptorship model allowed direct, continuous contact with a black physician with expertise in the field of psychiatry as well as in minority mental health, the overall experience was intense, highly educational, and rewarding. The experience also served to enrich my professional identity. The rotation, however, should not be a solitary, isolated experience designed only for the minority resident trainee. Such an approach would continue to perpetuate the homogeneous, dominant culture orientation that exists currently. Minority curriculum content should become a core component of all residency training programs in psychiatry; preferably, it should be incorporated early during the training experience and should include direct clinical experience, didactic courses, workshops, and distinguished lectures on an ongoing basis. Additionally, the need for continued research into minority mental health issues should be strongly emphasized and encouraged.

CONCLUSIONS

While the new generation of transcultural and transethnic psychiatric knowledge gains a legitimate place in the core curriculum content of psychiatric residency training programs, today's psychiatric residents continue to need special knowledge and skills to treat black populations. Attending workshops and lectures and taking preceptorships during special elective tracks continue to be an excellent temporary source of education about and experience with black psychiatric patient populations. The preceptorship format provides the most intensive educational process and allows for an experience tailored to the resident's previous experience with black populations. It also it allows the resident to experience the "real world" of a heterogeneous psychiatric patient population from a transethnic and transcultural perspective, as opposed to frequently found "ivory tower" experience, which gears residents to treat a homogeneous psychiatric population that, in reality, does not exist.

COMMENTARY

As my work became well known, I began to get requests to train psychiatric residents and medical students at the CMHC using the preceptor model of training that we developed for residents. We trained residents and/or medical students from the University of Illinois, University of Chicago, Chicago Medical School, Northwestern University, and Chicago School of Osteopathic Medicine. Additionally, we received requests to train University of Illinois psychology PhD candidates, University of Chicago social work students, Chicago School of Professional Psychology professional psychology PhD candidates, Chicago State University MA students, and others. CMHC has also had the occasion to serve as a psychology practicum site for out-of-state trainees, the most notable being Dr. Jacqueline Mattis, who was at the University of Michigan. Again, the content of this book is a testimony to the work I've done with a great deal of support from and partnership with many people. In many ways, it can serve as a training manual for some aspects of African-American health and mental health.

Training continues to be a major aspect of what we offer at the CMHC. We're able to train well because we provide a great deal of service to patients in various arenas. CMHC has researched its service outcomes, and we're able to advocate for service models because we know they work. It is yet another example of how we've discovered aspects of black mental health that were heretofore either unknown or unappreciated.

I'm extremely fortunate to have two senior vice presidents, Juanita Redd, MPH, MS, MBA, and Hayward Suggs, MS, MS, MBA. Because of their great deal of understanding about organizational dynamics, they've impressed upon me the need for training and coaching of our predominately African-American workforce. The CMHC trains people not only in evidence-based mental health interventions but also in how to work cooperatively on the job. Frequently, work goes undone not because of lack of know-how but because of "people mess" on the job. It's like having two people chained together and trying to run somewhere. If they have a personal conflict and one shoots the other's foot in anger, how far will they get? At the CMHC, we train people to negotiate and work together as a team, and the results have been remarkable.

The training must not be a one-shot deal, however. It must be ongoing and done annually, because staff come and go. This makes life very difficult for a nonprofit agency like the CMHC because you need staff on the line to generate income so that the agency can make payroll. To take staff off the line for training costs a great deal of money and prevents the staff from earning needed income. There will be a problem, though, if you're on the line and giving penicillin to people who come in with a heart attack. Heart attack patients need nitroglycerin or aspirin. Staff may need to be trained to understand this reality. Unfortunately, staff at most community-based organizations aren't doing evidence-based interventions proven to work with patients suffering from various psychiatric disorders. Thus, a great deal of training needs to be done to transmit those evidence-based interventions to staff in the field. As previously mentioned, this was one of the major findings in Dr. Satcher's groundbreaking mental health report and one that the CMHC has discovered how to fix. It's too bad that no one to date has given community-based organizations any money to help fix this problem, since such organizations provide a great deal of social service to those in need. It would be nice if what we do could be shown to work.

Recently, President Bush's New Freedom Mental Health Commission visited the CMHC because they had heard of my work and were extremely interested in the CMHC's training program. We make it a point in training our staff in evidence-based mental health interventions so that African Americans can get the benefit of new and modern technology. After all, our community-based organization sees a lot of poor patients who need help in addressing their problems in living, so why not give them the best science and humanity has to offer? The Commission's visit was interesting for me because I'd previously worked with various Commission staff members twenty years earlier. It just goes to show you— you never know who you'll bump into at critical moments later in life, so I always recommend doing your best work all the time.

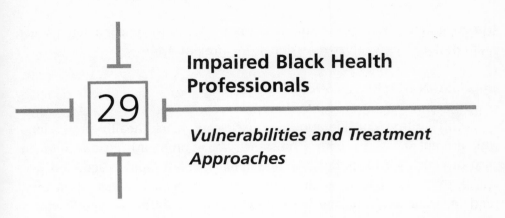

Impaired Black Health Professionals

Vulnerabilities and Treatment Approaches

The impaired black health professional (i.e., one with a substance abuse problem) is in a unique position in American society. Factors that contribute to this uniqueness include the small number of black health professionals, which limits resources for program development and referrals; overt and covert racism in society and in medical school curriculums; differences in black and white drug and alcohol abuse and suicide patterns; and upward mobility, which tends to isolate the black professional from black support systems. These factors need to be recognized by the health care profession. Bias-free investigations are needed to provide more information on ethnic differences so that impaired health professional programs and services may give more appropriate treatment.

INTRODUCTION

Although blacks represent 12% of the American population, only 2% of all physicians, 2% of all dentists, 3% of all pharmacists, and 1.7% of all veterinarians are black.[1] The position of the black professional in

Originally printed as Bell Carl C. Impaired black health professionals: vulnerabilities and treatment approaches. *J Natl Med Assoc.* 1986;78:925–930.

American society imposes unique features that must be considered when addressing black health professional impairment.

RACISM IN AMERICAN SOCIETY AT LARGE

The first consideration in discussing black health professional impairment (i.e. those with a substance abuse problem) must be the context in which the black health professional was born and raised, and lives currently. In 1986, black health professionals are acutely aware of the overt and covert forms of racism that still exist in the majority of American society and are aware that America's current race relations are only thirty-two years after the end of apartheid—in other words, since the 1954 decision to desegregate schools.

The overt forms of racism are made apparent from reports on current events,[1] and black health professionals are aware of these. For example, blacks are being burned out of their new homes in all-white neighborhoods. The Ku Klux Klan is still active, and the murder of black men by white men for associating with white women continues.

Black health professionals are also aware of the less violent forms that racism takes in American society, such as "mini-insults" and "micro-aggressions."[2,3] They are also aware of the subtle effects of "institutional racism," which may be defined as any cluster of norms (folkways, mores, principles, guidelines, rules, procedures, and laws) that have been formalized and accorded social recognition as an established way of doing things, but that promote racial discrimination, segregation, persecution, and dominance.[4] An example of an institutional procedure having inherent covert racism is a requirement of one's parents having been physicians in order to get into medical school. While this regulation would not exclude minorities specifically, only a few minorities would be able to gain medical school admission because there is a disproportionately small percentage of them whose parents are physicians.

The black health professional is constantly confronted with the stark realities of race relations in this country and must seek to cope with them in his/her nonprofessional interactions. It has been has been open to question whether the stress of experiencing direct effects of racism in housing, employment, and legal matters and the stress from awareness that racism places danger on one causes black health professionals to risk impairment. It has also been open to question whether the ever-present threat of being a victim of racism causes them to refute stereotypes of blacks by not engaging in "inferior" behaviors associated with impairment. Whether or not stress is used in a constructive or destructive manner[5,6] depends on the individual's makeup. Certainly, however, knowing that a white racist believes a black health professional is just a "nigger" and should be treated as such, becomes a source of stress for the black health professional. It indicates that one cannot acquire a social status high enough to remove the stigma of being black from some persons' minds. It should be apparent that every identifiable black person in this country because of his blackness has experienced having a dream deferred, the severe consequences of which black poet Langston Hughes writes about in his famous poem.[7] Certainly, this has an impact on blacks' development.

To be sure, racism experienced in the majority of American society would make any mindful black health professional hesitant to step forward and admit to society at large an impairment, since it might put the impaired black health professional at the mercy of a system that means him ill will. Most blacks are familiar with a criminal justice system that is more lenient with white criminals than with black ones. There are also anecdotal personal reports that state licensure boards have dealt more harshly with impaired black health professionals than with their white counterparts.

RACISM IN HEALTH PROFESSIONALS

While one may wish to believe that racism is a product of ignorance and poor education and should therefore not be found among health professionals, this is not the case. Thus, another consideration in discussing impaired black health professionals must be the context in which blacks are educated, as well as the racist practices that occur in their professional fields. An example can be found in medicine. The history of the exclusion of blacks from medical education is well-documented.[8] Affirmative action programs have tried to rectify the long-range effects of discrimination.[1] Such programs intended to make minority status a positive criterion for admission (previously, it had been used in an exclusionary manner), to

ensure financial aid and programs for special academic assistance, to provide safeguards like anonymous grading of examinations, and to provide
for a minority dean and ombudsman presence to guarantee a nondiscrim-
inatory educational environment. It is clear that in recent years, these
efforts have been dismantled. Shea and Fullilove[8] conclude that the commitment of medical schools to affirmative action has slackened. The dis-
mantling of affirmative action is a signal to the black health professional
that the medical profession at large means blacks no good will regarding
medical school admission and retention. This lack of good will is even
more evident when one considers that many of the objectives of the affirmative action programs developed by medical schools were being met. For
example, more minority physicians were made available to improve the
health care of the poor, physicians were supplied to underserved communities, and the number of physicians providing primary care was
increased.[9]

The perception that some whites have ill will toward black health
professionals is confirmed when blacks go to predominately white medical
schools. Bullock and Houston[10] reported on the perceptions of 31 black
medical students from five white medical schools and found that there was
a universal perception of racism in their educational context. As a result,
there was a general mistrust and avoidance of whites, and the black students felt more comfortable with other blacks. It is natural, then, that these
black students were also disheartened at the Bakke decision, which essentially said that affirmative action was no longer a legitimate consideration
for admission into medical school. While two thirds of the black students
were expecting racism and one third was not, there was generally shock
and anger at the phenomenon. Furthermore, the students had personally
observed discriminatory attitudes of white staff toward black patients.
Such witnessing of white health professional colleagues' ill will toward
blacks makes it difficult for an impaired black health professional to accept
a referral to a white treatment program.

Another area in which racism manifests itself in the medical education institution is in the curricular content of medical school and in post-
graduate training. To date, very little is taught about minority medical
issues in medical school and residency training programs. Occasionally,
there may be a course on racism in medicine, but the presence of such a

course is predicated on the interest of one or two faculty members. Most medical school faculty members teach medicine as though their future student physicians' patient population will be a homogeneous group: young, white, Anglo-Saxon, middle-class, Protestant men. In reality, the patient population is heterogeneous, having various cultures, ethnic groups, folk medicine beliefs, religious beliefs, disparate contact with noxious and carcinogenic stimuli, differing biologic responses to medication, and differing hygienic practices, all of which affect health, wellbeing, and responses to treatment of the various minority groups.

The lack of attention to minority curricular content represents an expression of institutional racism. Such omission transmits the covert message that the knowledge base needed for adequate response to minorities' health needs is not worthy of inclusion in medical school curriculums. The black health professional who observes this process will likely suspect that impaired physician programs, which may well suffer from this same "selective inattention," may not as a result be tailored to meet minorities' specific needs. For example, the overall white-to-black ratio for suicide is eleven to four, but black men aged 20–35 years have a suicide rate twice that of white men of the same age. It is the high number of whites over the age of 45 who commit suicide that makes the overall rate of white suicide greater than black suicide. For the impaired white health professional, those at greater risk of suicide are men over the age of 45, living alone, and on the downswing of life. If this profile is inappropriately extrapolated to black health professionals, it would cause impaired health professional programs to overlook the fact that older blacks tend not to be suicidal; it is the young, upwardly mobile black men who are at greater risk. There is evidence of different patterns of drug and alcohol abuse among blacks and whites,[11] but these differences (which may apply to impaired health professionals) might not be considered by impaired health professional programs and services.

Knowledge that information about minorities taught to medical students prior to the Civil Rights Movement was often full of stereotypes and racist, unfavorable, and degrading generalizations (some of them contrived) used as proof of the "inherent inferiority" present in blacks, may cause impaired black health professionals to avoid being identified. Specifically, they may view their impairment as ammunition for those who would say, "See, I told you blacks are incapable of professional training and status. Look at how the stress of professional status has impaired this one. It just proves that blacks cannot tolerate the stress of independence and that they were better off when they were dominated."

Black health professionals are also acutely aware of the difference in health care that blacks and whites obtain. Minorities are more likely to fall victim to the nation's major killers: cancer, cardiovascular and cerebrovascular diseases, chemical dependence, homicide, and accidents.[12] Amid such seeming indifference by the health services to their health issues, how could the impaired black health professional comfortably submit himself for treatment and not be somewhat wary of the type of treatment he will receive? It has been pointed out that there may be significant bias in the assessment of black psychiatric patients, which results in misdiagnosis and mistreatment.[13–20] Certainly, this would not inspire confidence in a psychiatrically impaired black health professional who was referred to a white psychotherapist.

If one accepts the hypothesis that racism persists in the health professions, then the issue of a black health professional who has recovered from impairment and is trying to reenter the practice of his profession, is of concern. Such a person has a double stigma, which in all likelihood makes reentry extremely difficult. The situation is further compounded if the recovered impaired black health professional is a woman.

BLACK HEALTH PROFESSIONALS: AN UPWARDLY MOBILE GROUP AT RISK?

Traditionally, blacks have had a low rate of suicide and suicide attempt[21,22]; however, Prudhomme[23] predicted that black suicide would increase as blacks make efforts to assimilate to white lifestyles. Clark[24] noted that while the suicide rate for Harlem was, on the whole, lower than that for New York City, there were three areas of Harlem where the suicide rate was almost twice that of the city as a whole. These were the middle-class areas, where blacks were striving to assimilate to white lifestyles. These and similar findings have led some researchers to hypothesize that there is a risk involved in the success black health professionals achieve.[25,26] Davis[27] and Gary[28] hypothesize that as blacks assimilate to white lifestyles, they lose their original support system, replacing it with a system allowing for desegregation but not integration, which leaves them at risk for egoistic and anomic suicide.[29] This accounts for the rising suicide rate in young blacks.

Dr. Schorer (personal communication, June 28, 1985) found that talking with a friend, spouse, or relative was the preferred way of handling stressful reactions in 180 medical students. Yet, the black health professional, who may not fit in with whites because of their racism, may not fit in with the majority of blacks either, due to his professional status. Clearly, he runs the risk of being a "marginal man." The isolation from family and friends many black health professionals experience when moving upward on the social and economic ladder may reduce their alternative of talking about their stress with family and friends.

Powell[30] has demonstrated that blacks in desegregated private schools have low self-esteem scores similar to those of ghetto blacks in Los Angeles and New York City; affluent blacks in parochial black schools in Nashville (where there are two black colleges and a black medical school) have high self-esteem scores comparable to those of whites in similar schools; and black students in segregated schools in the South have the highest self-esteem scores. These observations are attributed to readily identifiable role models, black culture in school, and the child's acceptance by peers and teachers in respectful black educational milieus. Significantly, Powell points out that desegregation does not necessarily mean integration, and that desegregation is a demeaning experience that erodes self-esteem.[30]

Griffith and Delgado[31] suggest that the black professional "not allow the white socialization process to separate him from his own intimate concept of himself and to obliterate his personal historical traditions." Gary and Berry[32] have noted that blacks having a strong sense of their blackness may prevent them from being victims of drug abuse. These findings have implications for prevention efforts aimed at reducing the number of impaired black health professionals. They suggest that promoting a strong, positive, ethnic identity while maintaining ethnic ties, despite professional status, will reduce suicide and drug abuse. It may well be that blacks who train at predominately black medical schools have a greater opportunity to develop a healthy black health professional identity and to learn coping skills for survival in their unique position in American society as "marginal persons." This hypothesis deserves further study.

The impaired black health professional may be at greater risk of suicide because of feelings of fatalism. Swanson and Breed[33] attribute this sense of being trapped and helpless as being at the root of suicide among blacks committing suicide when arrested (suicide is the greatest cause of death for everyone in jail). Durkheim[29] reported that fatalism motivated chained Africans being transported on slave ships to jump overboard to drown. Black health professionals who, because of their impairment get into legal difficulties such as licensure problems or malpractice litigation, may feel trapped or helpless. Because of a strong sense to avoid anything that resembles the trapped, helpless feeling inherent in enslavement, impaired black health professionals may be at greater risk of suicide. This unique aspect of impaired black health professionals must be addressed by impairment programs.

WHITE HEALTH PROFESSIONAL INTERFACE PROBLEMS

Whites experience problems in desegregated settings and during their interactions with black health professionals. They may become over-solicitous or distant out of concern that any time they criticize black health professionals, they will be perceived as being racist as opposed to giving legitimate critique. The identification process of a state medical society's impaired physician program may be hampered by these interracial interface difficulties. Furthermore, treatment using impaired health professional groups may be hampered by the black health professional being the "only one" in the group, an issue that may be inappropriately handled by "hallucinatory whitening"[34] (the pretense that there are no differences between white and black health professionals). To be effective, state medical society impaired physician programs must confront their discomfort in dealing with impaired black health professionals.

STATE OF THE ART:
BLACK HEALTH PROFESSIONALS' IMPAIRMENT PROGRAMS

The art of preventing, identifying, and treating impaired black health professionals has not been well explored, due to several reasons beyond the usual resistance to developing impaired health professional programs. First, there are fewer black health professionals who are members of minority health professional societies, which results in limited resources from which to develop programs. Likewise, there are problems in gathering enough impaired black health professionals to form a "critical mass," to work together. A limited number of black health professionals makes it difficult for them to start self-help groups for themselves. Smaller black health manpower pools limit referral resources for black health professionals who would feel more comfortable being treated by someone similar to them.

There is also a lack of a substantial knowledge base regarding black health professional impairment. In part, this is related to the cautious nature black health professionals have regarding any research on black issues, which is due to legitimate concerns about how such information will be interpreted and utilized. The health care profession has gone from using a racist portrayal of black mental health (and using racist research to justify discrimination and domination[19]), to having a selective inattention, to not finding any legitimate differences in the mental health of whites and blacks, to finally taking an honest, scientific look at black mental health. However, black health professionals are still aware of how any research on impaired black health professionals may be used against them.

Despite these impediments, some efforts in confronting the problems of black health professional impairment have occurred. In 1983, the National Medical Association's Annual Convention plenary session, coordinated by Dr. Calmez Dudley, addressed the issue of impaired physicians, and in 1985, Dr. Billy Jones coordinated the plenary session, "Lifestyle of the Physician: Indications for Stress Management." Collins[35] developed a stress management program at Howard University in an effort to prevent emotional or personal problems and to assist students with formal treatment, if indicated. He was instrumental in encouraging the Black Psychiatrists of America, which has about 500 members, to develop a national referral roster. It has become indispensable for referring impaired black health professionals to black psychiatrists.

SUMMARY

The impaired black health professional is in a unique position in American society. Factors that contribute to this must be considered in any health professional impairment program that seeks to aid these individuals. The issue of racism in American society at large must be broached, since impaired black health professionals may have concerns that they will receive harsher treatment from state medical boards and society at large, and that they will be at greater risk of losing their hard-earned social positions. There are still problems with black health professionals being fully integrated into white health professions. Both blacks and whites may have difficulties in the interracial interface, and these difficulties will impact the relationship between an impaired black health professional and the state health professional society's impaired professional programs and services.

The unique position of the black health professional may cause a greater risk of impairment, secondary to being isolated from black support systems. This possible isolation from black support systems must be considered in any impairment program attempting to help the impaired black health professional. Likewise, fatalistic motivations for committing suicide must be considered. These possible risks can be avoided by encouraging black health professionals to maintain ties with family, friends, and the black community despite the professional's upward mobility.

There is a dearth of information regarding the impaired black health professional. There are some indications that drug and alcohol abuse and suicide patterns differ in whites and blacks. The same may be true for impaired black and white health professionals. Bias-free investigations must fill this information gap to provide more appropriate impaired health professional programs and services for blacks.

Finally, the limited number of black health professionals and resources for them demand that all concerned health professionals band together to address the issue of the impaired health professional, regardless of ethnicity.

COMMENTARY

This article was included in this section because much of it deals with the racism that interferes with impaired black health professionals getting the same quality treatment as impaired European-American health professionals. When this paper was presented at the AMA's 7th National Conference on the Impaired Physician (quite different from the previous six), the conference leadership decided it would be good to establish linkages with other impaired professionals. As a result, they asked representatives from the African American, Asian, Native American, Hispanic, and women's medical associations to present on impairment issues peculiar to their members. They also made a similar request to dentists', pharmacists', and veterinarians' trade associations. Since the AMA conference would be in Chicago, the NMA asked me to represent our association, and I agreed. In my opinion, only the women's representative was very direct with the conference planning committee regarding women's issues. Everyone else was very gentle with the AMA. I saved my directness for my presentation that followed.

Since this article's publication, it's been my impression that again, not very much has changed. If anything, as the American economy has worsened, the drive to exclude black health professionals from medical practice has increased. Managed care efforts have largely excluded black physicians, who have a greater difficulty in complying with the information system demands that managed care require. I've followed the issue of impaired black professionals, and my observations have remained the same. Most often, impaired black health professionals are treated more harshly than their European-American counterparts. Recently, another "uneven playing field" has been revealed: the penalty for having a small amount of "crack" cocaine (an inner-city, lower socioeconomic drug) is much stiffer than having a large amount of powdered cocaine (a suburban, middle-class drug).

One major change that has occurred is the "war on drugs." As a result, drug addiction (a medical illness) has been criminalized. The new policy demands the incarceration of individuals caught using drugs and has caused the prison population to double, and in some states, even triple. Of course, the victims of this new policy are mainly poor, unemployed, African Americans. I think this is a travesty of justice and health care. There are at least two types of drug addicts in the country who benefit from drug treatment programs to have a recovery rate of about 85%: physicians and airline pilots. If we've devised a treatment that helps 85% of the patients who participate in that treatment, why are we incarcerating so many people for drug use? Where would the country be if instead of having a "war on drugs," we had a public health crusade to address the drug addiction epidemic? Where would we be if we directed all the resources spent building new prisons toward treatment and rehabilitation?

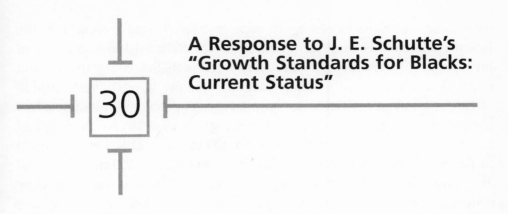

A Response to J. E. Schutte's "Growth Standards for Blacks: Current Status"

The article by Dr. J. E. Schutte entitled "Growth Standards for Blacks: Current Status" (*J Natl Med Assoc*. 1980;72:973–978) cleared up a question I have had for 11 years. In 1969, I did a study entitled "A Social and Nutritional Survey on the Children and Youth Center of Meharry Medical College of North Nashville, Tennessee" (*J Natl Med Assoc*. 1971;63:397–398), which surveyed the social and nutritional status of fifty lower socioeconomic black children attending a Meharry Medical College clinic. The results of the study were very startling; they contained some contradictory findings that I could not figure out.

The average number of individuals in the households of the children studied was 6.5, with an average monthly income of $222. The average amount of money spent on food during any given week for 6.5 people was $28.50. The fifty children studied had an average age of 9.6 years. They had an average birth weight of 6.7 pounds, with 8% having a low birth weight (less than 5 lb. 6 oz). Four percent of the patients had sickle cell hemoglobinopathy. Regarding nutritional parameters, 8% of the population had a hemoglobin value below 11 gm/100 ml (a range of 7.4–11gm/100 ml, and an average of 8 gm/100 ml). 10% of the patients had a hematocrit

Originally printed as Bell Carl C. Letter to the editor in response to an article by J. E. Schutte, "Growth Standards for Blacks: Current Status." *J Natl Med Assoc*. 1981;73:596–600.

value below 34%. With respect to vitamin levels (using criteria from the Interdepartmental Committee on Nutrition for National Defense), 10% of the sample had very low vitamin A serum levels (below 20 µg/100 ml) and 6% had deficient levels of serum vitamin A (below 10 µg/100 ml). A total of 16% had low or deficient vitamin A levels. Six percent of the sample had low vitamin C serum levels (below 0.5 mg/100 ml). Twelve percent had low serum protein levels (below 6.5 gm/100 ml) and 22% were classified as having deficient serum protein levels (below 6.0 gm/100 ml). A total of 38% had low or deficient serum protein levels. The study concluded by stating, "…50% of the population studied had low or deficient levels of one parameter, 8% had low or deficient levels of two parameters, and 6% had low or deficient parameters, which is a total of 64% of the population that exhibit deficient or low levels of nutrition" (Bell CC. A social and nutritional survey on the population of the Children and Youth Center of Meharry College of North Nashville, Tennessee. *J Natl Med Assoc.* 1971;63:397–398).

When the age- and sex-adjusted weight and height of these lower socioeconomic black children with poor nutritional status was compared with the age- and sex-adjusted weight and height of middle-class white children with acceptable nutritional status, there was no appreciable difference in the weight and height percentiles. According to the white growth standards percentile chart, my population had an average weight (sex and age adjusted) that corresponded to the 46th percentile, and an average height (sex and age adjusted) that corresponded to the 58th percentile (the 50th percentile being the average in the customary weight and height range).

When I re-examined my figures, I found that in contrast to the white standards, the growth charts for black boys and girls prepared by Spurgeon and Meredith revealed a more consistent reflection of my population's weight and height, considering their nutritional status. My population had an average weight (sex and age adjusted) that fell just above the lower limit of the average weight area in the Spurgeon/Meredith charts (estimated at the 41st percentile by my calculations) and an average height (sex and age adjusted) that fell below a median line bisecting the average height area of the Spurgeon/Meredith charts (estimated at the 46th percentile by my calculations).

I have evidence to explain the contradictory finding that nutritionally low or deficient lower socioeconomic black children have average weight and height percentiles, compared with middle-class white children of Northern European ancestry. Dr. Schutte's statement, "the inappropriate use of middle-class white standards could thus underestimate growth deficiencies among Black children," certainly would apply to my study. Had I not included nutritional data, the results could have been seriously misleading, since some political forces used my paper to attempt to elevate the quality of some public services for the residents of the area studied. Tthe study noted that a woman with two children received $105 per month from Aid to Dependent Children and that a woman with seven children received $120.

While it is important to note that my study was more internally consistent when using growth charts prepared for black boys and girls from lower socioeconomic families, I wonder how my population would rate in regard to weight and height percentiles when compared to middle-class black children with an acceptable nutritional status. Dr. Schutte's article supplies some data that my group's weight and percentiles may in fact be even lower when compared to black children from middle income families.

As Dr. Schutte points out, had there been percentile lines in the Spurgeon/Meredith charts and the charts for preschool children, my ability to compare groups would have been easier and more accurate. As it now stands, I have only an approximation, using 70% of my original sample (15 of the 50 children studied were under five years of age). In addition, I wonder if the five-year difference between my study and Meredith-Spurgeon's would account for an estimated 5% difference in age and sex adjusted weight percentiles and a 12% difference in sex- and age-adjusted height percentiles depending on whether or not one used a black lower socioeconomic growth chart verses a white middle-class growth chart. I tend to doubt that this is the case, though, and I suspect that the difference is due not to secular changes but to ethnic differences in growth.

All of this is to say that I am quite pleased to see that the JNMA continues to publish empirical scientific data gathered from observing blacks, which time and time again demonstrates that white standards do not adequately measure black parameters (which in no way implies that black parameters are inferior).

COMMENTARY

Though my original study spoke for itself, I had a puzzling question that would remain unanswered for a decade. Essentially, I couldn't understand at the time of the study why the poorly nourished African-American children of North Nashville had average or above-average heights and weights. I'd expected otherwise, considering that they were nutritionally deficient and that many had been born premature. Ten years after when I found the J. E. Schutte article, I finally learned that it wasn't my results but the standards that were faulty. I'd rated my African-American children's heights and weights using charts developed from middle-class white children's measurements. Through Schutte, I discovered that the heights and weights I'd recorded were in fact below average, but only when compared to wealthier African Americans.

We as African Americans are at a disadvantage when we evaluate ourselves on measures established with others in mind, or when we don't have any empirical, observable information about ourselves. Though Schutte's was a basic empirical study, I can't underscore enough the importance of performing such research on African Americans. I found Schutte's work so impressive that I wrote this letter to the JNMA editor commending their publication of the article.

My work has taught me some universal principles of health behavior change. I frequently point out how for years in efforts to promote good nutrition, the US promulgated their food pyramid with milk at the top. This is problematic, considering that milk causes bloating and gas for the vast majority of the world's population, which happens to be Non-white. Recognizing the universal principle that good nutrition is a must for all people on the planet is a noble consideration; however, it must be taken into account that different people have different dietary requirements.

I've recently found another article in addition to Schutte's that has finally examined the vitamin A levels in African-American children and compared them with those in European-American children (Ford ES, Gillespie C, Ballwe C, Sowell A, Mannino DM. Serum carotenoid concentrations in US children and adolescents. *Am J Clinical Nutrition.* 2002;76:818–827). As it turns out, after controlling for socioeconomic status, African-American children and adolescents have significantly higher concentrations of beta-cryptoxanthin (p < 0.001), lutein and zeaxanthin (p < 0.001), and lycopene (p = 0.006) concentrations but have lower alpha-carotene (p < 0.001) than do white children and adolescents. Again, using European-American standards to assess African-American children can lead one astray.

Back in 1971, I was surprised that only 16% of North Nashville's extremely poor, African-American children had vitamin A levels below 20 µg, which represented deficiency, by European-American standards. The finding that African-American children usually have higher vitamin A levels than European-American children suggests that many more of the poor black children I studied were deficient, by African-American vitamin A standards. As Dr. Satcher's Surgeon General's *Reports on Culture, Race, and Ethnicity* make clear, we have to figure out a way to include more diverse samples in our research studies. Otherwise, the health disparities within American society will continue, to everyone's detriment.

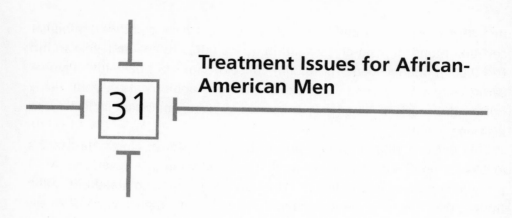

Treatment Issues for African-American Men

There has been a dearth of empirical and research literature on the treatment needs of African-American men.[1] Due to the diversity of socioeconomic status, education, and other experiences within the African-American community, it is difficult to make broad generalizations about African-American men and their treatment needs. However, one common experience that African-American men share is that of racism and discrimination. This article will review what is known about the treatment of African-American men and provide some current thoughts about African-American men's treatment issues.

REVIEW OF THE LITERATURE

Attitudes about psychiatric treatment of African Americans varied during two distinct periods in history: prior to and after the Civil Rights/Black Power Movement.

Before Civil Rights/Black Power Movement

Pinderhughes[2] outlines some of the themes exhibited by Negroes in psychotherapy prior to the 1960s, when the Civil Rights/Black Power

Originally printed as Bell Carl C. Treatment issues for African-American men. *Psychiatr Annals.* 1996;26:33–36.

Movement began, including a denial of problems, a vague commitment to therapy, transient paranoid feelings of persecution, repeated signs of distrust, and silence, or blocking. Adams admonishes white therapists to understand that the Negro patient will see them as threatening on many levels, due to not only parental transference issues but also very real racial and class matters.[3] Frank[4] and St. Clair[5] report on the difficulty of establishing rapport and securing a therapeutic relationship with Negroes because of their suspiciousness or submissiveness.

Adams notes that Negroes' inferiority feelings, resulting from forced isolation from the total culture, require consideration, as does the intense drive for upward social mobility in the Negro community.[3] St. Clair stresses the importance of dealing with hostility and self-esteem in Negro patients.[5] Adams[3] cautions that whites are frequently perplexed and uncertain in the presence of Negroes, causing them to respond to Negroes not as individuals, but as the Negro stereotypes with which they are familiar. Adams and others[3-5] suggest that therapists treating these patients need to examine their attitudes and feelings about race, and that they should possess a knowledge of the structure and cultural background of Negro social groups.[6]

After Civil Rights/Black Power Movement

Since 1967, Negroes have made an effort to change their relationship with whites in society. A change in their identity was reflected in their preference to be referred to as "black." Many blacks began to actively struggle with self-defeating patterns in themselves, examining confidence, self-esteem, assertiveness, and initiative. For blacks, to be "Negro" now meant being the bad, messy, aggressive, willful child. Being "black," on the other hand, meant being strong, resilient, mature, warm, emotional, sincere, honest, forthright, and attractive.

Pinderhughes[2] notes that accordingly, after the Civil Rights/Black Power Movement, the psychiatric treatment issues for blacks changed. The need to study problems arising from self-image and racial and social-class identification, and problems from handling anger toward whites became a concern in the treatment of blacks. Pinderhughes agrees with Calnek's assertion: "Currently, and perhaps for many years to come, Afro-

Americans are and will be torturously struggling to achieve self-identity and self-determination."[7] Pinderhughes[2] draws attention to the fact that biracial psychotherapy may present some special problems, and expands on the psychodynamic principles involved in this process. Calnek[7] focuses on optimizing treatment of black patients when the therapist is also black.

Writing about errors made in psychotherapy with blacks, Carter[8] notes that the inability of some therapists to confront anxieties about racial differences is crucial and notes that inquiry into the patient's feelings about working with someone of a different race should be raised as part of the initial contact. Carter[8] states that black patients also want to see evidence of assertiveness from their therapists and they want their therapists to respond to their real and pressing needs before moving to a more introspective approach to their problems.

Carter's hypothesis is honed out in a study by Wood and Sherrets.[9] They report that blacks rate administrative action, reality contact, and medication as significantly more important than whites do. This indicates that blacks seek relatively more direct and immediate types of services, although white and black patients are more alike than different in their service requests.

Siegel,[10] in reviewing the literature on how race affects clinical interventions between the white clinician and black patient, concludes that "despite much clinical speculation about the possible inability of white clinicians to help black patients, there is little evidence to suggest that this is the case as there is no research on therapeutic outcomes comparing black and white therapists with black patients." Empirical studies demonstrate that there are differences in service availability for blacks,[11-14] and that this availability might be predicated on the perceived undesirability of black patients and by class factors as well. These studies imply that because black patients may be excluded by white therapists, studying a white therapist's treatment efficacy with a black patient could be a moot point (i.e., a non-issue).

More Recent Research

Since Pinderhughes' seminal paper on the changing needs of blacks in treatment, there have been efforts to elaborate on the treatment needs of black men. Bell, Bland, Houston, and Jones[15] list concerns for therapists when treating blacks with dynamic psychotherapy: the need to dispel racial stereotypes and myths within the therapist, the need to address the significance of the black patient's race, the need to be sensitive to the patient's needs and reality, and the need to adjust to the black patient's expectations. Kupers[16] has written about transference and counter-transference when the therapist is white and the patient is black.

Jones, Gray, and Jospitre,[17] in a survey of 51 black and 42 white psychiatrists about their treatment of black patients (especially black men), found that 99% of the black psychiatrists and only 48% of the white psychiatrists were treating black patients. Several of the white psychiatrists reported not treating black patients because these patients were not being referred to them. Nine white psychiatrists were excluded from the study because they had little or no experience in treating black patients.

Jones and Gray[18] state, "white psychiatrists seem to have more difficulty relating to black male patients than to [black] female patients," and hypothesize that this may be because white psychiatrists expect black men to be threatening (i.e., they adhere to a common societal negative stereotype of black men). Another study[19] concludes that white therapists have a higher level of distress than do black therapists in cross-racial treatments and that some white therapists are over-solicitous or too distant with their black patients, or feel incapable of helping them.

Jones and Gray[20] report that the most frequent presenting problems of black men are depression and work-related issues. These observations are supported by researchers at the Institute of Social Research at the University of Michigan,[21] who found that men were significantly more likely than women to experience "a problem" or "depression."

Jones and his colleagues also report that conflict from aggression and passivity was the most frequent conflict encountered by the black male patients in their study (in contrast to high/low self-esteem being more problematic for black women[20]). They assert that black men often have conflicts in this area because society does not allow them the healthy expression of aggression, self-assertion, or passivity. This observation is underscored by Grier and Cobbs.[22] Jones and his colleagues suggest that the inappropriate channeling of aggressive drives and hostile feelings may lead to substance abuse, criminal activity (e.g., homicide), depression, and suicide. Finally, they assert that self-esteem is the second most frequent unconscious conflict area and hypothesize that this is because self-esteem is heavily influenced by external realities and by the negative stereotyping of black males.

African-American Men's Treatment Issues: 1995

Because overt discrimination is now illegal and courts have granted damages for emotional distress caused by racial discrimination,[23] the nature of racism has changed. It has become more covert.[24] Despite this change, Pierce[25] identifies racism as being akin to torture and terrorism. Therefore, racism continues to be a treatment issue for African-American men. Brantly,[26] in reviewing literature about the psychological effects of anti-black racism on black patients, underscores the continued importance of addressing racism in treating African-American men. However, because the nature of racism has changed, many African-American men are confused about racism. Drawing on Pierce's work, Bell[27] notes that African Americans are confused about it in at least four ways. First, while some whites accept African Americans as individuals, many harbor negative stereotypes about African Americans and merely tolerate their presence. Rejecting the genuine approbation of whites is as great an error as trusting a white person who harbors negative, racist stereotypes. African Americans cannot tell who is who and become uncertain if whites are tolerating or accepting them. Second, sometimes African Americans cannot distinguish between the supportive efforts of individual whites and the destructive action of whites as a group. This confusion can occur when an African American is truly accepted by an individual white person and consequently, erroneously begins to believe that racism no longer exists. Another hazardous puzzlement comes from figuring out when, where, and how to resist oppression, and when, where, and how to accommodate. Finally, African Americans have a difficult time determining when they are in control of their destiny versus when some external racist factors (sometimes visible and sometimes invisible) prevent their being in control. Where an African-American individual "draws the line" on these enigmas often has a far-reaching impact on how they are treated by other African

Americans who may have reached different conclusions about these conundrums.

Considering these recent issues, Brantly's[26] suggestion that a therapist should help the patient explore his coping mechanisms and develop more productive ways of dealing with the anxiety triggered by racism is still timely. During treatment, African-American men should be made aware of the four areas of confusion about racism in an effort to determine how the individual is managing these complex issues. Considering Pierce's observation that micro-insults and micro-aggressions cause very subtle but powerful erosions in self-esteem,[24] Brantly's proposal—that patients with self-esteem problems will have these problems exacerbated by racial confrontations—is especially cogent.[26] Brantly believes that the therapist who underestimates the impact of racism on a fragile defensive structure designed to protect the patient from a real external assault on his sense of self will be counter-therapeutic. He recommends that the therapist help the black patient develop a coping style that allows the patient to admit the existence of racism but that does not let it be seen as the dominant force in life. The person's self-esteem should be supported or developed so that it cannot be "dissolved by narrow-sighted racist perceptions"[26] (i.e., the patient should be helped to develop self-pride). Brantly also proposes that black patients do not need therapists who will over-identify with them; rather, therapists should help them see more clearly. Carter[8] concurs, adding that the therapist must not be too intimidated or apologetic because of an insufficiency of interracial experiences.

Jones and his colleagues[1,17,18,20] hypothesize a societal etiology for black males' conflicts from aggression and passivity. Jenkins and Bell[28] believe this kind of conflict may have to do with early exposure to violence and other forms of traumatic stress. Consequently, exposure to violence, as either a witness or victim, needs to be explored in the treatment of African-American men.

What African-American Men Need from their Therapists

A review of the empirical and research literature on the treatment of African-American men reveals that African-American men need therapists to do the following:

◆ Confront anxiety surrounding racial issues and explore their own issues pertaining to race.[29]

◆ Understand and are sensitive to issues of culture, class, family structure, educational levels, and social activities, thereby avoiding stereotyping.

◆ Understand barriers and frustrations about denied access as well as the need to achieve and be upwardly mobile.

◆ Understand the need for strong racial and class identity as well as for group identification and mutual dependence.

◆ Have the capability to be active and assertive, when appropriate, and attend to the real needs of the patient in an immediate and direct manner.

◆ Understand why some African-American men would be distrustful of people in authority why they would have transient paranoid, persecutory, and suspicious feelings as well.

◆ Understand why some African-American men might feel vulnerable and inferior and also feel a need to be submissive and passive.

◆ Understand self-image issues that some African Americans bring to treatment, including concerns about skin color, hair texture, facial features, body types, etc.

◆ Understand the special issues of establishing rapport with African-American men.

◆ Understand the need to explore potential problems of anger/hostility, self-esteem, confidence, assertiveness, initiative, and the need for external approbation.

◆ Understand that some African-American men will have a continuous, torturous struggle with self-identity and self-determination and that they will be confused about various aspects of racism.

◆ Understand the difficulties of working with African-American men, depending on whether the therapist is African American or white.

COMMENTARY

Psychiatric Annals had invited Dr. Terry Kupers to guest edit a special issue focusing on the topic, "Men's Issues in Treatment," and he invited me to write this article. When writing it, I relied on Dr. Pierce's work on racism. Most importantly, I drew on the work of Charles Pinderhughes, another psychiatric hero of mine, on psychotherapy issues of treating blacks. Frequently, I am concerned that young mental health professionals don't build upon the work of their elders. This is an error I have sought to avoid at all costs.

Dr. Pinderhughes presented an insightful experiment in March 1980 at joint BPA/New York Medical College conference, "Training in Mental Health Services for Black Populations," in Port Chester, New York. He asked everyone in the room to stand up. There were 30 African-American psychiatrists, 20 European-American psychiatrists, 5 Latino-American psychiatrists, and 5 Asian-American psychiatrists present. Next, Dr. Pinderhughes asked those who could trace their origin family's language, religion, and country to sit down. Only two of the African-American psychiatrists sat down. Eighteen of the European-American psychiatrists and all of the Latino-American and Asian-American psychiatrists sat down. Dr. Pinderhughes then theorized that the two African-American psychiatrists who sat were from Africa and that the 28 left standing were the products of slavery that had stripped them of their sense of connectedness. He went further to theorize that the 18 European-American and all the Latino-American and Asian-American psychiatrists who'd sat were from families who'd immigrated from their country of origin and had retained their connectedness. Finally, Dr. Pinderhuges hypothesized that the two European-American psychiatrists left standing were orphans, and they in fact were.

He pointed out that the orphan's sense of connectedness was similar to that of the African Americans in the group. With this type of insight, it isn't surprising that Dr. Pinderhughes has done a great deal of work on how stereotypes develop.

So far, this article has received much positive attention. Dr. James Carter, an exemplary African-American psychiatrist in North Carolina, published a summary of it in *Epikrisis*, a newsletter he edits from the North Carolina Governor's Institute on Alcohol and Substance Abuse, Inc. The Chicago School of Professional Psychology has published a modified version of many of the thoughts contained in the article as well. It was also a part of the Proceedings from their 1996 Cultural Impact Conference, during which I delivered a major lecture on the same subject.

This article has also opened up speculations for further study. Dr. Hugh Butts, who is editing a book on racism, African Americans, and post-traumatic stress disorder (PTSD), asked Dr. Johnny Williamson and me for help. Our paper was presented in Philadelphia at the 2003 annual meeting of the NMA. Dr. Butts wanted me to focus specifically on the relationship between racism, PTSD, and African-American children. So far, though, I haven't been able to find a case of an African-American child with PTSD caused directly by racism, and I've never had such a child referred to me. What I have seen is countless children with PTSD caused by witnessing violence, being victim of violence, having a terminal illness, being in both man-made and natural disasters, and having been in a war. Despite this reality, I believe that racism can damage African-American resistance to stress. Of course, I also believe that racism can "steel" African Americans against stress as well. These questions raised by the specter of racism will remain unanswered until, as I've said before, African Americans develop the administrative, methodological, and statistical skills to study these issues.

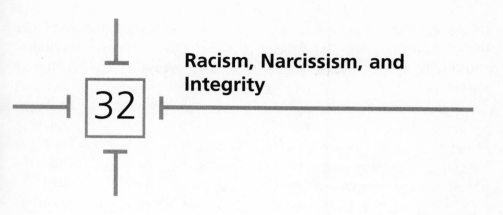

Racism, Narcissism, and Integrity

Recently there has been much literature pertaining to the psycho-dynamics of narcissism and its relation to psychopathological and normal psychic functions. While these models of the mind are primarily aimed at understanding individual behavior in the therapeutic relationship, they are also useful in clarifying one's thinking about racism, which can be approached both from an individual and social viewpoint. The author demonstrates that the racist individual suffers from a defect in narcissistic personality development, which precludes the subsequent development of such qualities as creativity, empathy, and integrity.

INTRODUCTION

Racism is the practice of racial discrimination, segregation, persecution, and domination based on a feeling of racial differences or antagonisms, especially with reference to supposed racial superiority, inferiority, or purity. In a half-hearted attempt to deal with racism, our society has made discrimination and segregation illegal, but this action only deals with overt, empirical behavior. Beneficial though this attempt may be, it allows

Originally printed as Bell Carl C. Racism, narcissism and integrity. *J Natl Med Assoc.* 1978;70:89–92. Presented at the 82nd Annual Convention of the NMA, Los Angeles, CA, August 1977.

a more pervasive and substantial type of racism to perpetuate—covert racism, which is subtle and difficult to prove. Covert racism is a psychological attitude and as such, should fall under the scrutiny of psychiatry as a psychopathological symptom of a personality disturbance. Integrity and the personality disturbance denoted by racism may be said to be on a continuum at opposite poles because integrity implies respect, while racism is a form of disrespect. A person who deserves respect is usually able to give it as well. To be clear, respect implies courtesy, showing consideration for others, and avoiding molesting or intruding upon others.

Recently, there has been much literature pertaining to the psychodynamics of narcissism and its relation to psychopathological and normal psychic functions. While these models of the mind are primarily aimed at understanding individual behavior in the therapeutic relationship, they are also useful in clarifying one's thinking about racism. The racist individual suffers from a psychopathological defect of developmental processes involving narcissism, which precludes the subsequent development of such qualities as creativity, empathy, wisdom, and integrity. Kohout's work on narcissistic personality disorders,[1] Masterson's work on borderline adolescence,[2] and Kernberg's work on borderline personality organization[3] deal with theoretical and developmental aspects of basic defects in racists, in addition to the murderer, child molester, and other behavioral types characterized by a basic lack of respect.

The infant begins with a fragmented self. In other words, it has an unrelated set of psychic structures and functions, as well as a set of drives that the mother needs to take care of. As the mother soothes these drives—a function she can perform only with the aid of an empathetic linkage with the child—the child begins to coalesce in relation to the mother. This process is called symbiosis. As the mother's inevitable separation from the child and her moments of unempathetic contact begin to impact the child, the child must tolerate this frustration (hopefully because of the nurturing received in earlier life) and maintain his sense of self. If on the other hand, the mother-child connection has been unempathetic, or if the child perceives the mother-child separation to have been too traumatic, a defect in relatedness occurs. In addition, there will be the accompanying tendency to function on or regress to the fragmented, agitated, and enraged early level of functioning. It is this lack of experience with empathetic linkage that characterizes the racists I have treated. It has been traced to the original paradigm of interpersonal relatedness—the mother-child relationship. One does unto others what has been done unto him.

Likewise, the murderous person's family history reveals unempathetic parental figures who dehumanized him as a child with unpredictable and violent behavior, the result of projecting onto the child unacceptable parts of the parents' personality. Abusive parents have familial histories of parental abuse, expectations of the child meeting their needs, a sense of self-righteousness, a feeling of owning the child and that he is their property, and a high degree of ambivalence towards love and rage. The murderous person, then, learns to totally dehumanize others in his mind. Characteristically, my murderous patients did not recognize their victims as persons with feelings. This is a clear indicator of having no respect for human life, which I feel is inherent in the psychological make-up of the racist.

In attempting to do intensive psychotherapy with racist individuals, one finds striking similarities between such patients and murderers, child abusers, child molesters, and sadists. The racists I have treated all had similar histories; in fact, their major motivation for seeking treatment revolved around frustration tolerance and impulse control. Although it is conceivable that patients with symptoms of dyscontrol may be racists, all racists do not necessarily have symptoms of dyscontrol. I have never seen a racist who has highly respected the perceived inferior's territory. This lack of respect does not always lead to the racist perpetuating violence against that perceived inferior, but it can lead to a violation of basic human rights. Such a disposition implies grandiosity, lack of self-boundaries, and dehumanization, all of which are theoretically and clinically characteristic of narcissistic personality disorder. The level of grandiosity in racism can be demonstrated by a white borderline patient I once encountered. Upon seeing me, a black, entering his clinic, this patient entered a state of agitation and narcissistic rage because he felt I had invaded his territory. He ran to me and within inches from me, ordered me to get out of his face. He was halfway down the hall before I realized what had happened. Territoriality or boundaries are paramount for racists because of their lack of self-definition and tendency to extend their boundaries, which thus motivates them to make anything foreign a stimulus for protective action.

It is interesting to note that treating a patient's underlying narcissistic personality disorders through the application of empathy relieved the symptoms of racism regardless if the patient was black, white, or Hispanic. It is only the narcissist who cannot see perceived inferiors as whole people after he has been thoroughly exposed to them. This is due to the narcissist's internal fragmentation. Persons with this type of psychological disorder are attentive only to those characteristics (real or imagined) that are important to them and pay little attention to other attributes that the perceived inferiors may possess. On the other hand, a person whose racist attitudes are secondary to cultural indoctrination can relinquish his attitudes with some exposure to perceived inferiors, as this type of racism is mainly due to ignorance and not narcissistic personality disorder. The difference with the racist attitude resulting from a defect in narcissistic development is in the degree of hostility directed toward the perceived inferiors. For example, the narcissistic racist who discusses miscegenation with the therapist and goes home afterwards might not beat up a perceived inferior who passes him on the street, but he does tear up his home in a fit of rage.

One of the clearest models of the narcissistic personality disorder is present in the Hollywood movie, *Play Misty for Me*. Briefly, it is a story about a disc jockey who makes it clear to one of his female fans that she should not get attached because their relationship is purely transitory. She chooses not to let him go, so she shows up in his house one day with his dinner prepared. He bewilderingly accepts the dinner but tells her to get lost, since he has begun to feel imposed on. The next day, while the fan sees him being interviewed by a female television executive for a job, she flies into a jealous rage based on her narcissistic assumption that he is her man. Again, the disc jockey tells her she has no claim on him and tells her to go away. She pays little attention to his sense of independence and eventually fragments, becomes livid with narcissistic rage, and nearly kills several people. It is precisely this imposing tendency that is characteristic of the racist with an underlying narcissistic personality disturbance.

The issue of narcissism in blacks is more complex in terms of racism. I can understand a black person's need to identify with whites to identify with a culture that has "made it" (by white standards) and as a defense typical of victims; i.e., identification with the aggressor. Fanon once stated, "It is the racist who creates his inferior."[4] Therefore, it is extremely difficult to distinguish black racism from a reaction to white racist practices. Langston Hughes dealt with this issue in his celebrated poem, "Dream Deferred."[5]

A black friend of mine once told me his solution to white racism, one that I suspect is adopted by many who are subjected to racism and which has become part of a culture's mores. He told me that at the age of twelve he decided he would be free, so he went out into the world. After a sufficient number of "brick walls," he decided that since he could not be free on the outside, he would be free on the inside. I suspect this attitude is the source of "soulfulness," which has been defined as being full of deep feelings.

The white racist's need to identify with blacks is a much more complicated issue. While on one hand blacks have much to offer, such as "soul," slang, humor, empathy, wisdom, style, and color, these are usually derided by whites, who closely associate such attributes with the "inferior being." However, whites spend millions on suntans, are masters of cultural burglary and plagiarism, and have a historical reputation for entrusting their children to black women.

One must ask why the identification with the victim. It is useful to look at the model of sadomasochistic character disorder, which revolves around anal struggles. I would say that we live in a very asinine anal society; therefore, the question is no longer "to be or not to be" but "to have or not to be." The narcissist believes that somehow, extending self-boundaries to personal property (be it one's children, wife, new car, slaves, etc.) will in some way bolster his false grandiosity, which has a narcissistic base. I suspect that the majority culture of this country has a collective unconscious awareness that it is an affect-less, sterile, unempathetic milieu that emphasizes achievement and hoarding. As a result of this unconscious awareness, the majority becomes ambivalent toward the groups in this culture that have not sold their souls. Grier and Cobbs point out in their book, *The Jesus Bag*,[6] that the conscience of America rests in the hands of empathetic groups such as blacks.

As a black psychiatrist treating black patients, I find myself more aware than my white counterparts of the turning inward that black people do to be free by developing soulfulness and an inner world of humor, creativity, empathy, etc. White psychiatrists are more willing to attribute a reactive depression (secondary to lack of work) to a defect in character structure and dispense a minor tranquilizer rather than do nothing, expose social action, or empathize with the victim's plight. Marx's comment, "Religion is the opium of the people," seems consistent with another message in *The Jesus Bag*, specifically that religion has kept black folks content with having dreams deferred by expecting a reward in heaven. As it seems that psychiatry is fast becoming a modern religion since religion provides meaning and psychiatry is now doing so, it might be more appropriate to say that "psychiatry is the opium of the people," an opinion many would support. However, neither religion nor psychiatry needs be such, any more than an acute psychotic episode need be uninsightful and unproductive, or any more than the racism that has caused black folk to turn inward need be a totally negative experience. I think the evidence for this belief is reflected by the integrity, empathy, wisdom, creativity, and humor present in people who have experienced religion or racism in a constructive, growing manner. I once saw a whole trainload of black folks prevent a young white girl from getting off at the wrong stop and give her explicit instructions on getting to her location safely.

Kohut once observed, "Wisdom is achieved largely through man's ability to overcome his unmodified narcissism and it rests on his acceptance of the limitations of his physical, intellectual, and emotional powers."[7] Furthermore, he stated, "Man's capacity to acknowledge the finiteness of his existence and to act in accordance with this painful discovery may well be his greatest psychological achievement..."[7] From my personal and clinical experience, it is abundantly clear that black folks are always facing "the finiteness of their existence"; however, their ability "to act in accordance with this painful discovery" varies from individual to individual.

I saw an 11-year-old black child who, despite having lived in housing projects and having a reading score on a first-grade level, showed no signs of a reading disability and lost only two of thirteen tic-tac-toe games we played, with the other eleven resulting in a draw. I asked this youngster the standard question of three wishes, to which he replied, "To move out of the projects, get a job when I am old enough, and learn something in school." When questioned further about his first wish, he replied in a matter-of-fact fashion, "There is too much death there." I asked what he meant by that, and he gave me a rundown of that week's occurrence of death and violence. A 66-year-old woman had been murdered on the stairwell over $1.65, and a four-year-old girl had been raped, all since Monday, and the week was only half over (it was a Wednesday when I saw him).

I saw another patient, around 16 years of age, because he needed to get a clean bill of health (he had been in psychotherapy for about seven years, beginning at age nine). I asked him the nature of his difficulty that led him into therapy, and he told me that he had been afraid to grow up. Further exploration revealed that this fear had seized him during the height of the Vietnam War. The etiology was that he had apparently concluded that young black men were sent to Vietnam to die; thus, he was determined to forestall his death by not growing up. The point is that, as the victims of racism, blacks are much more likely to have to turn inward or introspect than the majority racist population, and thereby have a greater possibility either to develop what Kenneth Clark referred to as "over-compensatory grandiosity"[8] or to develop empathy, integrity, wisdom, humor, and creativity.

I suspect that in order to have integrity, a person has to see death and not fear it. If one does not stand for something (i.e. have integrity), he/she will fall for anything. People with integrity may be afraid, but their integrity allows them to have courage, which is the opposite of fear. Dealing with this inevitably involves relying on some aspect of faith, whether through belief in a philosophy or religious tenets. Accompanying this attitude of tranquility, despite the realization of one's own death, are feelings of compassion, empathy, or what has been called brotherly love. The most familiar example of developing integrity based on the realization of a finite existence secondary to a racist form of oppression is "I've Been To The Mountain Top,"[9] the speech Martin Luther King, Jr., delivered in Memphis on April 3, 1968, ironically the night before his death. King talked about the parable of the Good Samaritan, in which a man talks to Jesus about how he had been beset by robbers and laid injured on the road to Jericho. Neither a Levite nor a priest who passed him stopped to help. It was a Samaritan who finally stopped and administered first aid. Dr. King talked about why the others had not taken this compassionate approach, speaking as well about his and Mrs. King's visit to Jerusalem and their experience of the road to Jericho. He remarked:

> That's a dangerous road. In the days of Jesus it came to be known as the "Bloody Pass." And you know, it's possible that the robbers were still around. Or it's possible that they felt that the man on the ground was merely faking. And he was acting like he had been robbed and hurt, in order to seize them over there, lure them there for a quick and easy seizure. And so the first question that the Levite asked was, "If I stop to help this man, what will happen to me?" But the good Samaritan came by. And he reversed the question: "If I do not stop to help this man, what will happen to him?"
>
> That's the question before you tonight. Not, "If I stop to help the sanitation workers, what will happen to all of the hours that I usually spend in my office every day and every week as a pastor?"
>
> The question is not, "If I stop to help this man in need, what will happen to me?"
>
> "If I do not stop to help the sanitation workers, what will happen to them?" That's the question.[9]

Later in the speech, Dr. King gives us a clear view of his having faced and accepted his own mortality secondary to his own character structure, religious upbringing, and experience with the racist attitudes so prevalent in this country. This recognition and the constructive adaptation of this experience concerning helplessness in the face of death is the companion of the good Samaritan attitude that precludes a racist orientation. He said:

> And then I got into Memphis. And some began to say the threats or talk about the threats were out. What would happen to me from some of our sick white brothers?
>
> Well, I don't know what will happen now. We've got some difficult days ahead, but it doesn't matter with me now. Because I've been to the mountain top. And I don't mind. Like anybody, I would like to live a long time. Longevity has its place. But I'm not concerned about that now. I just want to do God's will. And He's allowed me to go to the mountain. And I've looked over. And I've seen the Promised Land. I may not get there with you. But I want you to know tonight, that we as a people will get to the Promised Land. And I'm happy, tonight, I'm not worried about anything.

I'm not fearing any man. Mine eyes have seen the glory of the coming of the Lord.[9]

In conclusion, there appears to be a continuum of the ability to respect another's being with a cluster of features at each end. On one hand is the cluster so characteristic of the racist features of grandiosity—lack of empathetic linkage in terms of either having to give or having received empathy as a child; poor self-boundaries, with a tendency to intrude upon or molest others; and an underlying mood of fragmentation with anxiety, agitation, and rage. On the opposite end of the spectrum lies the cluster of characteristics commonly associated with integrity: wisdom, humility, empathy, creativity, peacefulness, and a feeling of brotherly love.

COMMENTARY

In this article, I discussed the dynamics of how an unresolved sense of narcissism can cause a person to treat others in an extremely unempathic manner such as through racism and murder. At the time, my understanding of the various motivations for homicide was not very sophisticated. Like nonprofessionals, I had the misconception that murderers belong in a single category of persons with problems in their narcissistic development. My understanding of the motivations for violence were improved when I first wrote about homicide in "Interface Between Psychiatry and the Law on the Issue of Murder" (see Chapter 10) and when I began to explore the acquired biologic causes of violence in "Coma and the Etiology of Violence, Part 1" (see Chapter 11).

Another aspect of Kohut's work that attracted me was his emphasis on the other side of psychopathology, which I've always though of as "psychocreativity." As a result, this article also focused on integrity. My early notions about how integrity, empathy, wisdom, creativity, humor, and spirituality could be developed from various subtle or traumatic stresses were later developed in "States of Consciousness" (see Chapter 18) and "Black Intrapsychic Survival Skills" (see Chapter 19), and further in the next chapter.

Nothing in this paper can be proven by scientific methods because of the subjective nature of the material. Instead, there must be an internal measure similar to evaluating varying shades of emotions like anger, happiness, fear, etc. This intuitive, metaphoric type of "knowing" isn't considered as valid as the empirical or logical type of "knowing." I disagree with this.

This article was noticed by *The Journal of Continuing Education in Psychiatry*'s editor, Gene Usdin, MD, and I was requested to summarize it for publication in the journal's "Psychiatric Digest" section. I was pleased to learn that the Digest was being "translated into three languages for increased circulation in Europe," because it was the first time my work went international—every young author's dream. However, I was disappointed that brothers and sisters in the African Diaspora were not targeted markets. Since my work had appeared in the JNMA, there was some hope that people of color around the world would see it.

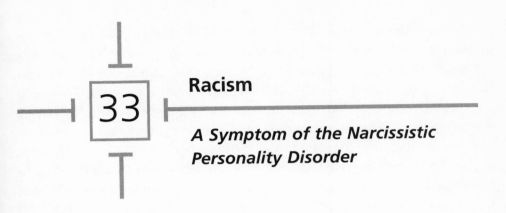

Racism

A Symptom of the Narcissistic Personality Disorder

Despite criticism that psychoanalytic models are not applicable to social phenomena, knowledge of the dynamics of narcissistic development aids in understanding a particular kind of racist. Specifically, racist attitudes may be indicative of a narcissistic personality disorder, or of a regression to primitive narcissistic functioning secondary to environmental forces. The differentiation between the narcissistic racist, the stress-induced racist, and the socially misinformed racist is discussed, utilizing clinical paradigms discovered in psychotherapy. Life experiences and religion are discussed as possible aids in transforming primary into secondary narcissism.

INTRODUCTION

In reviewing the literature on racism, one finds a wide spectrum of etiologic agents cited as the cause for racist attitudes in individuals. At one end of the spectrum is the view that racist attitudes are induced by enculturation, while at the other are those who feel that psychologic (personality and intrapsychic) factors are responsible.[1,2] Also found in the literature

Originally printed as Bell Carl C. Racism: a symptom of the narcissistic personality disorder. *J Natl Med Assoc*. 1980;72:661–665. Presented at the 132nd Annual Meeting of the APA, Chicago, IL, May 1979.

is what is believed to be a more reasonable or eclectic approach.[3-6] The proponents of the model of racism as a social ill in which cultural patterns are institutionalized and internalized by socialization feel that the solution to racism lies in politics and social change, not in the interpretive techniques of psychiatry.[7,8] Despite the fact that values and attitudes can be generated from social indoctrination, it is also recognized that while a person is a product of society, he is also a product of his individuality.

The questions remain: what characteristics cause an individual to accommodate to racist views that are in direct opposition to a democratic, free society's values? What causes a person raised in a racist family and social group to genuinely relinquish racist values and practice brotherhood? What causes a young man who has never previously demonstrated viciousness in his earlier life to commit atrocities against women and children because they belong to a different racial group? I suspect that the answers to these questions lie in the consideration of the vicissitudes of narcissism, its effect on the individual, and the individual's response to groups and stress.

THE NARCISSISTIC RACIST

There are as many different reasons why one commits a racist act since many etiologic agents are proposed for racism. However, on examining the intrapsychic dynamics of racist behavior, one clear feature is manifest—a lack of empathy for the perceived inferior race. Already, it has been noted that the individual's psychopathology influences his response to group pressure and that in many instances, racist beliefs can serve psychopathic needs.[4] It should be clear that there is a kind of racist individual who reveals the same type of psychopathology (narcissistic personality disorder[9,10] or borderline syndrome[11,12]) found in the murderer, child molester, rapist, child abuser, and in a sadomasochist.[13] For the narcissistic racist, racism is primarily a symptom of a narcissistic personality disorder (a personality disorder diagnosis does not relieve the person of responsibility for his behavior in terms of the legal consequences). This personality disorder has been examined by Allport,[1] Adorno.[2] Kohut states:

All instances of narcissistic rage have, nevertheless, certain features in common because they all arise from the matrix of a narcissistic or pre-narcissistic view of the world. It is this archaic mode of experience that explains the fact that those who are in the grip of narcissistic rage show a total lack of empathy toward the offender.[14]

Clearly, this is the state of being for someone who commits any overt, racist act.

The DSM-III contains a description of the narcissistic personality disorder that is also classic of the racist individual. The criteria are as follows:

A. Grandiose sense of self importance or uniqueness [this fits the racist's supposed racial superiority].

B. Preoccupation with fantasies of unlimited success, power, brilliance, beauty, or ideal love [clearly, the wish to dominate another racial group fits here as well as the Malthusian principles of the "rightness whiteness" and the Teutonic standard of white beauty[15]].

C. Exhibitionistic: requires constant attention and admiration [e.g., wearing white sheets or swastikas].

D. Responds to criticism, indifference of others, or defeat with either cool indifference or with marked feelings of rage, inferiority, shame, humiliation, or emptiness [e.g., the phenomena of white backlash and the feeling that blacks are being pushy].

E. Two of the following:

1. Lack of empathy: inability to recognize how others feel [racists could not possibly recognize how their "inferiors" feel; otherwise, they would not behave in such an unempathic manner].

2. Entitlement: expectation of special favors with reactions of surprise and anger when others don't comply [e.g., racists are always surprised and angry when the "inferiors" do not accede to their wishes].

3. Interpersonal exploitiveness: takes advantage of others to indulge his own desires or for self-aggrandizement, with disregard for the personal integrity and rights of others.

4. Relationships characteristically vacillate between the extremes of overidealization and devaluation [e.g., the characterization of blacks as primitive, yet expressing extreme cultural plagiarism, such as in the suntan phenomenon].[16]

Kohut reports that "the most violent forms of narcissistic rage arise in those individuals for whom a sense of absolute control over an archaic environment is indispensable..."[14] It is this need for a sense of absolute control that the racist feels justifies his self-given right to violate another's "territory" through either physical attack, segregation, or discrimination. The "territory" (in this country) is, for example, the individual's right to adequate health care, education, and housing wherever he can afford it.

THE STRESS-INDUCED RACIST

It has long been said that man's greatest psychological achievement is to come to grips with his own limitations, the greatest being that no one lives forever. This issue is clearly related to the vicissitudes of narcissism. Facing this issue prematurely is probably enough to induce regression to an earlier phase of narcissistic development (i.e., before primary narcissism can transform into secondary narcissism).

In examining patients who have suffered residual consequences from exposure to life-or-death circumstances, there is clear evidence that most of them regressed to a narcissistic level of functioning. A life-or-death struggle provides sufficient stress to cause a number of patients the same type of difficulty one of Kohut's patients demonstrated. Specifically, that patient's "insufficiently idealized superego could not provide him with an adequate internal supply of narcissistic sustenance and he needed external approbation in order to maintain his narcissistic balance. He became, therefore, inordinately dependent on idealized figures in his environment whose praise he craved."[14] This accords with Angela Davis' observation that "because it was drummed into the heads of US soldiers that they were confronting an inferior race, they could believe that raping Vietnamese women was a necessary soldierly duty."[17]

In practice, one can identify a transient form of narcissistic rage (characterized by "the need for revenge, for righting a wrong, for undoing a hurt by whatever means"[14]) which was a product of a stressful situation and which given time and narcissistic gratification can allow a re-establishment of narcissistic equilibrium.[18] This transient rage occasionally takes the form of transient racist behavior, which involves either stress or the need to be mirrored and be grandiose.

There are some forms of racist behavior that occur in response to stress and are not due to a chronic personality disorder characterized by committing chronic racist acts.

THE SOCIALLY MISINFORMED RACIST

A great number of studies point to a socially induced form of racism. This indicates that racism in this country is institutionalized and as such can be adopted by those in the culture who are not necessarily suffering from individual psychopathology. Certain racist individuals have a cognitive schemata that causes them to believe their race is superior and believe that to subjugate other races through discrimination and segregation is no more inhumane than doing the same to animals.

The moral hypocrisy and ethical inconsistency experienced by the socially misinformed racist is felt to be a source of cognitive dissonance that can induce a change in the cognitive schemata, which says that the racist's race is superior. Eliminating racism by making discrimination and segregation illegal has been attempted. The subtle intention of this jurisprudence is that forcing people together and guaranteeing minorities their rights will give socially misinformed racists the opportunity to familiarize themselves with different racial types. Theoretically, such education should eventually eliminate a great number of myths about racial differences and thus destroy the base of social aspects of racism; yet, people still tenaciously cling to their racist ideas. This leads one to suspect that an intrapsychic dynamic plays a part in their beliefs.

Allport discusses the phenomenon of the demagogue and the types of people who tend to adopt their philosophy because of an internal need associate themselves with a powerful being. Kohut describes this same need from a psychoanalytic perspective when he states:

> Yearning to find a substitute for the missing or insufficiently developed psychic structure, such persons are forever seeking, with addiction-like intensity, and often through sexual means (the clinical picture may be that of a perversion), to establish a relationship to people who serve as stand-ins for the omnipotent idealized self-object; i.e., to the archaic precursor of the missing inner structure. In everyday life and in the analytic transference the self-esteem of such persons is therefore upheld by their relationship to archaic self-objects.[19]

In the black community, this type of person is referred to as someone who always needs a cosigner to make a decision.

If the man behind the institution is a narcissist of the grandiose fashion, as was Hitler, then a racist institution is bound to be established. As Emerson stated, "The institution is but the shadow of a man." Kohut describes such people:

> They seem to combine an absolute certainty concerning the validity of their ideas with an equally absolute lack of empathic understanding for large segments of feelings, needs, and rights of other human beings and for the values cherished by them. They understand the environment in which they live only as an extension of their own narcissistic universe.[19]

There appears to be two types of socially misinformed racists. There are those with an underlying narcissistic personality disorder. They require a merger with the archaic self-object in order for their unempathic feelings and behavior to emerge. There are also those who are simply socially misinformed at an early age and who, with adequate exposure, may be placed in a sufficient state of cognitive dissonance to cause them to relinquish their ignorant beliefs.

RELIGION AND LIFE'S EXPERIENCES IN TRANSFORMING PRIMARY NARCISSISM

Persons who lack racist attitudes tend to also lack features of unmodified narcissism. In his chapter, "Tolerant Personality," Allport observes that the character structure most opposed to the prejudiced per-sonality has empathic ability and self-insight—things the narcissist lacks. He does not need to have some "great person" co-sign his behavior and self-esteem. In discussing the man who has attained an average state of mental health Kohut states:

> And, in particular, there will again be empathic contact with oth-ers which will prevent the development of a sense of absolute moral superiority over the fellow man. When comparing his own performance with the performance of others, the judgment of the non-messianic person will be influenced by his empathic under-standing of the fact that others, too, experience limited failures and success in the moral sphere, and thus no unrealistic feelings develop that the self is perfect and that the selves of other people are in essence corrupt.[14]

To be able to relinquish attitudes, a cognitive schemata, or a racist indoctrination, a person has to be fairly comfortable in regard to narcissis-tic balance. We must be aware that in order to attain an enlightened state, our thought processes do not belong to the core of our selves. The ability to see one's thoughts as not self (insight gained from introspection) is relat-ed to transforming narcissism by gaining subsequent greater empathic abil-ity and creativity. Inability to do this would explain the fact that despite increased exposure to other races, some whites have still clung to their racist views. If bigots were not so narcissistically attached to their thoughts as part and parcel of their being, they might be able to be creative, defer their judgment, and become aware that the belief of a race as superior or inferior is a "red herring."

Just as the capacity for introspection influences the development of insight (which in turn aids in the transformation of primary narcissism), the individual's life experiences also influence his/her narcissism. Blacks in this country have numerous experiences that impinge upon their narcis-sistic development: a black child is twice as likely to die in the first year of life as a white one; because black children have a higher rate of maternal mortality than do white children, the chance that a black child will grow up without his mother is three or four times that of a white child; blacks die six years younger than do whites; blacks are more likely to die from the leading causes of death than are whites; blacks are less likely to be hospitalized than are whites; cancer deaths are increasing two times faster for blacks than for whites; the unemployment rate for blacks has been double that of whites for the past two decades; black family incomes average only 52% that of white families; less than half of black folks will earn a high school diploma; and 27% of black families will have incomes below the poverty level.[20,21]

It should be obvious that blacks face death and annihilation daily, which puts special stress on their coming to grips with the vicissitudes of narcissism. Furthermore, the manner in which blacks deal with the narcissistic vulnerability imposed on them by racist elements in American culture varies from time to time and person to person, depending on circumstances and individual development. One negative mechanism used by the black American subculture to handle this stress is the individual outburst of narcissistic rage, which results in the high homicide and suicide rates in the black community. Another self-limiting style of handling vulnerability is the compensatory grandiosity described by Kenneth B. Clark in *Dark Ghetto*.[22] In terms of coping with narcissistic vulnerability through archaic self-object merger, it is surprising how many black persons decry social injustice but who prefer doing business with a white rather than black professional because they have more confidence in the white one. A less negative form of coping is introspection, as evidenced by blacks' preoccupation with the "blues" and by the comfort obtained through the empathic delivery and content of such songs. Blacks also have a highly developed style of creativity and humor, commonly labeled as "soul."

These coping styles may be soothing in terms of giving narcissistic gratification and comfort, but blacks who so adapt seldom get proper credit in society. Their development of such coping styles may sometimes preclude and sometimes aid in the development of other styles of coping with narcissistic vulnerability, which take the form of social activism. It is important to mention that the transformation of narcissism, which aids the individual in the development of initiative, can also be used to change the social circumstances responsible for the vulnerability.

Religion may aid in transforming primary narcissism via its emphasis on introspection and attaining altered states of consciousness (the reservoir of creativity). Specifically, compassion, empathy, wisdom, brotherhood, and unity with all living things are desirable results of such religious practices. Clearly, people like Dr. Martin Luther King, Jr., and Mahatma Gandhi reached such states. Like life's other experiences, however, religion is a double-edged sword. It can also be used to gratify the unfilled need of merger with the archaic omnipotent self-object. It can serve as a haven for the narcissistic person. This may have tragic consequences for religious followers if the leader develops difficulty with grandiosity, as was seen in Jonestown. Be this as it may, this use of religion may be a necessary phase in the transformation of primary narcissism into secondary or modified narcissism.

CONCLUSION

While a number of etiologic factors appear to be involved in the genesis of racism, there seems to be some justification in understanding racist behavior by examining the intrapsychic dynamics of narcissistic personality development. There are individuals whose narcissistic development is fixed at an early developmental level. They express their intrapsychic pathology through the production of various psychic derivatives characterized by a total lack of empathic capacity and extreme amounts of narcissistic rage. Racism (the belief of racial superiority and thereby, the right to dominate other races) is one psychic derivative through which narcissism may manifest itself. Stress-induced racism appears to be related to the shift in narcissistic balance secondary to the attack on the self (by far the greatest narcissistic injury is death) before it has had sufficient time to mellow. It would appear that this form of racism is not necessarily related to a relatively fixed narcissistic imbalance but is rather due to a regressive push. There is also a kind of racist who may be described as socially misinformed because his/her racist beliefs stem from socialization that has been internalized. Some in this group can be re-educated to have a more realistic value system; however, there are others whose need for an archaic self-object merger will cause them to do or believe practically anything. Obviously, those in the latter category have a narcissistic personality base beneath their ardent belief in their racial superiority, as advocated by their idealized leaders.

Finally, blacks, because of their vulnerable position, can develop either a grandiosity or destructive narcissistic rage secondary to a total lack of empathy from a racist society, or they can psychologically survive by developing their empathy, wisdom, and creativity.

Introspection is one answer for survival in intragroup conflict. Religion as a means of introspection may be invaluable, although it may also cause a merger with the archaic self-object. The ability to give and receive empathic linkage satisfies the narcissistic component long enough for the individual to pause from needing gratification to viewing in a different light the circumstance, thought, or affect. This produces flexibility and creativity, which allows the individual to choose a life philosophy based on the ideology, not the man behind it. As the old Zen proverb states, "Follow the path the master took, not the master."

COMMENTARY

After publishing "Racism, Narcissism, and Integrity" (see Chapter 32), I decided to study the issue of racism further, the result being this article. It was based on a paper presented in 1979 at the 132nd Annual Meeting of the APA. During that time, the APA required that presentations at their conference be submitted to and reviewed for publication in the *American Journal of Psychiatry*. Needless to say, the process by which journals accept or reject articles on issues of race is controlled by a primarily European-American editorial board. This process has always fascinated me. I've always suspected that a great deal of it is based on politics rather than science or philosophy. When I submitted my paper, it was rejected because the reviewer felt it seemed to be "a confused application of Kohut's work." This experience confirmed my suspicion about the politics behind acceptance of articles by primarily European-American editorial boards. The JNMA published the article instead.

I sent Dr. Kohut, with whom I'd previously corresponded, a copy of "Racism, Narcissism and Integrity." He responded that he'd been making efforts to understand some of the social issues I raised in my essay. After his response, I was inspired to send him a copy of this article as well. He wrote back: "I am very glad to see this evidence of the applicability of many of my thoughts outside of the area from which they were derived." He ended his letter to me by asking that I keep him on my mailing list to send him more interesting contributions that I produced.

My work on racism came in handy during a discussion that occurred after I presented "Impact of Violence on African-American Youth" at the Public Forum, "Creation of a Self: Color and Trauma in the Life of a Child," sponsored by the American Psychoanalytic Association in New York City, December 19, 1997. Several young African-American analysts in training were present. They were quite interested in learning that Kohut and I had corresponded about the relevance of my applying his narcissism theories to racism. I hope that my efforts will spur these young analysts and the American Psychoanalytic Association to do more research on racism.

I would later learn that my articles on racism were influential in ways I never was aware. In 1981, when the Committee of Black Psychiatrists of the APA gave Mr. Andrew Young, the former Ambassador to the UN, the Solomon Carter Fuller Award, I had the opportunity to discuss this article with him. Mr. Young and I had similar views on how stress could develop an individual's spirituality. He provided some insight I had overlooked in the article. He reminded me that despite the numerous attempts on Dr. King's life, he'd witnessed Dr. King grapple with these constant threats and take a spiritual path rather than crumble under the pressure.

In late 1996, Dr. Edward Dunbar of the Department of Psychology, University of California, asked me to participate in his session on racism at the 1997 American Psychological Association Convention in Chicago. He sent me several articles he'd been working on regarding racism. To my surprise, he'd referenced both my articles on racism and its relationship to narcissism. In corresponding with Dr. Dunbar, I learned that my early work had helped him develop psychological tests to identify persons with racist characteristics (Dunbar E. Symbolic, relational, and ideological signifiers of bias motivated offenders: toward a strategy of assessment. *Am J Orthopsychiatry*. 2003;73:2; Dunbar E. The assessment of the prejudiced personality: the Pr scale forty years later. *J Personality Assessment*. 1995;65:270–277; Dunbar E. The relationship of DSM diagnostic criteria and Gough's prejudice scale: exploring the clinical manifestations of the prejudiced personality. *Cultural Diversity and Mental Health.* 1998;3:247–258). He's also improved on my three categories of racist motivations by developing a more sophisticated categorization of psychopathologic causes of prejudice.

I was also instrumental in putting the study of racism on the research agenda for the DSM-V, which will be published in 2010 (First MB, Bell CC, Cuthbert B, Krystal JH, Malison R, Offord D, Reiss D, Shea T, Widiger T, Wisner K. Personality disorders and relational disorders: a research agenda for addressing critical gaps in DSM. In: Kupfer DJ, First MB, Regier DA, eds. *American Psychiatric Association Research Agenda for DSM-V.* Washington, DC: American Psychiatric Press, Inc.; 2002:123–199). In this chapter, we suggest that racism is an extremely complex phenomenon and that it might be a symptom of different disorders such as paranoia or paranoid schizophrenia (we don't know since patients with those diagnoses have never been asked about their attitudes toward racial differences). I also suggest that racism might be an indication of a narcissistic personality disorder. Further, I suggest that racism may be best thought of as a relational disorder, where racial beliefs of different people conflict so much that interpersonal difficulties develop between them despite the absence of any individual psychopathology. Finally, I note that racism might not indicate a symptom of a psychiatric disorder, a personality disorder, nor a disorder manifesting in a relationship. I note that it may simply be a learned behavior and that it should be treated as such (i.e., negatively sanctioned rather than treated).

The problem is that regardless of where one stands with making racism a psychiatric diagnosis that should be in DSM-V or not, the reality is that no one has done any scientific research to determine the complexity of racist behavior, nor has anyone researched how we should handle it, depending on its origins. I suspect that like violence, racist attitudes, values, and behaviors have complex beginnings and solutions.

More recently, in 2004, Dr. Chester Pierce at Harvard University has been facilitating national conversations on whether racism should or should not be considered a mental disorder. He has been calling together mental health, social science, political science, and anthropologic associations, as well as other organizations, to discuss this thorny topic. My sense is that he has assigned me the role in leading this conversation, as my "unpacking" the complexity of the various potential psychiatric and social motivations behind racist behavior makes sense and gives us an opportunity to address this public health scourge.

Section Six

HEALTH

AND

WELLBEING

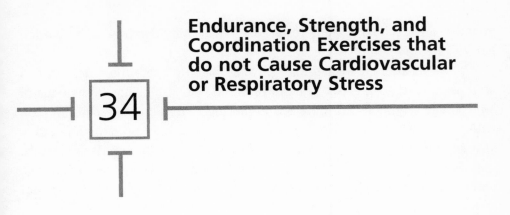

Endurance, Strength, and Coordination Exercises that do not Cause Cardiovascular or Respiratory Stress

34

In an attempt to maintain physical health, the author studied various exercises and, after six years of research, has gained knowledge of a form of exercise that increases endurance, strength, and coordination without cardiovascular or respiratory strain. This paper introduces five exercises, outlines their physiology, and proposes some aspects of their mechanisms of action.

INTRODUCTION

In recent years, there has been an increased interest in how the somatic sphere of physiology affects an individual's general physical and mental health. There have been numerous reports that somatic manipulation, whether through spinal manipulation (osteopathic spinal alignment), massage,[1,2] acupuncture,[3-8] acupressure,[9-12] or physical exercise[13] (running,[14,15] yoga,[16,17] Tai Chi,[2,18-23] etc.), aids in the relief and prevention of numerous human ailments. Running has been reported to relieve nonpsychotic depression.[14] Acupuncture has been reported to relieve

Originally printed as Bell Carl C. Endurance, strength, and coordination exercises without cardiovascular or respiratory stress. *J Natl Med Assoc.* 1979;71:265–270.

migraine headaches,[10] Meniere disease,[9] narcotic withdrawal,[24] cerebral palsy,[7] operative pain,[5,6] etc.

In an attempt to maintain physical health, the author has studied various exercises. After six years of research, the author has knowledge of an exercise regimen that increases endurance, strength, and coordination without cardiovascular or respiratory strain. In addition, this regimen may produce health benefits not found from participation in standard Western exercises. The purpose of this article is to introduce five of these exercises, outline their physiology, and propose some aspects of their mechanisms of action.

HISTORICAL BACKGROUND

Western exercise has traditionally been divided and classified by the effects produced on the body.[1,13,25] Strength exercises are performed by placing maximum tension on the muscles for brief periods of time. Strength exercises can be further divided into isometrics, in which there is muscular contraction exerting force against an immobile resistance, and isotonics, in which there is a muscular contraction against a movable resistance (e.g., dynamic tension and weight lifting).[13] Endurance exercises are performed by placing a medium amount of tension on the muscles for long periods of time, which imposes a mild cardiovascular and respiratory strain secondary to "oxygen debt."[1,13,25,26] Skill, coordination, and speed exercises are performed with minimal weight with the intent of building neuromuscular habits through numerous slow, purposeful repetitions.[1,25] Flexibility exercises are designed to increase the range of motion in the joints.

While these exercises are beneficial, they also have certain drawbacks. The endurance exercises (e.g., running, jumping rope, medium weight-lifting with high repetitions) and strength exercises have been strongly associated with pneumonia, shin splints, muscular tears, overfatigue, and ligament pulls.[1,27,28] Furthermore, such exercises pose a problem for patients who have compromised cardiovascular and/or respiratory functions. Warnings should be issued to people aged over 40–50 years who have not kept in physical condition and who wish to engage in strenuous exercises.[1]

On examining the history of Eastern exercise, one finds a departure from the traditionally "hard," strenuous, Western exercises to "soft," relaxing forms of exertion. These exercises have their historical root in India where for centuries, yoga has been the somatic manipulation that maintains strength and health. Yoga is characteristically and primarily a "passive" exercise in terms of body motion, as it tends to focus on static body postures, breathing techniques, and meditation. The primary focus of yoga is flexibility and psycho-physiologic control. The techniques of yoga are aimed at cleansing what in Sanskrit are called "nadis."[16] This allows a freer flow of life's "prana," or vital energy, which is generated from breathing. Yogic masters claim that this increase of "intrinsic energy" is responsible for their greater-than-average longevity and better physical and mental health. This "intrinsic energy" is quite different from the "extrinsic energy" from muscular strength developed through strength and endurance exercises.

In 520 AD, a Buddhist monk from India crossed the Himalayan mountains and introduced the practice of Zen and "sinew changing and marrow washing" exercises into the Chinese Taoist exercise system for longevity.[18,29,30] The fusion of these Indian and Chinese exercises developed into present-day Tai Chi, an exercise system that stimulates the body's acupuncture points so that "chi" ("intrinsic energy") can flow freely throughout the body, thereby producing longevity and health. In Japan, people practice Akido,[31] another form of internal or "soft" exercise clearly based on similar principles. In addition to the "soft," primarily intrinsic forms of Eastern exercise, there are also forms of Eastern exercise that are quite hard, strenuous, and extrinsic in nature, such as karate and certain forms of yoga that emphasize stress postures.

The author has had the opportunity to know and study with teachers of both the "hard" and "soft" schools of exercise. While both schools contain some "soft" and "hard" aspects, on the whole, teachers of the "hard" schools have many more "old" injuries that result from the strenuous nature of their discipline. Invariably, one of their major joints (hip, knee, elbow, shoulder) develops a limited range of motion or ligament weakness from a previous tear. Teachers from the "soft" schools are on average much more flexible in all their joints and are free from aches and pains from old injuries. Physical examination has made clear that they are the healthier of the two groups (Sexton T, Lee R, Sligar W, et al., personal communication, 1974; Tohei K, personal communication, 1975; Kuo LY, personal observation, 1978; Nam TH, personal communication, 1975; Hu GL, personal communication, 1976; Dunning W, personal communication, 1974). Furthermore, the author has met several teachers who have changed from the "hard" to "soft" school due to older age and frequency of injuries in "hard" exercise regimes.

FIVE "SOFT" EXERCISES

While there are numerous "soft" exercises that can be presented, the following five are among the simplest to communicate via writing. They are peculiar (i.e., different from Western calisthenics) in several ways. They are not strenuous and should be done with as little muscular tension as possible; however, the amount of work accomplished is comparable to that in the more exhausting Western forms of exercise. Great emphasis is placed on coordination of breathing with the physical movements. The breathing is diaphragmatic, and the intra-abdominal pressure produced should be as low in the pelvis as possible. This means that the chest remains static while the abdomen protrudes with inhalation and retracts with exhalation. If placing one hand on the epigastric area and one on the suprapubic area, there should be protrusion of the suprapubic area, as opposed to the protrusion of the epigastric area or both. The end of each exhalation or inhalation should coincide with cessation of movement or with a change in the direction of body motion.

The spine, including the slightly lordotic curvature of the lower back, should remain straight, which is accomplished by tucking in the pelvis from its forward tilting position.[32] This causes the subjective feeling of removing the upper body weight from the lower back and finding the total body weight on the heels. This will also produce a shortening of the distance between the costal cartilage arch of the tenth rib and the anterior superior iliac spine.

Finally, the exercises are done slowly so that no cardiovascular or respiratory strain is produced.

Exercise 1. The plantar surface of the foot is raised by dorsiflexion while flexing the hand and forearm in unison. It is important not to protrude the buttocks when up on the heels. As this motion is performed, inhalation is accomplished (Figure 1A). The forearms are flexed only to the point at which they are parallel to the floor. Next, with the onset of exhalation, the foot is plantar flexed and the forearms, wrists, and fingers are extended in unison. The arms remain at the sides (Figure 1B).

FIGURE 34.1. Exercise 1

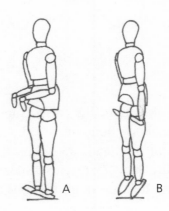

A   B

Exercise 2. All of the weight is placed on one leg. The hips are tucked in and the other leg is slightly flexed with the toe touching the ground to aid balance (Figure 2A). The arms are at the sides. With exhalation, the weight on the leg is lowered slowly, and the arms are loosely raised until they are parallel to the floor. While the plantar surface of the "weightless" leg touches the floor, it should remain "weightless" (Figure 2B). Next, with inhalation, the leg bearing the weight is extended and the body is raised to the initial position as the arms are dropped slowly to the sides. The exercise is then repeated standing on the other leg.

This exercise is done gently with as little tension in the arms and abdomen as possible. A mild burning sensation of the anterior thigh muscle is likely as the muscular work limit is reached. There is no need for concern, though, since this sensation abates with cessation of the exercise. These exercises produce none of the cramps nor the immobile, stiff, soreness characteristic of Western exercises.

Exercise 3. This is probably the most difficult of the five exercises. Yet, if done properly, there should be no strain or extreme exertion. The weight is placed on one leg. The raised leg's thigh and leg are flexed so that the raised leg's foot is adjacent to the knee of the standing leg (Figure 3A).

FIGURE 34.2. Exercise 2

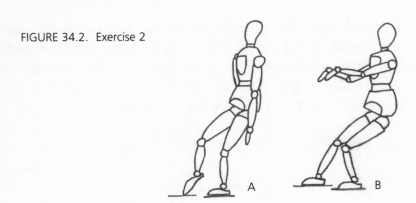

With exhalation, the raised foot steps forward approximately two feet. The upper body bends forward as the arms swing forward, with the dorsal surface of the hands sweeping the ground. The chest should touch the thigh (Figure 3B). Next, with inhalation, the body is propelled back by extension of the forward thigh to a position similar to the starting position (the difference is that the forearms and wrists are flexed at the sides, Figure 3C). Finally, with exhalation, the leg is extended with the foot dorsiflexed, while the arms drop gently to the sides (Figure 3D). There should be no tension in the stomach or upper body, but rather minimal tension in the pelvic muscles and anterior thigh. With inhalation, the leg returns to the starting position, and the cycle is repeated.

FIGURE 34.3. Exercise 3

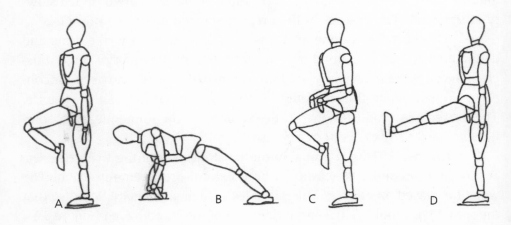

Exercise 4. This focuses primarily on the arms and should be done slowly. It is performed by extending both arms out to the sides, parallel to the floor, with the shoulders down and palms up (Figure 4A). The hips are tucked in but not locked forward. The thighs are spread apart, the knees push outward, the legs are perpendicular to the floor, and the feet are straight forward, with body weight on the heels. The spine is straight, and the distance between the edge of the tenth costal cartilage and the anterior superior iliac spine is slightly shortened. With exhalation, the palms are pronated and the extended arms are lowered approximately 30 degrees (Figure 4B). Next, with inhalation, the palms are supinated and the arms are raised to their original position (Figure 4B). For maximum benefit, the shoulders should be down, with the arms as relaxed as possible. This should produce a slightly uncomfortable pulling feeling from the tips of the fingers to the shoulders.

Figure 4C illustrates four errors common in this exercise: (1) pointing the feet outward, (2) protruding the buttocks, which results in a slightly lordotic spine with the upper body weight falling on the weakest part of the spine, L4 and L5, (3) raising the shoulders, (4) not fully extending the arms and fingers (however, the elbows should not be locked).

FIGURE 34.4. Exercise 4

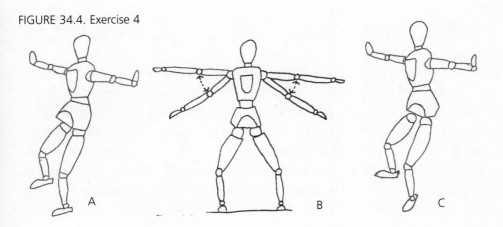

A　　　　　　　　　　　　　　　　B　　　　　　C

Exercise 5. This focuses on the waist and should be done gently and slowly. The position of the lower body is the same as in Exercise 4, and the arms hang loosely between the thighs (Figure 5A). Coinciding with exhalation, the pelvis is tucked in (not to the point of being locked forward), and the distance between the ribs and hips is greatly shortened. This results in the hands being lowered to the knees and the lower back being straightened (Figure 5B). With inhalation, the upper body is raised. When performed properly, a warming sensation should be produced in the lower abdomen.

FIGURE 34.5. Exercise 5

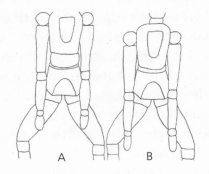

DISCUSSION

There are several major advantages that the preceding regimen has over more strenuous, Western exercises. The five exercises described can be done at any age regardless of physical condition (assuming that the practitioner is ambulatory and has no range-of-motion limitations) because they are gentle enough not to produce physical stress. If done on a daily basis, the practitioner is not so fatigued the next day that he/she is weak and "dragging." The exercises produce neither muscular cramps from over-work nor the immobilizing muscular stiffness associated with Western exercises. Furthermore, it has been this author's experience that the exercises described here produce greater endurance with fewer difficulties, even though Western endurance exercises are intended to put the athlete's body in condition, i.e., the homeostatic mechanisms of physiology (electrolyte balance, cardiovascular dynamics, respiratory dynamics, etc.) have a greater capacity to adjust to long periods of stress.

Before the author began these exercises, he was able to perform 500 rope jumps a day (equivalent to about three miles of jogging) and regain oxygen balance in one minute. It was not possible to increase the number of jumps, because the resulting leg fatigue would cause misses. After the first week of performing these exercises, the author could easily exceed 1,000 rope jumps. Now I am able to jump with 10-lb. weights on each leg for an hour or put my 80-lb. daughter on my shoulders and do 60 two-leg squats and 30 one-leg squats on each leg.

In teaching these exercises to other athletes (i.e., persons whose physiologic homeostatic mechanisms have adjusted to exercise to the point that his/her sweat is almost entirely free of salt),[1] the consensus is that in increasing endurance, these exercises are superior to "hard" ones. In addition, they do not cause the damage to the body that traditional Western exercises do. They promote coordination due to their slow, deliberate nature, which in turn increases strength secondary to a greater number of "motor units" (anterior horn cell and muscle fiber) working in concert and proper sequence. Finally, these exercises do not require the warming-up necessary to prepare the body for performing strenuous exercise without risking injury.

PHYSIOLOGIC DYNAMICS OF "SOFT" EXERCISES

Recently, there has been experimental evidence that relaxation during exercises produces decreased oxygen consumption.[39] The results of this research are as follows:

> Oxygen consumption averaged 0.763 liters/min/m^2 in the subjects working at a fixed work intensity before eliciting the relaxation response. While continuing to exercise at this work intensity, but simultaneously eliciting the relaxation response, subjects decreased their oxygen consumption to 0.730 liters/min/m^2 ($p = 0.05$). When subjects stopped using the technique that elicited the relaxation response, oxygen consumption increased to 0.748 liters/min/m^2 at this same load.[33]

The respiratory quotient remained unchanged, as did the heart rate. The relaxation response used was a simple non-cultic technique that focused attention on breathing. The physiologic changes present during the relaxation response are consistent with decreased sympathetic nervous system activity. There are decreases in respiration rates and minute ventilation.

Arterial blood pH and base excess decrease slightly. Arterial blood lactate decreases markedly. The authors conclude:

> Decreased oxygen consumption at a fixed work intensity was associated with the simultaneous elicitation of the relaxation response. It therefore leads to an improved efficiency of the oxygen transport system during exercise. The decreased oxygen consumption should enable increased work at a given level of oxygen consumption or prolonged work at a diminished level of oxygen consumption. In subjects with compromised cardiac-respiratory function, the simultaneous elicitation of the relaxation response with work should lead to a greater exercise tolerances.[33]

Clearly, the endurance exercise derives most of its energy from anaerobic metabolism, i.e., glycolytic breakdown of glucose or glycogen to pyruvic acid, which is further converted to lactic acid. When glycogen is split into pyruvic acid, each mol of glucose in glycogen yields three mols of adenosine triphosphate (ATP). Most energy required for strenuous activity lasting for more than thirty seconds is derived from glycolysis. After the exercise, oxidative metabolism reconverts five sixths of the lactic acid into glucose, and one sixth goes to pyruvic acid, which is degraded and oxidized in the tricarboxylic acid cycle.

The oxygen debt and "air hunger" experienced after strenuous exercise aids to convert the lactic acid back into glucose and reconvert decomposed ATP and creatine phosphate back to their original states. The "soft" exercises discussed are able to derive their energy from aerobic metabolism. One significant difference between the sources for aerobic and anaerobic energy is that the anaerobic is dependent on carbohydrates, while the aerobic can utilize carbohydrates, fats, and proteins.[26] This difference may account for the greater efficiency of the "soft" exercises over the "hard."

HEALTH BENEFITS FROM "SOFT" EXERCISES

Initially, the author pursued exercise techniques to maintain good physical health. Traditional, "hard" Western exercises did this very well; however, they did not relieve the chronic postnasal drip and sinusitis that the author developed six years ago. The author regularly ingested 8 milligrams of chlorpheniramine and 50 milligrams of phenylpropanolamine HCl in a timed-release capsule at bedtime in order to prevent bronchitis and sinusitis. After performing "soft" exercises, the author was quite pleased to discover that they did in fact relieve nasal difficulties, as claimed in "soft" exercise manuals[2,18,–23]. Presently, the author no longer needs antihistamine medication for his sinus symptoms.

Several quite similar case histories have been found. While clear scientific evidence that "soft" exercises have a health benefit very different from that of traditional Western exercises cannot be presented, one particular case history illustrates peculiar therapeutic benefits from the exercises presented in this paper.

The case is that of a 35-year-old black woman who prior to engaging in "soft" exercises had a history of chronic menstrual difficulties and allergic rhinitis. Since the onset of her menses at age 14, she had had irregular cycles, ranging 35–52 days. The duration of her periods were about seven days, usually with a heavy flow. Accompanying her periods was severe abdominal and leg cramping and water retention difficulties. She had her first child at age 22 and shortly thereafter took birth control pills for two years. The contraceptives regulated her cycle to 28 days and decreased the severity of the abdominal and leg pains to minor ones, but the water retention problems remained.

For the following two years, she stopped taking "the pill" and returned to having an irregular menstrual frequency (35–52 days) with severe menstrual cramps. During this time, she was quite physically active (regular college physical education classes, golfing, roller skating three times a week, etc.). Although her muscles were toned, the quality of her periods remained the same. She became pregnant for the second time and had a miscarriage secondary to severe hay fever, respiratory distress, and allergic rhinitis.

She returned to birth control pills and was again relieved of some symptoms for three years. Due to what was diagnosed as a form of endometriosis, she had two dilation and curettages and discontinued using "the pill." She became pregnant shortly thereafter and following the second delivery, reported that the frequency of menstruation was 35–42 days, with abdominal and leg cramps plus swelling. However, the cramps were not so severe as in the past, and the use of propoxyphene HCl, aspirin, phenacetin, and caffeine or codeine was no longer necessary.

At the time of the interview, it had been five years since her last pregnancy. During this time, she continued to suffer from moderate cramps and fluid retention. She reported that she had been once placed on a medication that relieved the fluid retention and cramps, but that she had discontinued taking it since she "doesn't like to take pills." After six months of being engaged in "soft" exercises, she reported that since the first month, she has had regular 28-day cycles without menstrual pain and without the use of birth control pills. She stopped exercising for one month due to the "flu" and reported that though the cycle for that month had been 28 days, she had experienced some minor abdominal pain.

This patient also had severe allergy problems that developed when she moved to Chicago. She was found to be allergic to trees, wool, dust, mold, feathers, fur, goldenrod, and ragweed. She has no allergy to eggs or penicillin, but she developed a slight rash with sulfa. She has had chronic severe sinus headaches for which she has taken pseudoephedrine, triprolidine, chlorpheniramine, etc. (in addition to having a miscarriage secondary to these problems). Since engaging in "soft" exercises, she has been free of headaches and allergy medication, which she previously had to take year-round. She still has a slight postnasal drip. She reports that her energy levels are higher and that she has more endurance.

CONCLUSIONS

There may be said to be two classifications of exercise: "soft" and "hard." The "hard" exercises are devoted to developing muscular strength and endurance, which is known as "extrinsic energy." The "soft" exercises are devoted to developing "intrinsic energy," which in addition to increasing strength, endurance, coordination, and flexibility, may also have some therapeutic value. The "hard" exercises are strenuous and produce cardiovascular and respiratory strain, while the "soft" exercises are gentle and as such, do not strain the vital functions. They therefore have a wider range of use than do "hard" exercises. The mechanisms of action of these "mystical," "soft" exercises are gradually being discovered as Western science explores ancient Eastern practices. While the benefit of "soft" exercises has not been scientifically documented as superior to that of "hard" exercises, empirically, the author has found them to be superior and has therefore presented them here for further scrutiny.

Swami Rama of the Himalayan International Institute states:

> All human beings have the inner potential and resources to be completely healthy. We must understand these inner resources and use them as much as possible in order to have perfect health. Our health is very important, but we seldom realize this until we no longer enjoy good health. Only when we lose our natural resistance do we pay attention to our health. Finally, we realize that the mental aspect of health is more important than the physical, and that the spiritual aspect of health is of greater importance than either of these. Once we know and obtain the keys to a healthy life by paying attention to our physical being, we become aware that all our activities are governed from within through our conscious and unconscious minds. But when we start paying attention to the various zones of our minds and learn to transcend them, there comes another, more subtle level of our being. This particular level I call 'spiritual health.' Those who understand this level practice the art of living and being.[34]

COMMENTARY

Many physicians, especially psychiatrists, concern themselves only with pathology, or diseases of the body/mind. Having always been concerned with maintaining a proper balance, I've always thought this single-mindedness to be a tragic error. Therefore, I've consistently sought to maintain symmetry in my work by focusing not only on the mind but also on health and wellbeing. This quest for equilibrium led me to study various forms of exercise. After years of research and direct personal experience, I believe that the Chinese system of exercise holds the greatest health benefits.

George Hu, a Tai Chi teacher trained by Master Wang Yen-nien, taught me the exercises described in this article. The article's title boasted that these exercises didn't cause respiratory or cardiovascular stress but would increase endurance, strength, and coordination. It wasn't until a decade later in 1989, though, that I realized how efficient they really were. A marathon runner friend of mine, Leroy Tyree, had heard me talking about these exercises and decided to put me to the test. He challenged me to a 15-kilometer race about two weeks before the event. I felt training for the race by running was unnecessary since I felt the Chinese exercises I was doing would provide me with enough endurance. Anyway, I don't run, except for an occasional five or ten kilometer run (two or three a year). I follow the philosophy of Green Neal, MD, a medical school classmate of mine, who once jokingly explained to me why he didn't run. He believed that God gave everyone a certain limited number of heartbeats, and that exercise would only use them faster than needed, causing premature death. He avoided exercise like the plague. When I was in the Navy, I used to run barefoot at least three miles a day, but after catching a slight case of pneumonia from running in the rain one summer, I gave it up.

At any rate, since I had only two weeks to prepare for the 15-kilometer race, I ran three 3–5-mile runs just to make sure I wouldn't die during the middle of it. Right before the race, a race coordinator advised the runners to drink plenty of water to prevent dehydration, so I drank about a quart. During the first two miles, I realized the error of having drank so much water—I developed some disturbing gastrointestinal discomfort that slowed me down a great deal.

I finished the race in 82 minutes, an average of 8'49" per mile, and I'm told that running even nine minute miles for 10 miles for someone who isn't trained is pretty good. My friend beat the pants off me, but it was clear that my exercise regime did develop a great deal of endurance. Since I was also in the habit of jumping rope for 30–45 minutes a day, three times a week, I, unfortunately, couldn't be sure if my endurance was due to the Chinese exercises or jumping rope.

My answer came four years later when Leroy Tyree again challenged me to another ten-mile race two weeks before the run. This time I was doing only the "soft" Chinese exercises and not jumping rope. To prepare, I ran three miles three times before the run. My gym shoes lacked resiliency, so I brought a new pair a few days before the race. I did much better this time, since I had enough experience to know not to drink any water before the run. Because a quart of water wasn't sloshing around in my stomach, I was able to stay within six to nine feet of my friend. In the last two hundred yards of the race, my new gym shoes chaffed a blister on my foot the size of a golf ball. The pain caused me to slow down, and my friend pulled away from me. I realized that this was probably the last time I was going to engage in this ridiculous heartbeat-depleting activity, and if I didn't beat him this time, I'd never get another chance! I began to sprint and managed to quickly close the wide lead he'd gained on me. He beat me by just four feet. This time I had averaged 8'40" per mile, which I was reassured was quite good for someone over 45 who rarely ran. I'd even reduced by a minute and a half the time it took me to run the same ten miles I'd run four years before. My victory was due to the Chinese exercises I'd written about in 1979 that had given me endurance.

I still do these exercises regularly. My experience is that my endurance, strength, and coordination have continued to improve. I have more energy to live and work. I've noted also that my tolerance to heat and cold has increased. Furthermore, my tolerance to pain has improved, and as will be shown in the next article, this attribute can come in handy at times.

Lately, I've stepped up my efforts in this area. We at the CMHC have a video explaining how to do the exercises, and it's quite easy to pop the tape into a VCR and exercise along. At the end of the tape, we offer a more academic explanation (essentially drawn from the next article) about why the exercises work. As previously mentioned, I've come to realize that the cultivation of "chi" is an Asian strategy to cultivate resiliency and is furthermore an effort to cultivate an "indomitable fighting will."

Accordingly, the CMHC has embarked on a goal to develop a Wellness Institute where we'll teach these exercises along with other forms of resilience/resistance training. I think I've learned enough about these exercises, so critical in my success and in my endurance, to begin sharing them with the general public. I'm the first person to realize that I need to learn much more, so I continue to study Southern Praying Mantis Chi Kung under Wilbert Rimes, who learned the exercises from Sifu Henry Poo Yee. We're convinced that these exercises can be very beneficial for elderly practitioners. I doubt if many of them are in shape to do some of the more strenuous exercise programs being marketed. The idea of funding a Wellness Institute is rather foreign in the African-American community, so in order to keep such a program running, we must find the capital to market it. In the not-for-profit world, this is especially true, considering that most community-based, not-for-profit mental health centers focus on deficits rather than strengths or building strengths.

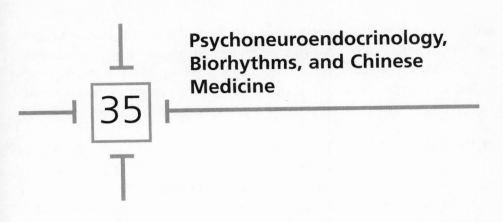

Psychoneuroendocrinology, Biorhythms, and Chinese Medicine

35

The discovery of an endogenously formed opioid substance in the body that is intimately related to corticotrophin and thus a major consideration in the body's response to stress already has demonstrated the impact that psychoneuroendocrinology can have on the practice of medicine. The psychoneuroendocrinologic system is characterized by a daily rhythm. Because of this rhythmic variation, the body is in different physiologic states at different times of the day. This has raised some important questions for clinical practice. Western medical science and Chinese medicine are compared, and suggestions are made on how to best utilize the knowledge currently being gained in psychoneuroendocrinology and biorhythms.

INTRODUCTION

Corticotrophin (ACTH) is a large polypeptide produced in the pituitary. It causes the adrenal cortex to increase the production of adrenocortical hormones such as cortisol. ACTH has been found to follow a rhythmic pattern of release known as circadian (one cycle of release being approximately 24 hours). It is the intent of this chapter to review some

Originally printed as Bell Carl C. Psychoneuroendocrinology, biorhythms and Chinese medicine. *J Natl Med Assoc.* 1981;73:31–35.

important physiologic changes produced by ACTH rhythms and to examine how this naturally occurring phenomenon might be used to improve the practice of medicine. Finally, the knowledge of modern medicine, with regard to biological rhythms, is discussed in relationship to the phenomenologic art of Chinese medicine, which originated in 200 BC.

PHYSIOLOGY OF ACTH

In recent years, there has been increasing documentation that ACTH production is influenced by a circadian rhythm, resulting in higher levels of ACTH being available to the body in the morning hours than in the afternoon or evening. Krieger and Allen, using immunoassay techniques, have demonstrated that ACTH is highest in the hour preceding awakening (6:30–7:30 a.m.), at a level of approximately 12.5 µg/hour. Between 10:00 and 11:00 a.m. and 9:00 and 10:00 p.m., ACTH levels were 4.7 µg/hour and 1.6 µg/hour, respectively.[1] As a result of the morning increase in ACTH production, cortisol also has been shown to be in high concentrations in plasma between 6:00 and 8:00 a.m., at a level of about 12 ± 2 µg/100 ml.[1-4] Plasma cortisol levels decline to 5 ± 1 µg/100 ml from 6:00 to 8:00 p.m.[2-4] There is a variation in plasma cortisol concentration of 50% (it has been reported that this variation may be as high as 70%[5]). As ACTH has been shown to increase production of cortisol, it is generally held that this rhythmic pattern of cortisol is caused by the rhythmic production of ACTH.

ACTH has been shown to be produced by the cleavage of a larger precursor peptide known as "big ACTH," which in addition to ACTH contains beta-lipotrophin.[6] It is interesting to note that the end third of beta-lipotrophin has an amino acid sequence that contains both enkephalin and beta-endorphin, two substances that replicate opiate activity in the body. It has been shown that approximately equimolar concentrations of ACTH and beta-endorphin are released simultaneously in the body.[4]

The production of ACTH (and therefore, beta-endorphin) appears to be regulated by several factors. ACTH and beta-lipotrophin (rises in parallel with beta-endorphin) are released in human subjects by hypoglycemic stress.[7] Pain has been associated with an increase in ACTH level.[8] Depression tends to cause an increase in cortisol and failure of suppression from dexamethasone, suggesting increased ACTH in such patients.[9] Finally, job pressures and noon meals appear to influence cortisol circadian rhythms and thus may also influence ACTH production.[10,11] However, since many of these factors are still unclear, the author will look at the early morning high level of ACTH, beta-lipotrophin (thus beta-endorphin), and cortisol and examine how this naturally occurring, light-regulated circadian rhythm could be of clinical use.

PHYSIOLOGIC STATE OF THE BODY IN THE MORNING

To a great extent, the physiologic state of the body in the morning is regulated by the increased production of ACTH, which stimulates the production of cortisol. Cortisol has a generalized effect on body metabolism and causes gluconeogenesis, leading to an increase in liver glycogen and blood glucose, which in turn causes an increase in insulin secretion. Cortisol also increases blood amino acids, which may be the most important function of this hormone, and results in the reduction of protein stores of the body (with the exception of those in the liver). It is well known, for instance, that the different cells continually synthesize a multitude of chemical substances from amino acids. Since the normal concentration of amino acids in the body fluids totals only 30 μg percent, mobilization of amino acids from the tissues might play a valuable function in providing an available supply of amino acids for damaged cells in time of need.[8]

In the liver, cortisol stimulates the deamination of amino acids, protein synthesis, the formation of plasma proteins, and the change of amino acids into glucose. Cortisol causes the mobilization of fatty acids from adipose tissue, increasing unesterfied fatty acids in plasma and making them available for energy use. Finally, cortisol blocks the process of inflammation and prevents fluids from leaking into damaged areas, thus blocking inflammatory responses to allergic reactions.

In observing the physiologic state of the body in the morning hours, one finds a manifestation of high biologic levels of ACTH, beta-lipotrophin (thus beta-endorphin), and cortisol. In the early hours of the morning (3:00–6:00 a.m.), the liver has used up much of its glycogen due to the lack of food intake during the night. As is true with most of the other amino acids, tyrosine concentrations reach a high point at 10:00 a.m. It is interesting to note that this pattern is not dependent on whether or not an individual is receiving a high- or low-protein diet. The same holds true for the glycogen rhythm, regardless if the individual is on a starvation diet. Triglycerides are also at their highest level at 6:00 a.m.

In addition to these biochemical parameters, vital signs may change. The respiratory rate is usually increased, and blood pressure tends to be lower. Individuals documented to have hypertension may show high blood pressure levels at 6:00 p.m. but have normal levels at 8:00 a.m. A person taking a glucose tolerance test in the morning may be seen to be "normal," but if that individual receives the same test in the afternoon, the results may indicate that he/she is "diabetic." Probably as a result of the early morning release of beta-endorphin, individuals are more insensitive to pain, noise, taste, and smell in the morning (sensory acuity is at its maximum at 3:00 a.m., when corticosteroid levels are at the lowest, after which it decreases as steroid levels rise). Finally, since histamine levels show the reverse pattern of release of cortisol, histamine levels are at their lowest for the day in the early morning.[5]

As a result of this different physiologic state of the body in the morning, responses to various medications change. Aspirin has its longest half-life in the body when taken at 7:00 a.m. The effects of antihistaminic medication last longest with morning dosages (17 hours); when antihistamines are taken in the evening, the effects last only for a few hours. When given to asthmatic patients in the morning, dexamethasone has its greatest effects in increasing lung vital capacity and increasing one-second forced-expiratory volume. It has been shown that there is a circadian responsiveness of the pituitary gland to exogenously administered steroids.[12] If 0.5 mg of synthetic cortisone is injected at 8:00 a.m., there is a transient drop in blood cortisol levels, but if the same dose is given at midnight, cortisol production tends to be suppressed for 24 hours.[5]

CHINESE MEDICINE AND CIRCADIAN RHYTHMS

The Yellow Emperors' classic on internal disease (200 BC) was the first book on acupuncture.[13] The Chinese were more concerned with the system of forces in the body causing physiologic homeostasis and illness rather than with the scientific elaboration of anatomy or organ systems. As a result, their conceptualizations tend to be symbolic of bodily processes. They conceptualized the existence of a life energy (chi), which they felt activated all bodily processes. Through regulation of chi, the Chinese physician sought not only to combat disease but more importantly, to prevent it.

In addition to laws representing the interplay between the energy of one "organ" and another, there was a law called "midday-midnight,"[13] which described the rhythm of life's energy. This law proposed that the chi flowed through twelve energy channels (acupuncture meridians) at regular times over a period of 24 hours. Thus, it was felt that there existed a daily rhythm that determined when organs received their maximum or minimum chi, or energy supply. With this knowledge, an acupuncturist would coordinate his treatments with the time of day yielding best results. From this evidence, it is clear that ancient Chinese had phenomenologic understanding of circadian biorhythms, which they utilized to treat and prevent illness better. The law of "midday-midnight" (Chinese biological clock pattern) has many parallels with the circadian rhythm patterns demonstrated in modern Western laboratories.

The acupuncture meridian cycle (i.e., the path of life's energy in the course of a day) begins with the "lungs," since the chi enters there first. Chi is supplied by digestion of food and water in the "stomach" as well and is transferred from the "stomach" by the "spleen" to the "lungs." From the "lungs," the chi enters the lung meridian (recorded as most active from 3:00–5:00 a.m.) and is transmitted to its "coupled organ," the "large intestine" (an "organ" is coupled to another "organ" when the stimulation of one "organ's" meridian has a stimulatory effect on the other's meridian). From the large intestine meridian (highest peak 5:00–7:00 a.m.), the vital energy is transferred to the stomach meridian (most active 7:00–9:00 a.m.). From there, the chi moves on to the "stomach's" "coupled organ," the "spleen" (most highly energized 9:00–11:00 a.m.).

As a result of this metaphoric understanding of circadian rhythms, the Chinese felt that the best time to do breathing exercises was early in the morning from 3:00–7:00 a.m., when the lung meridian and its coupled organ (large intestine) meridian were most active. It was best to eat when the stomach meridian, and its coupled organ (spleen) meridian were most active, 7:00–11:00 a.m. According to Chinese medicine tenets, these were optimal times to increase the body's chi and thus prevent illness.

Chinese physicians recommended that in order to remain healthy, one should do Tai Chi exercises,[14] "soft" aerobic exercises designed to generate and distribute chi in the body, in the early morning. Using modern knowledge of the physiologic state of the body in the morning, nothing could make more sense. While the body is resting in the morning, the blood (rich in amino acids, free fatty acids, beta-endorphin, and cortisol) perfused the body at a very slow rate compared with when the body is active. At rest, the blood flows through the muscles at 4–7 ml/100 gm of muscle, while during extreme exercise, the amount of blood flow may reach as high as 100 ml/100 gm, a 15–20-fold increase. This apparently is due to the fact that strenuous exercise causes all muscle capillaries to open, compared with only 3% being open at rest. In addition, strenuous exercise may increase blood pressure 50–70%, thus doubling available blood supply to muscles.[8] In addition, exercise causes an increase in body temperature, which in turn causes an increase in perfusion to the skin in an attempt to regulate body heat.

Clearly, "soft" exercises, which do not produce oxygen debt, also increase the blood perfusion to the body but have an additional advantage. Strenuous exercise derives most of its energy from anaerobic metabolism— blood glucose is converted from glycogen into lactic acid. After exercise, oxidative metabolism reconverts five sixths of the lactic acid into glucose, and the remaining one sixth is oxidized in the tricarboxylic acid cycle. "Soft" exercises, while increasing blood perfusion, derive their energy from aerobic metabolism and thus derive their energy not only from carbohydrates (as does anaerobic exercise) but from fats and proteins as well. Therefore, "soft" exercises performed in the morning not only cause increased perfusion of nutrient- and hormone-rich blood but also promote metabolism that can best utilize those ingredients. Brandenberger and Follenius found that "physical exercise in man produces an increase in cortisol concentration affecting the normal diurnal pattern and reverses the morning decline in plasma cortisol concentrations."[15] Several other studies have demonstrated a rise in plasma cortisol in response to athletics.[16,17]

Regarding the Chinese concept of eating when the stomach meridian is most active (7:00–9:00 a.m.), it has been shown that "500 gm of liver eaten at 8:00 a.m. led to a very swift rise of amino acid levels. Yet, the same protein meal eaten at 8:00 p.m. did not elevate blood levels of amino acids above the fasting value generally found at that time."[5] Finally, further linkage between Chinese medicine and ACTH/beta-endorphin has been shown by Chapman at Johns Hopkins. Chapman demonstrated that the analgesic effect of acupuncture was destroyed when patients were given an opioid blocker, which suggests that an endogenous opioid mechanism results from this ancient Chinese procedure.[18]

CONCLUSION

The discovery of the formation of an endogenously formed opioid (beta-endorphin), which is closely related to the body's stress hormones, ACTH and cortisol, has already caused the expanding field of psychoneuroendocrinology to have a considerable impact on medicine. While there is considerably more to be learned, sufficient data is available to improve the present quality of medical care. The Chinese had an understanding of body physiology and biorhythms and sought to harmonize their medical treatment with the natural laws of the body. Administering medication without taking into account the body's biorhythms may well cause a disruption of the body's natural rhythms. This will result in an illness more chronic and severe than that with which the patient initially presented himself to the physician.

An illustrative case is that of a 23-year-old black woman referred to this author by her dermatologist, who thought she might improve if attention was given to the psychosomatic component of her illness. Her history revealed that the dermatologist had attempted to control her dermatitis with oral steroids, in a pattern that did not mimic the normal circadian rhythm of cortisol. Her reaction to this regimen was total disruption of her normal biological rhythms: her sleeping pattern was disturbed, she often felt tired and irritable during times when she usually felt relaxed and calm, and she began to develop a Cushing-like syndrome. As a result, the prednisone was discontinued, and she was given diphenhydramine hydrochloride, 50 mg three times a day, with the psychiatric referral.

With the author's understanding of biorhythms, the patient was asked to reduce the dosage of diphenhydramine to 25 mg at 6:00 a.m. and

50 mg at 6:00 p.m. The patient subsequently reported that her itching was substantially reduced, despite her taking one half as much medication.

Other precepts that follow from a rudimentary knowledge of biorhythms include (1) advising patients seeking to lose weight to exercise in the morning, when the body's biorhythm allows fat to be more easily metabolized and (2) advising patients with allergic problems to take advantage of early morning high biologic levels of cortisol by increasing the perfusion of this steroid-rich blood to the body. As modern medicine continues to unravel the mysteries of psychoneuroendocrinology and biorhythms, the ancient claims of Chinese medicine and Tai Chi of ability to cure allergies, asthma, neurodermatitis, hypertension, and mental illness may be found to not have been so farfetched, and it may be discovered that those "primitive" people knew more than they are generally credited with knowing.

COMMENTARY

This article was the result of my continued study of the benefits of the "soft" Chinese exercises and Chinese medicine. Essentially, the exercises I was advocating for in Chapter 34 were a form of acupuncture exercises, since they caused stimulation of the acupuncture meridians in the human body. In many ways, the exercises represent the prevention aspects of Chinese medicine, as they are designed to maintain health and wellbeing. Since there is a strong theme of biologic rhythms in Chinese medicine, I decided to investigate how Western knowledge of the body's biologic rhythms is related to the exercises. The article was theoretical, as I didn't have the time or resources to do any scientific, empirical studies to prove what I was proposing. There is still much scientific work that needs to be done to test my hypothesis.

I may not have any hard scientific proof that doing "soft" Chinese exercises at sunrise increases one's blood levels of beta-endorphin or increases one's ability to burn more fat, but I do have several personal experiences that have convinced me it is true. A couple of years after I wrote this article, I fractured a bone in my finger. It was particularly difficult to set because the break was diagonal along the length of the bone. The orthopedic surgeon wanted to give me an injection in the finger so I wouldn't feel any pain while he tried to set the fracture. It was clear to me that if he gave me that shot, it would cause the tissues in my finger to swell, making the chances of him fixing my finger without surgery very slim. I told him that I wouldn't take a local anesthetic but would deal with the pain the best way I could. Reluctantly, he agreed. A half hour later, my finger was set and in a cast, with no need for surgery. Because of all of the nerves that cover the bone, the doctor was impressed that I could tolerate the pain. Bone pain is quite severe. He asked me my method, and I told him that I'd done some lower diaphragmatic breathing that I'd learned from Tai Chi exercises. The only thing I'd felt while he was pulling on my finger to set it was a sense of heat coming from the middle of my palm. I'd never done anything like that before. I suspect that my ability to tolerate the pain was related to the increased levels of beta-endorphin that I have developed over the years.

There is another benefit to the exercises that I wrote about, which I did not fully appreciate until years later. Many people are appropriately concerned with their amount of body fat, but they don't know how to get rid of it. I was watching a PBS show called "Fit or Fat" with Covert Bailey. He clearly explained how anaerobic exercises like sprinting used sugar as a source of energy while aerobic exercises like jogging used fat as a source of energy. It became apparent to me that the "soft" Chinese exercises I was recommending were some of the best fat-burning exercises in existence, as they are aerobic.

Half of our body fat is underneath the skin, and the other half is in the muscles. Doing a thousand sit-ups a day won't get rid of the fat around the stomach. Laying down on the side and doing a thousand sideways leg lifts won't get rid of the fat on the sides of the legs. This is because when you exercise the abdominal or adductor muscles of the thigh, they don't burn only the fat closest to them as an energy source; they use fat from all over the body. Thus, the fat under the skin of the abdomen or thighs will never be reduced until all the fat in the body is reduced. Unfortunately, neither the abdominal muscles, nor the abductor muscles on the sides of the thighs, are large enough to reduce whole body fat. The main way to burn large amounts of total body fat is to exercise the muscles from the waist to the knee, because these muscles are the largest in the body. Tai Chi "soft" exercises specialize in this variety of exercises. They are especially beneficial if done in the morning, when the body's sugar supply is depleted and when the body has to get its energy from the body's fat and protein.

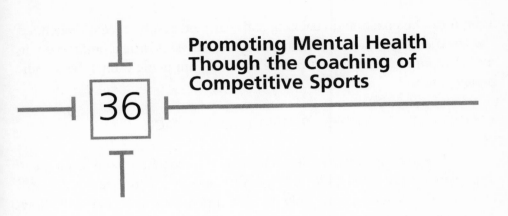

36

Promoting Mental Health Though the Coaching of Competitive Sports

Competitive sports can have a negative or positive impact on an athlete's mental health, and an athlete's coach plays a large role in determining this. The coach's goal should be to help athletes realize that developing human potential is equally as important as winning. This article highlights guidelines to assist coaches in instructing and mentoring athletes.

INTRODUCTION

The role of coach carries with it a great responsibility that goes far beyond winning games, as it can nurture or destroy an athlete's human potential by virtue of the direction the coach chooses to take. A healthy coach is an instructor-mentor who uses sports as a vehicle to tutor individual competitors or players on his/her team. One of the qualified coach's ultimate goals is to provide guidance for developing useful life skills such as leadership. In addition to having significant influence over school athletes, the coach and coaching staff are frequently in charge of a "subculture" that has intimate contact with a core of student or school leaders.

Originally printed as Bell Carl C. Promotion of mental health through coaching of competitive sports. *J Natl Med Assoc*. 1997;89:517–520. Presented at the 101st Annual Convention and Scientific Assembly of the NMA, Chicago, IL, July 27–August 3, 1996.

Therefore, the coach and coaching staff can potentially have an extended influence on the school and community milieu. This article outlines some of the important lessons that can be learned from being trained by a competent coach.

VALUES AND ATTITUDES OF THE HEALTHY COACH

The healthy coach understands that as a coach, he/she has a great responsibility for developing the human resources of the team's players. This includes developing not only physical and mental skills that will allow the athletes to win at competition, but also skills to enhance physical health, intellectual growth, character development, spirituality, and maturation. Hence, the adept coach realizes that one of his/her goals is to foster the appropriate development of aggression. The sensible coach also promotes teamwork and interdependence in players who participate in team sports. For competitors in individual sports, the coach is concerned with nourishing a sense of independence and self-reliance. The able coach attempts to instill confidence, inner peace, courage, ethics, initiative, discipline, concentration, and a sound respect for nutrition, training, a drug-free body, and a balanced lifestyle in their athletes, all of which have a profound impact on self-image. Finally, the proficient trainer seeks to promote efforts toward self-fulfillment and self-actualization.

Healthy coaches appreciate that leadership is necessary in groups and families as well as in individual tasks and that while the need to lead is innate, leadership must be learned. Coaches perceive leadership training as a way to learn self-motivation, positive expectancy, problem-solving skills, decision-making skills, and communication and listening skills, while making worthwhile contributions to others. The complete coach understands that a goal-less player is dissatisfied and discontented; however, being goal-oriented (i.e., self-leadership produces purposeful behavior), a competitor may be unsatisfied but happy to be struggling. Additionally, the sound coach understands that success is the progressive realization of a person's own worthwhile predetermined goal and is not to be evaluated by comparisons. Such coaches seek to influence their players' goal-setting behavior and encourage their players to be in competition with themselves. They also seek to remove factors that will inhibit the competitors' ability to provide leadership themselves, which will move them toward their goals.

LEADERSHIP INHIBITORS

Fit coaches are aware of leadership inhibitors and how they interfere with reaching aspirations. They understand that basic needs are prioritized, with biologic needs (food, drink, and shelter) having the highest priority over higher-level basic needs of safety and security, love and social connection, esteem, and self-fulfillment. This implies that if basic biologic needs are not satisfied, leadership is stifled because the higher needs, which drive leadership, are not given attention. Quality trainers are concerned with ensuring that their players' basic biologic needs are satisfied.

Sound coaches realize that the need for social acceptance also can block leadership. Being conditioned to derive acceptance from others versus gaining approbation from self-esteem can block motivation to change. One of the major sources that cultivates a need for social acceptance is family influence, which seeks to pressure individuals in positive or negative directions; fortunately, however, behavior is learned and can be unlearned. Competent coaches teach their athletes that sports participants should never give their individuality completely to the group nor accept mediocrity as the norm. Ergo, proper training of athletes urges them to place their personal missions over the goal of social acceptance. Such guidance helps the athlete bypass weekend parties to study so they can maintain the grade point average necessary to stay on the team.

Outstanding coaches understand that petty emotions that lead to bitterness, jealousy, hatred, malice, fear, and doubt need to be discouraged, as they divert individuals from setting constructive goals for themselves. The same holds true for procrastination. Similarly, people can relive past failures and develop an unwholesome attitude to failure. We pay a heavy price for our fear of failure; it is a powerful obstacle to growth since it assures the progressive narrowing of the personality and prevents exploration and further experimentation. Failure can become so entrenched in memory that it creates a motivational block because of the association with embarrassment, fear, and doubt. The total personality is threatened because the embarrassment is so acute that the athlete would rather not try again. Sound coaches instruct that growth is a painful process and that it is better to have tried and failed than to not have tried at all. Coaches teach that a player should react to failure with curiosity, not with fear or pain—it is the difference between seeing a lesson in life or feeling punished.

The instructor/mentor coach aspires to remove these leadership impediments from the athlete's life, as such efforts can have positive, far-reaching consequences. Because people will act like who they think they are, self-concepts also can form a restrictive barrier to success. Sports persons cannot achieve more than they think they can, because anything beyond the self-concept will not be tried. This causes them to become their own worst enemy. Capable coaches seek to alter their players' ideas about themselves and try to teach athletes that "an individual who thinks he or she can and a human being who thinks he or she can't are both correct."

LESSONS TO BE TAUGHT BY AND LEARNED FROM HEALTHY COACHES

Self-Motivation. This is one of the skills athletes can cultivate from being involved with competitive sports under the tutelage of a healthy coach. Such coaches know that desires coming from belief and expectation are strong motivating forces that propel one toward his/her goals. They comprehend that the world stands aside for people who make their own choices and steps on those who let others choose for them.

Self-motivation can be developed by using visualization to crystallize expectation and belief. First, however, an athlete must know his/her needs and desires and must know how to convert them into action. To properly motivate, one must appeal to the strongest desire. Motivating through fear of punishment, restriction of privileges, or social disapproval is disadvantageous because fear sometimes loses effect when the form of punishment is known or commonplace. Further, motivating through fear discourages voluntary fellowship. If a player is fearful, his/her effectiveness decreases because of all the energy expended by fear. There are also limitations of leading that offers incentives (the opposite of motivation from fear) in exchange for performance, because the prizes are no longer motivating once the appetite is filled. Leading with attitudes and values is the only truly useful type of motivation for personal and group leadership.

Such leadership is based on an understanding of human nature—people love to learn and master rather than be lazy.

Successful leaders practice self-motivation and then use that knowledge to motivate and lead others. They see their motivational blocks, recognize how they block, and then remove them. Their self-insight then can be used to help others remove their impediments. Proficient coaches supply their players with opportunities to rehearse their self-motivation capacity.

Positive Expectancy. Exemplary coaches fathom that competitors cannot have positive expectations about themselves until they are conversant with themselves. An individual's relationship with him/herself is a strong factor in his/her personal expectations. A deficit in self-awareness will cause players to search for themselves, resulting in a waste of energy. Another important aspect of the awareness athletes have of themselves is self-reliance, which is developed by visualizing a problem, solving it, and benefiting from the solution. Needing self-confidence causes a loss of energy due to doubt and causes a contender to be irresponsible and fearful. Self-confidence is power and comes from "know how," which comes from experience, which comes from willingness to subject oneself to fearful experiences. Self-respect occurs when people choose high values and live by, rather than up to, them. Self-acceptance occurs when one is aware of and acknowledges one's own strengths and weakness. This skill is crucial, as a person must know his/her weaknesses to strive to change them. Thus, self-acceptance implies self-improvement.

Leadership Essentials. Sound coaches understand that there are several leadership essentials. Their athletes must know themselves to know what they want and where they stand. Such knowledge helps to crystallize thinking around short- and long-range goal-setting. Short-range goals are good confidence builders that help form success habits and broaden vision, while long-range goals take foresight and need intermediate steps. In order to choose a goal, one must indulge in self-analysis.

Written plans and deadlines are also crucial to leadership. A realistic plan of action that puts theory into action is necessary, as visualized plans lead to crystallized thoughts, and consciousness creates memory. Written plans keep things clear and prevent goals from being lost. Further, writing stimulates visualization. It is a reference and reminder, conserving time and energy and giving an overall view of goals to decrease conflict. It helps keep track of plans, eliminate distractions, overcome procrastination, and keep a sense of progress and expectancy.

Another integral component is the desire for leadership. A leader must have a need for action, and plans must have emotion. Supreme self-confidence is also needed since competitors must be assured of being able to change their attitude and then their behavior. Finally, good leaders need unshakable determination, as they cannot afford to live in the shadow of public opinion, dogmatism, or blind stubbornness. Worthy coaches teach these leadership essentials by displaying these talents to their protégés and giving them an opportunity to rehearse this expertise.

Problem Solving. Suitable coaches realize that attitudes about problem solving make or break a player. To engage in effective problem solving, competitors must have awareness of the problem to objectively define it. If a person tries to define it subjectively (i.e., with his/her emotions involved), then he/she becomes a part of the problem instead of the solution. Competent problem solving involves being time-conscious, which often requires setting a deadline and deciding on available information. Vision is another key component to adept problem solving, since a contender must be able to envision a goal to reach it. Also indispensable in working out impediments are being inquisitive—the feeling of needing knowledge, knowing how to get data, and knowing what to look for. Finally, the ability to be creative and brainstorm about the predicament are imperative in problem solving.

Competitive sports provide fertile training grounds for all these aspects of problem solving. In addition, truculent sports furnish an opportunity for developing creative leadership. Such leadership demands trying the untried and relating the unrelated. It demands that conceptual skills be honed, along with a willingness to innovate and see things in unusual ways, permitting open-mindedness, and preventing jumping to the obvious. This state of mind is uninhibited with culture and convention, allowing the creative athlete to face the future and change without stress. For the creative leader, stress in fact heightens interest and causes self-competitiveness. The ability to remain calm under stress comes from confidence that stress shall be overcome and that with improvisation, things will go well. Finally, sports afford the prospect of testing a person's ability for critically analyzing the steps to settle a quandary, objectively choose a course, and implement a decision.

Decision-Making. An integral part of problem solving is becoming a decision-maker. Making decisions is an outward manifestation of internal leadership abilities. The best decision comes from using common sense, intellect, confidence, and dedication. Making a half-hearted endorsement leads to failure. Advance preparation and knowing one's self leads to making good decisions. It is the compulsive who over-think decisions and make them too quickly. The fearful do not make decisions at all. Good decision makers refuse to be pressured, consider one decision at a time, and decide from evidence as opposed to inspirations (this does not rule out intuition). Deciding involves accepting the risk of a bad outcome and should always include an alternative. Wishy-washy decisions do not work, but this is different from the decided way to a goal. A decision should be matched with an action; if the decision is wrong, the skillful problem-solver will change it. Competition in sports renders myriad circumstances to practice making arduous decisions, and competent coaching can amplify a player's facility at constructing conclusions.

Communication. Finally, a person must be able convey ideas to lead; thus, communication is the sum and substance of leadership. Instructor/mentor coaches know how to be heard and how to hear, as they understand good communication is an exchange of feelings and attitudes. Competent coaches realize that the art of listening entails understanding that if you want another's attention, you must give him/her yours. Coaches model such skills for their athletes. They understand that ideas can be powerful things.

CONCLUSIONS

This article has outlined themes gleaned from sports training governed by enlightened coaches who seek to pass on their sagacity. These coaches realize that to do less is to abandon the greatest responsibility of their profession. Such educators search for the purpose and meaning in life and find within themselves the spring of motivation to contribute unique things. They attract people with understanding and empathy, which motivates others to search for their own potential for success. Successful coaches find vitality in the opportunities around them, see challenges where others see threats and problems, look to the fruits instead of the toils of their labors, and look to the future rather than the present. They have no fear of the future and are dedicated to the philosophy of change, growth, and development, because they acknowledge that one can maintain the momentum to keep on leadership's course only by setting progressively higher goals.

COMMENTARY

Knowing my interest in sports medicine, Dr. Jeanne Spurlock asked me to present a paper at the 101st Annual Convention of the NMA, where she'd present some of her clinical work revealing how competitive sports have a negative influence on adolescent development.

While being aware of the negative potential of competitive sports, I've always tried to develop the positive aspects. When I was an instructor at Martial Arts Systems, Inc., from 1973 to 1985, I used to talk with my Judo instructor, Willard Dunning, about leadership. Trained in Japan, he gave me a great deal of information about the topic. Because of my martial arts training, I'd given the lecture, "Stress and Sports," at Jackson Park Hospital's Sports Medicine Conference, June 5, 1981. This gave me the opportunity to interface with "healthy coaches" such as Larry Hawkins, then at University of Chicago, and Dennis Green, then at Northwestern University. Our discussions confirmed that competitive sports could have a constructive outcome for youth. I also had the opportunity to be a clinician at the Chicago Forum, Youth Fitness and Sports Program, presented by the President's Council on Physical Fitness and Sports. This allowed me to develop my thoughts further.

In 1996, fifteen years later, I finally put my thoughts on paper in this article. After I wrote it, I had several insights. For one, I'd never realized how much my martial arts training had impacted my professional life. I've been President/CEO of a successful business for seventeen years, yet have never had any formal management training. In an effort of self-education, I'd been reading various management books and had hired various management consultants. To be honest, I wasn't learning anything new. Since writing the paper, I've realized why. Martial arts training had already provided me a course in leadership, problem solving, decision-making, and communication.

Reading management books did give me useful information—they helped me understand where America is regarding management philosophy. Bullying is the predominating management style in the country, whether on the sports field or in business. Fortunately, W. Edwards Deming studied Japanese management and returned to the US with a message that there was a better way than management through intimidation. Reading management books by Peter F. Drucker, Max Depree, Stephen R. Covey, and Peter M. Senge confirmed that the way we were doing business at the CMHC made sense. Most importantly, our on-the-job results told the CMHC management team that we were on the right track. I've also had two of the best senior vice-presidents, Juanita L. Redd, MPA, MBA, and Hayward Suggs, MS, MBA, to help me and educate me about management systems.

One of the major challenges facing the country is how to infuse evidence-based practices into everyday practice. As President/CEO of the CMHC, I brought evidence-based practices to the CMHC staff for years. The staff seemed to receive the evidence-based practices with enthusiasm, but they would never utilize the practices in caring for patients. I finally took the problem to the CMHC operations team, who began to give the staff ongoing training in negotiations, being effective on a team, navigating change, taking risks, and developing business plans. We believe this training allows African-American mental health providers to perform their missions more effectively and puts the CMHC in a better position to "Save Lives—Making a Difference."

Afterword

Writing this afterword has been one of my most difficult tasks. The problem is that an afterword seems like the final word. How does one ever get down to final words and answers that complete the discussion in a field as complex as psychiatry? At a recent Chicago Institute of Medicine lecture, it was explained that "simple" is a recipe, "complicated" is a moon rocket, and "complex" is raising a child. Thus, I'm in a field in which there are no final words or answers. The most we can do is recognize where we are at a given time. Once we know where we are, we must also understand that there's a vast amount of truth and wisdom yet to be discovered. Further, if we're honest with ourselves, we'll admit that the truth and wisdom we've discovered is as old as human existence. The only difference between the human species in 2004 and thousands of years ago is that our technology is more advanced, but the basic process of being human remains the same. So, for now, here's my "afterword."

I've recently realized that a major problem with psychiatry is that it's too focused on what we were trained to do. It sometimes feels like psychiatry is stuck in a box that only recognizes diagnosis and treatment. Unfortunately, being in this box precludes psychiatrists from involving themselves with prevention and from focusing on strengths and characteristics of resilience and resistance. These are just as much a part of the human condition as is the psychopathology we were trained to identify and treat. Fortunately, some of us are blessed enough to be on the fringe, which allows us to occasionally leave the box and get a different perspective. This brings new paradigms and models that benefit the human condition. I recall Dr. Boris Astrachan, former Chairman of Psychiatry at the University of Illinois at Chicago, who helped promote me to the rank of Professor there, telling me that I'm on the fringe. Psychiatrists are already on the fringe of society because we address the ills of those who are on the fringe by virtue of their psychopathology, but at the time, Dr. Astrachan's comment didn't make me feel good. Being on the fringe of the fringe, if you will, by virtue of being ahead of your time, is a lonely existence. It's an existence I've never cherished, because most people tarnish psychiatrists with the same stigma with which society tarnishes psychiatric patients. The very people you've dedicated your life to helping call you crazy behind your back, simply because you aren't in their box and they don't understand what you see.

I also recall Dr. Astrachan telling me that the fringe was the best place to be because I could bring new ideas and have a great deal of innovative influence. I've often wondered why I find myself at the seat of power since I'm usually the "odd man out," and based on the depth and breath of my work, haven't really belonged in many rooms. With time and experience, I've learned that my being the "odd man out" has contributed greatly to the creativity, humor, leadership, and productive dynamic tension in the room, and that we all have walked out more enriched. So, being on the fringe of the fringe has been a curse but also a huge blessing.

I hope that this book can help others to "Dream the Impossible Dream." If anyone needs further inspiration, I suggest locating that song and listening to it repeatedly, as I believe it contains some of the answers for developing "kokoro" (indomitable fighting spirit, in Japanese).

References

CHAPTER 1:
Black-on-Black Murder: A Community Psychiatry Response

1. Nickens H. Report of the Secretary's Task Force on Black and Minority Health: a summary and presentation of health data with regard to blacks. *J Natl Med Assoc.* 1986;78:577–580.
2. Koop CE. *Surgeon General's Workshop on Violence and Public Health: Source Book.* Washington, DC: National Center on Child Abuse and Neglect; 1985.
3. Walker ML. Trauma prevention. *J Natl Med Assoc.* 1986;78:489–491.
4. Mazique EC. National Medical Political Action Committee. *J Natl Med Assoc.* 1986;78:138.
5. Attorney General's Task Force Report on Family Violence. Washington, DC: US Department of Justice; 1984.
6. Bell CC. Coma and the etiology of violence, part 1. *J Natl Med Assoc.* 1986;78:1167–1176, 1986.
7. Bell CC. The need for accreditation of correctional health care facilities. *J Natl Med Assoc.* 1984;76:571–572.

CHAPTER 2:
Preventive Strategies for Dealing with Violence among Blacks

1. Freed HM. Subcontracts for community development and service. *Am J Psychiatry.* 1972;129:568–573.
2. Freed HM, Schroder DJ, Baker B. Community participation in mental health services: a case of factional control. In: Miller L, ed. *Mental Health in Rapid Changing Society.* Jerusalem, Israel: Jerusalem Academic Press; 1972.
3. Koop CE. *Surgeon General's Workshop on Violence and Public Health: Source Book.* Washington, DC: National Center on Child Abuse and Neglect; 1985.
4. University of California at Los Angeles and Centers for Disease Control. *The Epidemiology of Homicide in the City of Los Angeles 1970–79.* Atlanta, GA: Centers for Disease Control; 1985. Dept of Health and Human Services, PHS.

5. Stark E, Filtcraft A. Medical therapy as repression: the case of the battered woman. *Health and Medicine.* 1982;Summer/Fall:29–32.

6. Okun L. *Woman Abuse: Facts Replacing Myths.* Albany, NY: State University of New York Press Albany; 1986.

7. Police Foundation. *Domestic violence and the Police: Studies in Detroit and Kansas City.* Washington, DC: Police Foundation; 1977.

8. Rynearson EK. Psychological effects of unnatural dying on bereavement. *Psychiatr Annals.* 1986;16:272–275.

9. American Psychiatric Association. *Diagnostic and Statistical Manual of Mental Disorders.* 3rd ed. Washington, DC: American Psychiatric Association; 1979.

10. Jennett B, Teasdale G. *Management of Head Injuries.* Philadelphia, PA: FA Davis; 1981.

11. Ramos SM, Delany HM. Freefalls from heights: A persistent urban problem. *J Natl Med Assoc.* 1986;78:111–115.

12. Clark K. *Dark Ghetto.* New York: Harper & Row; 1965.

13. Lewis DO, May E, Jackson LD. Biosocial characteristics of children who later murder: a prospective study. *Am J Psychiatry.* 1985;142:1161–1167.

14. Lewis DO, Pincus JH, Feldman M. Psychiatric, neurological, and psychoeducational characteristics of 15 death row inmates in the United States. *Am J Psychiatry.* 1986;143:838–845.

15. Bell CC, Thompson B, Shorter-Gooden K, Shakoor B, Dew D, Hughley E, Mays R. Prevalence of coma in black subjects. *J Natl Med Assoc.* 1985;77:391–395.

16. Linnolia M. Alcohol abuse linked to brain changes causing violence. *Behavior Today Newsletter.* 1986;17:6–7.

17. Allen NH. Homicide prevention and intervention. *J Suicide and Life Threatening Behavior.* 1981;11:167–179.

18. Stengel R. When brother kills brother. *Time.* 1985;September:32–36.

19. Staver S. MD stresses physician role in stopping murder. *Am Med News.* 1986;July 31.

20. Freed HM. The community psychiatrist and political action. *Arch Gen Psychiatry.* 1967;17:129–134.

21. Attorney General's Task Force Report on Family Violence. Washington, DC: US Department of Justice; 1984.

22. Lystad M, ed. *Violence in the Home: Interdisciplinary Perspectives.* New York: Brunner/Mazel; 1986.

23. Bell CC. Coma and the etiology of violence, part 1. *J Natl Med Assoc.* 1986;78:1139–1167.

24. Bell CC. Coma and the etiology of violence, part 2. *J Natl Med Assoc.* 1987;79:79–85.

25. Lion JR, Bach-y-Rita G, Ervin FR. The self-referred violent patient. *J Am Med Assoc.* 1968;205:503–505.

26. Lion JR, Bach-y-Rita G, Ervin FR. Violent patients in the emergency room. *Am J Psychiatry*. 1969;125:1706–1710.

27. Lion JR, Bach-y-Rita G. Group psychotherapy with violent outpatients. *Intl J Group Psychotherapy*. 1970;20:185–191.

28. Rose HM. *Black Homicide and the Urban Environment*. Washington, DC: Government Printing Office; 1981. United States Dept of Health and Human Services, NIMH.

29. Dennis RE, Kirk A, Knuckles BN. *Black Males at Risk to Low Life Expectancy: A Study of Homicide Victims and Perpetrators*. Washington, DC: Center for Studies of Minority Group Mental Health; 1981. NIMH grant 1-R01 MH36720.

CHAPTER 3:
Stress-Related Disorders in African-American Children

1. Jenkins EJ, Thompson B. Children talk about violence: preliminary findings from a survey of black elementary children. Presented at the Association of Black Psychologists Annual Convention, Oakland, CA, August 13–17, 1986.

2. Bell CC, Jenkins EJ. Traumatic stress and children. *J Health Care Poor Underserved*. 1991;2:175–188.

3. Bell CC, Jenkins EJ. Community violence and children on Chicago's Southside. *Psychiatry: Interpersonal and Biological Processes*. 1993;56:46–54.

4. American Psychiatric Association. *Diagnostic and Statistical Manual of Mental Disorders*. 4th ed. Washington, DC: American Psychiatric Press; 1995.

5. Amaya-Jackson L, March JS. Post-traumatic stress disorder in children and adolescents. *Child and Adolescent Psychiatric Clinics of North America*. 1993;2:639–654.

6. Hammond WR, Yung BR. Preventing violence in at-risk African-American youth. *J Health Care Poor Underserved*. 1991;2:359–372.

7. Richters JE, Martinez P. The NIMH community violence project 1: children as victims of and witnesses to violence. *Psychiatry*. 1993;56:7–21.

8. Orsofsky JD, Wewers S, Hann DM, Fick AC. Chronic community violence: what is happening to our children? *Psychiatry*. 1993;56:36–45.

9. Fitzpatrick KM, Boldizar JP. The prevalence and consequences of exposure to violence among African-American youth. *J Am Acad Child Adolesc Psychiatry*. 1993;32:424–430.

10. Jenkins EJ, Bell CC. Violence exposure, psychological distress and high risk behaviors among inner-city high school students. In: Friedman S, ed. *Anxiety Disorders in African-Americans*. New York, NY: Springer Publishing; 1994:76–88.

11. Bell CC, Davis K. Is psychoanalytic therapy relevant for public health programs? *Psychiatr Times*. 1994; 11:31–34.

12. Sizemore CC, Pittillo ES. *I'm Eve.* New York, NY: Jove Publications; 1978.

13. Shore JH, Tatum EL, Vollmer VM. Psychiatric reactions to disaster: the Mount St. Helen's experience. *Am J Psychiatry.* 1986;143:590–595.

14. Burton D, Foy D, Bwanausi C, Johnson J, Moore L. The relationship between traumatic exposure, family dysfunction, and post-traumatic stress symptoms in male juvenile offenders. *J Trauma Stress.* 1994;7:83–93.

15. Goenjian AK, Pynoos RS, Steinberg AM, Najarian LM, Asarnow JR, Karayan I, et al. Psychiatric comorbidity in children after the 1988 earthquake in Armenia. *J Am Acad Child Adolesc Psychiatry.* 1995;34:1174–1184.

16. Angelou M. *I Know Why the Caged Bird Sings.* New York, NY: Random House; 1969.

17. Davidson J. Issues in the diagnosis of post-traumatic stress disorder. In: Oldham JM, Riba MB, Tasman A, eds. *Review of Psychiatry.* Vol. 12. Washington, DC: American Psychiatric Press; 1993.

18. Fullilove M, Fullilove R. Post-traumatic stress disorder in women recovering from substance abuse. In: Friedman S, ed. *Anxiety Disorders in African Americans.* New York, NY: Springer Publishing; 1994:89–101.

19. Pynoos R. Exposure to catastrophic violence and disaster in childhood. In: Pfeiffer CR, ed. *Severe Stress and Mental Disturbance in Children.* Washington, DC: American Psychiatric Press; 1996:181–208.

20. Murphy L, Pynoos RS, James CB. The trauma/grief focused group psychotherapy module of an elementary school based violence prevention/intervention program. In: Osofsky, ed. *Children in a Violent Society.* New York, NY: Guilford Press; 1997:223–255.

CHAPTER 4:
The Role of Psychiatric Emergency Services in Creating Alternatives to Hospitalization in an Inner-City Population

1. Borus JF. Community mental health and the deinstitutionalized patient. *Weekly Psychiatry Update Series, Parts 1 and 2;* 1977.

2. Levison DJ, Astrashan BM: Organizational boundaries: entry into the mental health center. In: *Administration in Mental Health.* NIMH; Summer 1974.

3. Borus JF: The coordination of mental health services at the neighborhood level. *Am J Psychiatry.* 1975;132:1171–1181.

4. *Region 2 Street and Coding Guide.* Illinois Department of Mental Health; 1972.

5. Ghetto psychiatry: Harlem version, parts I and 2. *Psychiatr Annals.* 1974;4(4&5).

6. Lazare A, Cohen F, Jacobson AM, et al. The walk-in patient as a customer: A key dimension in evaluation and treatment. *Am J Orthopsychiatry.* 1972;42:872–883.

7. Whittington HG, Zaburck R, Grey L: Pharmacotherapy and community psychiatric practice. *Am J Psychiatry.* 1969;126:133–136.

8. Anderson WH, Kuehnie JC, Catanzano DM: Rapid treatment of acute psychosis. *Am J Psychiatry.* 1976;133:1076–1078.

9. Mann PL, Chen CH: Rapid tranquilization of acutely psychotic patients with intramuscular haloperidol and chlorpromazine. *Psychosomatics.* 1973;14:59–63.

10. Ayd F: The depot fluphenazines: a reappraisal after 10 years' clinical experience. *Am J Psychiatry.* 1975;132:491–500.

11. Orlinsky DE, Howard KI: Communication rapport and patient progress. *Psychotherapy: Theory, Research and Practice.* 1968;5:131–136.

12. Navaco RW: The functions and regulations of the arousal of anger. *Am J Psychiatry.* 1976;133:1124–1128.

13. Morcornity E: Aggression in human adaptation. *Psychoanal Q.* 1973;42:226–232.

14. Herz MI, Endicott J, Spitzer RL: Brief versus standard hospitalization: the families. *Am J Psychiatry.* 1976;133:795–801.

15. Weissmann M: Prognostic factors in attempted suicide. *Am J Psychiatry.* 1974;131:987–990.

16. Tucker GJ: Psychiatric emergencies: evaluation and management. In: Freedman DX, Dryud JE, eds. *American Handbook of Psychiatry.* Vol. 5, 2nd ed. New York: Basic Books; 1975:567–592.

CHAPTER 5:
Security Procedures in a Psychiatric Emergency Service

1. Lazare A, Cohen F, Jacobson AM, et al. The walk-in patient as a customer: a key dimension in evaluation and treatment. *Am J Orthopsychiatry.* 1972;42:872–883.

2. Farnsworth D. Dangerousness. *Psychiatr Ann.* 1977; 7: 55–70.

3. Guze S, Woodruff R, Clayton P. Psychiatric disorders and criminality. *J Am Med Assoc.* 1974;227:641–642.

4. Bell C. Interface between psychiatry and the law on the issue of murder. *J Natl Med Assoc.* 1980;72:1093–1097.

5. Madden D, Lion J, Penna M. Assaults on psychiatrists by patients. *Am J Psychiatry.* 1976;133:422–425.

6. Whitman R, Armao B, Dent O. Assault on the therapist. *Am J Psychiatry.* 1976;133:426–429.

7. Increased violence in psychiatric patients, male and female, refuted in a large study. In: *Roche Report: Frontiers of Psychiatry*. 1980;10:12–13.

8. Bell C. The role of psychiatric emergency services in aiding community alternatives to hospitalization in an inner-city population. *J Natl Med Assoc*. 1978;70:931–935.

9. Bell C. States of consciousness. *J Natl Med Assoc*. 1980;72:331–334.

10. Cornfield C, Fielding S. Impact of the threatening patient on ward communications. *Am J Psychiatry*. 1980;137:616–619.

11. Lion J, Madden D, Christopher R. A violence clinic: three years' experience. *Am J Psychiatry*. 1976;133:432–435.

12. Levy P, Hartocollis P. Nursing aids and patient violence. *Am J Psychiatry*. 1976;133:429–431.

13. Bell C. Analysis of the political sophistication of the black psychiatrist. *Black Psychiatrists of America Newsletter*. 1974;3&5.

14. Marcovitz E. Aggression in human adaptation. *Psychoanal Q*. 1973;42:226–232.

15. Griffith E, Griffith E. Duty to third parties, dangerousness, and the right to refuse treatment: problematic concepts for psychiatrist and lawyer. *Calif Western Law Review*. 1978;14:241–274.

16. Soloff PH. Physical restraint and the nonpsychotic patient: clinical and legal perspectives. *J Clin Psychiatry*. 1979;40:31–34.

17. Gutheil TG. Restraint versus treatment: seclusion as discussed in the Boston state hospital case. *Am J Psychiatry*. 1980;137:718–719.

18. Holinger PC: Violent deaths among the young: an epidemiological study of recent trends in suicide, homicide and accidents. *Am J Psychiatry*. 1979;136:1144–1147.

19. Man P. Are 'dangerous' patients dangerous? *Legal Aspects Med Pract*. 1979;7:46–48.

CHAPTER 6:
The Need for Psychoanalysis is Alive and Well in Community Psychiatry

1. Fenichel O: *The Psychoanalytic Theory of Neurosis*. New York: WW Norton; 1954:24, 136, 144–151, 44, 127.

2. Thomas A, Sillen S. *Racism and Psychiatry*. New York: Brunner/Mazel; 1972:136.

3. Jones B, Lightfoot O, Williams D, et al. Problems of black psychiatric residents in white training institutes. *Am J Psychiatry*. 1970;127:798–803.

4. Freud S, Breuer J. *Studies on Hysteria (1893–1895)*. Standard ed., vol. 2. London: Hogarth Press; 1955:90, 219, 173, 6, 24, 265, 14, 18.

5. Freud S. *On the Theory of Hysterical Attacks (1886–1899)*. Standard ed., vol. 1. London: Hogarth Press; 1955:153.

6. Cameron N. *Personality Development and Psychopathology*. Boston: Houghton Mifflin; 1963:341.

7. Feighner J, Robins E, Guze S, et al. Diagnostic criteria for use in psychiatric research. *Arch Gen Psychiatry*. 1972;26:57–63.

8. Comer J. What happened to minorities and the poor. *Psych Annals*. 1977;7:80–85.

9. Cannon M, Locke B. Being black is detrimental to one's mental health: myth or reality. *Phylon*. 1977;38:408–428.

CHAPTER 7:
Preventive Psychiatry in the Board of Education

1. Freedman A, Kaplan H, Sadock B. *Modern Synopsis of Comprehensive Textbook of Psychiatry*. Baltimore: Williams and Wilkins; 1972:687–692.

2. Sticknev S. Schools are our community mental health centers. *Am J Psychiatry*. 1968;124: 1407–1414.

3. Federal Register. Department of Health, Education, and Welfare; August 23, 1977;42:424–478.

4. Steegmann A, White H. *Examination of the Nervous System: A Student's Guide*. 3rd ed. Chicago: Year Book Medical Publishers, Inc.; 1970:182–216.

5. Masterson J. *Treatment of the Borderline Adolescent: A Developmental Approach*. New York: J. Wiley and Sons, Inc.; 1972:37–48.

6. Cantwell D, ed. *The Hyperactive Child*. New York: Spectrum Publishers; 1975:17–48.

7. Shaw C, Lucas A. *The Psychiatric Disorders of Childhood*. 2nd ed. New York: AppletonCentury-Crofts; 1970:161–190.

8. Bender L. *A Visual Motor Gestalt Test and Its Clinical Use*. New York: American Orthopsychiatric Association; 1938:57–97.

9. Mykelburst H, Johnson D. *Learning Disabilities: Educational Principles and Practices*. New York: Grune-Stratton; 1967:26–46.

10. Bookert C. Address of the retiring president: equal opportunity for all. *J Natl Med Assoc*. 1979;71:85–86.

11. Barber J. President's inaugural address: health status of the black community. *J Natl Med Assoc*. 1979;71:87–90.

12. Bell C. A social and nutritional survey of the population of the children and youth center of Meharry Medical Colleges of North Nashville, Tennessee. *J Natl Med Assoc*. 1971;63: 397–398.

CHAPTER 9:
Treating Violent Families

1. Report of the Secretary's Task Force on Black and Minority Health, Vol. 1: Executive Summary. Washington, DC: Government Printing Office; 1985. US Dept of Health and Human Services publication PHS 0-487-637.

2. Centers for Disease Control. *Homicide Surveillance: High-Risk Racial and Ethnic Groups—Blacks and Hispanics, 1970 to 1981*. Atlanta, GA: Centers for Disease Control; 1986.

3. Bell CC. Preventive strategies for dealing with violence among blacks. *Community Ment Health J*. 1987;23:217–228.

4. Okun L. *Woman Abuse: Facts Replacing Myths*. Albany, NY: State University of New York Press Albany; 1986.

5. Levinger G. Sources of marital dissatisfaction among applicants for divorce. *Am J Orthopsychiatry*. 1966;26:803–807.

6. Fields M. Wife-beating: facts and figures. *Victimology*. 1977;2:643–647.

7. O'Brien J. Violence in divorce-prone families. *J Marriage and the Fam*. 1971;33:692–698.

8. Parker B, Schumacher DN. The battered wife syndrome and violence in the nuclear family of origin: a controlled pilot study. *Am J Public Health*. 1977;67:760–761.

9. Mowrer E, Mowrer H. *Domestic Discord*. Chicago: University of Chicago Press; 1928.

10. Sanders D. Marital violence: dimensions of the problem and modes of intervention. *J Marriage and Family Counseling*. 1977;3:43–55.

11. Rounsaville B, Weissman M. Battered women: a medical problem requiring detection. *Int J Psychiatry Med*. 1978;8:191–202.

12. Stark E, Filtrcraft A. Medical therapy as repression: the case of the battered woman. *Health and Med*. 1982;Summer/Fall:29–32.

13. Straus M. Gelles R, Steinmetz S. *Behind Closed Doors: Violence in the American Family*. New York, NY: Doubleday/Anchor; 1980.

14. Goodwin J. Family violence: principles of intervention and prevention. *Hosp Community Psychiatry*. 1985;36:1074–1079.

15. Schulmar FA. *A Survey of Spousal Violence Against Women in Kentucky*. Publication 792701. Washington, DC: Government Printing Office, Law Enforcement Assistance Administration; 1979.

16. Teske R, Parker M. *Spouse Abuse in Texas: A Study of Women's Attitudes and Experiences*. Huntsville, TX: Criminal Justice Center, Sam Houston State University; 1983.

17. Boudouris J. Homicide and the family. *J Marriage and the Family*. 1971;33:667–676.

18. Gelles R. *The Violent Home.* Newbury Park, CA: Sage Publications Inc; 1987.

19. Straus M. Domestic violence and homicide antecedents. *Bull NY Acad Med.* 1986;62:446–465.

20. Block CR. *Lethal Violence in Chicago over Seventeen Years: Homicides Known to the Police, 1965–1981.* Chicago: Illinois Criminal Justice Information Authority; 1985.

21. Hollinger P. *Violent Deaths in the US: An Epidemiologic Study of Suicide, Homicide, and Accidents.* New York, NY: Guilford Press; 1987.

22. Barnhill L. Clinical assessment of intrafamilial violence. *Hosp Community Psychiatry.* 1980;31:543–547.

23. Reid W, Calis G. Evaluation of the violent patient. In: Hales R, Frances A, eds. *Psychiatric Update: The American Psychiatric Association Annual Review,* vol. 6. Washington, DC: American Psychiatric Press Inc; 1989:491–509.

24. University of California at Los Angeles and Centers for Disease Control. *The Epidemiology of Homicide in the City of Los Angeles 1970–79.* Atlanta, GA: Centers for Disease Control; 1985. Dept of Health and Human Services, PHS.

25. Kraus JF, Sorenson SB, Juarez PD, eds. *Research Conference on Violence and Homicide in Hispanic Communities.* Los Angeles, CA: UCLA Publication Services; 1988.

26. Bell CC. Black-on-black homicide: the implications for black community mental health. In: Smith-Ruiz D, ed. *Mental Health and Mental Illness Among Black Americans.* Westport, CT: Greenwood Press; 1990.

27. Griffith E, Bell CC. Recent trends in suicide and homicide among Blacks. *J Am Med Assoc.* 1989;262:2265–2269.

28. Wolfgang ME, Ferracuti F. *The Subculture of Violence: Towards an Integrated Theory in Criminology.* New York, NY: Methuen; 1967.

29. American Psychiatric Association. *Management of Violent Behavior: Collected Articles From Hospital and Community Psychiatry.* Washington, DC: Hospital Community Psychiatry Service; 1988.

30. Brizer L, Crowner M, eds. *Current Approaches to the Prediction of Violence.* Washington, DC: American Psychiatric Press Inc; 1989.

31. Barnhill LR. Basic interventions for violence in families. *Hosp Community Psychiatry.* 1980;31:547–551.

CHAPTER 10:
Interface between Psychiatry and the Law on the Issue of Murder

1. Bell CC. States of consciousness. *J Natl Med Assoc.* 1980;72:331–334.

2. Becker LE. Durham revisited: psychiatry and the problem of crime. *Psychiatr Annals.* 1973;3(8&9):6–57, 6–73.

3. Freedman A, Kaplan H, Sadock B. *Modern Synopsis of Comprehensive Textbook of Psychiatry.* 706–714.

4. Malmquist CP. Empirical problems in the selection of the insanity defense. *Psychiatr Annals.* 1974;4:48–66.

5. Farnsworth D. Dangerousness. *Psychiatr Annals.* 1977;7:55–70.

6. The mind of a murderer. *Med World News.* 1973;14:39–45.

7. Lunde DT. Our murder boom. *Psychology Today.* 1975;9:35–42.

8. Langberg R. Homicide in the United States, 1950–1964. *Vital and Health Statistics.* Series 20, no. 6. Washington, DC: Government Printing Office; 1967.

9. Davis V. *Crime.* New York: Time-Life Books; 1976:58.

10. Guze S, Woodruff, Clayton P. *Psychiatric disorders and criminality. J Am Med Assoc.* 1974;227:641–642.

11. Man P. Are 'dangerous' patients dangerous? *Legal Aspects Med Pract.* 1979;7:46–48.

12. Interview with Louis J. West, MD, on the violent patient/causes and management. *Practical Psychiatry.* 1974;2:1–4.

13. Tanay E. Psychiatric aspects of homicide prevention. *Am J Psychiatry.* 1972;123:7.

14. Cannon M, Locke B. Being black is detrimental to one's mental health: myth or reality? *Phylon.* 1977;38:408–428.

CHAPTER 11:
Coma and the Etiology of Violence, Part 1

1. Report of the Secretary's Task Force on Black and Minority Health, Vol. 1. Executive Summary. Washington, DC: Government Printing Office; 1985. US Dept of Health and Human Services, DHHS publication PHS 0-487-637.

2. When brother kills brother. *Time.* Sept. 16, 1985:32.

3. Minority health ADAMHA concern. *Alcohol, Drug Abuse, and Mental Health Administration News.* 1985;11:6.

4. Koop CE. *Surgeon General's Workshop on Violence and Public Health: Source Book.* Washington, DC: National Center on Child Abuse and Neglect; 1985.

5. Rynearson EK. Bereavement after homicide: a descriptive study. *Am J Psychiatry.* 1984;141:1452–1454.

6. Allen NH. Homicide prevention and intervention. *Suicide Life Threat Behav.* 1981;11:167–179.

7. Jason J, Flock M, Tyler CW. Epidemiologic characteristics of primary homicide in the United States. *Am J Epidemiol.* 1983;117:419–428.

8. Meredith N. The murder epidemic. *Science.* 1984;5:42–47.

9. Attorney General's Task Force on Family Violence. Washington, DC: US Department of Justice; 1984.

10. Tanay E. Psychiatric aspects of homicide prevention. *Am J Psychiatry*. 1972;123:7.

11. Taylor PJ, Gunn J. Violence and psychosis, 1: risk of violence among psychotic men. *Br Med J*. 1984;288:1945–1949.

12. Hillard JR, Zung W, Ramm D, et al. Accidental and homicidal death in a psychiatric emergency room population. *Hosp Com Psychiatry*. 1985;36:640–643.

13. Bell CC, Thompson B, Shorter-Gooden K, et al. Prevalence of coma in black subjects. *J Natl Med Assoc*. 1985;77:391–395.

14. Papez JW. A proposed mechanism of emotion. *Arch Neurol Psychiatry*. 1937;38:725–743.

15. Kluver H, Bucy PC. Preliminary analysis of functions of the temporal lobes in monkeys. *Arch Neurol Psychiatry*. 1939;42:979–1000.

16. Bard P, Mountcastle V. Some forebrain mechanisms involved in expression of rage with special reference to suppression of angry behavior. *Res Publ Assoc Res Nerv Ment Dis*. 1948;27:362–399.

17. Glusman M. The hypothalamic "savage" syndrome. *Res Publ Assoc Res Nerv Ment Dis*. 1974;52:52–92.

18. Brady JV, Nauta WJH. Subcortical mechanisms in emotional behavior: affective changes following septal forebrain lesions in the albino rat. *J Comp Physiol Psychol*. 1953;46:339–346.

19. King FA. Effects of septal and amygdaloid lesions on emotional behavior and conditioned avoidance responses in the rat. *J Nerv Ment Dis*. 1958;126:57–63.

20. Reis DJ. Central neurotransmitters in aggression. *Res Publ Assoc Res Nerv Ment Dis*. 1974;52:119–148.

21. Goldstein M. Brain research and violent behavior. *Arch Neurol*. 1974;30:1–35.

22. Symonds C. Concussion and its sequelae. *Lancet*. 1962;1:1–5.

23. Windle WF, Groat RA, Fox CA. Experimental structural alterations in the brain during and after concussion. *Surg Gynecol Obstet*. 1944;79:561–572.

24. Ommaya AK, Gennarelli TA. Cerebral concussion and traumatic unconsciousness: Correlation of experimental and clinical observations on blunt head injuries. *Brain*. 1974;97:633–654.

25. Van Woerkom TCA, Teelken AW, Minderhoud JM. Difference in neurotransmitter metabolism in frontotemporal lobe contusion and diffuse cerebral contusion. *Lancet*. 1977;1:812–813.

26. Veneer HL, Swine H. Sequelae in post-traumatic psychosis. *Psychiatr Q*. 1941;15:343–349.

27. Skolnick MH. Trauma as a factor in dementia praecox. *J Mich Med Soc*. 1937;36:563–565.

28. Gordon A. Delayed mental disorders following cranial traumatism and their psychopathological interpretation. *J Nerv Ment Dis*. 1933;77:259–273.

29. Jellinger K, Seitelberger F. Protracted posttraumatic encephalopathy: pathology, pathogenesis and clinical implications. *J Neurol Sci*. 1970;110:51–94.

30. Strich SJ. Diffuse degeneration of the cerebral white matter in severe dementia following head injury. *J Neurol Neurosurg Psychiatry*. 1956;19:163–185.

31. Gronwall D, Wrightson P. Cumulative effect of concussion. *Lancet*. 1975;2:995–997.

32. Merskey H, Woodforde JM. Psychiatric sequelae of minor head injury. *Brain*. 1972;95:521–528.

33. Rimel RW, Giordani B, Barth JT, et al. Disability caused by minor head injury. *Neurosurgery*. 1981;9:221–228.

34. Rutherford WH, Merrett JD, McDonald JR. Sequelae of concussion caused by minor head injuries. *Lancet*. 1977;1:1–4.

35. Jennett B. Early complications after mild head injuries. *NZ Med J*. 1976;84:144–147.

36. Kay DWK, Kerr TA, Lassman LP. Brain trauma and the post-concussional syndrome. *Lancet*. 1971;2:1052–1055.

37. Savan AS. Depression after minor closed head injury: role of dexamethasone suppression test and antidepressants. *J Clin Psychiatry*. 1985;46:335–338.

38. Rimel RW, Giordani B, Barth JT, et al. Moderate head injury: completing the clinical spectrum of brain trauma. *Neurosurgery*. 1982;11:344–351.

39. Levin HS, Grossman RG, Rose JE, et al. Long-term neuropsychological outcome of closed head injury. *J Neurosurg*. 1979;50:412–422.

40. Kwentus JA, Hart RP, Peck ET, et al. Psychiatric complications of closed head trauma. *Psychosomatics*. 1985;26:8–17.

41. Lishman WA. The psychiatric sequelae of head injury: a review. *Psycho Med*. 1973;3:304–318.

42. Davidson K, Bagley CR. Schizophrenia-like psychoses associated with organic disorders of the central nervous system: a review of the literature. *Br J Psychiatry*. 1969;4(suppl):113–184.

43. Symonds CP. Mental disorder following head injury. *P R Soc Med*. 1937;30:1081–1094.

44. Mapother E. Mental symptoms associated with head injury. *Br Med J*. 1937;2:1055–1061.

45. Schilder P. Psychic disturbances after head injuries. *Am J Psychiatry*. 1934;91:155–188.

46. Shapiro LB. Schizophrenic-like psychosis following head injuries. *Ill Med J*. 1939;76:250–254.

47. Bonner CA, Taylor LE. Traumatic psychoses. *Am J Psychiatry*. 1936;92:763–770.

48. Aita JA, Reitan RM: Psychotic reactions in the late recovery period following brain injury. *Am J Psychiatry*. 1948;105:161–169.

49. Hoch P, Davidoff E. Preliminary observations on the course of the traumatic psychoses. *J Nerv Ment Dis*. 1939;90:337–343.

50. Hillborn E. Schizophrenia-like psychoses after brain trauma. *Acta Psychiatr Neurol Scand*. 1951;60(suppl):36–47.

51. Bender L. Children and adolescents who have killed. *Am J Psychiatry*. 1959;116:510–513.

52. Jacobs D. Evaluation and management of the violent patient in emergency settings. *Psychiatr Clin North Am*. 1983;6:259–269.

53. Anderson WH. Psychiatric emergencies. In: Wilkins EW et al., eds. *Emergency Medicine*. Baltimore: Williams & Wilkins; 1983.

54. Levin HS, Grossman RG. Behavioral sequelae of closed head injury. *Arch Neurol*. 1978;35:720–727.

55. Strecker EA, Ebaugh FG. Neuropsychiatric sequelae of cerebral trauma in children. *Arch Neurol Psychiatry*. 1924;12:443–453.

56. Blau A. Mental changes following head trauma in children. *Arch Neurol Psychiatry*. 1936;35:723–769.

57. Lishman WA. Brain damage in relation to psychiatric disability after head injury. *Br J Psychiatry*. 1968;114:373–410.

58. Goethe KE, Levin HS. Behavioral manifestations during the early and long-term stages of recovery after closed head injury. *Psychiatr Ann*. 1984;14:540–546.

59. Thomsen IV. The patient with severe head injury and his family. *Scand J Rehabil Med*. 1974;6:180–183.

60. Lezak MD. Living with the characterologically altered brain injured patient. *J Clin Psychiatry*. 1978;39:592–598.

61. Brooks DN, McKinlay W. Personality and behavioral change after severe blunt head injury: a relative's view. *J Neurol Neurosurg Psychiatry*. 1983;46:333–344.

62. Jarvie HF. Frontal lobe wounds causing disinhibitions. *J Neurol Neurosurg Psychiatry*. 1954;17:14–32.

63. Casson IR, Sham R, Campbell EA, et al. Neurological and CT evaluation of knocked-out boxers. *J Neurol Neurosurg Psychiatry*. 1982;45:170–174.

64. Casson IR, Siegel O, Sham R, et al. Brain damage in modern boxers. *J Am Med Assoc*. 1984;251:2663–2667.

65. Casson IR, Siegel O, Ames W. Chronic brain damage in boxing. *Hosp Med*. 1985;1:19–30.

66. Kaste M, Vilkki J, Sainio K, et al. Is chronic brain damage in boxing a hazard of the past? *Lancet*. 1982;2:1186–1188.

67. Mawdsley CT, Ferguson FR. Neurologic disease in boxers. *Lancet*. 1963;2:795–801.

68. Spillane JD. Five boxers. *Br Med J.* 1962;5314:1205–1210.

69. Johnson J. Organic psychosyndromes due to boxing. *Br J Psychiatry.* 1969;115:45–53.

70. Corsellis JAN, Bruton CJ, Freeman-Browne D. The aftermath of boxing. *Psychol Med.* 1973;3: 270–303.

71. LaCava G. Boxer's encephalopathy. *J Sports Med Phys Fitness.* 1963;3:87–92.

72. Critcheley M. Medical aspects of boxing, particularly from a neurological standpoint. *Br Med J.* 1957;5014:357–362.

73. Pilleri G, Poeck K. Sham rage-like behavior in a case of traumatic decerebration. *Conf Neurol.* 1965;25:156–166.

74. Malamud N. Psychiatric disorder with intracranial tumors of limbic system. *Arch Neurol.* 1967;17:113–123.

75. Zeman W, King FA. Tumors of the septum pellucidum and adjacent structures with abnormal affective behavior: an anterior midline structure syndrome. *J Nerv Dis.* 1958;127:490–502.

76. Sweet WH, Ervin F, Mark VH. The relationship of violent behavior to focal cerebral disease. In: Garattini S, Sigg E, eds. *Aggressive Behavior.* New York: Wiley; 1969.

77. Mark VH, Sweet WH. The role of limbic brain dysfunction in aggression. *Res Publ Assoc Res Nerv Ment Dis.* 1974;52:186–200.

78. Gastaut H. So-called "psychomotor" and "temporal" epilepsy. *Epilepsia.* 1953;2:59–91.

79. Gibbs FA. Abnormal electrical activity in the temporal regions and its relationship to abnormalities of behavior. *Res Publ Assoc Res Nerv Ment Dis.* 1958;36:278–294.

80. Bingley T. Mental symptoms in temporal lobe epilepsy and temporal lobe gliomas. *Acta Psychiatr Neurol.* 1958;33(suppl 120):112–135.

81. Nuffield EJA. Neurophysiology and behavior disorders in epileptic children. *J Ment Sci.* 1961;107:438–458.

82. Ounsted C. Aggression and epilepsy in children with temporal lobe epilepsy. *J Psychosom Res.* 1969;13:237–242.

83. Davis E. Explosive or episodic behavior disorders in children as epileptic equivalents. *Med J Aust.* 1959;46:474–481.

84. Treffert DA. The psychiatric patient with an EEG temporal lobe focus. *Am J Psychiatry.* 1964;120:765–771.

85. Liddell DW. Observations on epileptic automatism in a mental hospital population. *J Ment Sci.* 1953;99:732–748.

86. Serafetinides EA. Aggressiveness in temporal lobe epileptics and its relation to cerebral dysfunction and environmental factors. *Epilepsia.* 1965;6:33–42.

87. Taylor DC. Aggression and epilepsy. *J Psychosom Res.* 1969;13:229–236.

88. Stevens JR. Psychiatric implications of psychomotor epilepsy. *Arch Gen Psychiatry*. 1966;14:461–471.

89. Rodin EA. Psychomotor epilepsy and aggressive behavior. *Arch Gen Psychiatry*. 1973;28:210–213.

90. Flor-Henry P. Ictal and interictal psychiatric manifestations in epilepsy: specific or nonspecific? *Epilepsia*. 1972;13:773–783.

91. Flor-Henry P. Psychosis and temporal-lobe epilepsy: A controlled investigation. *Epilepsia*. 1969;10:363–395.

92. Small JG, Small IF, Hayden MP. Further psychiatric investigations of patients with temporal and non-temporal lobe epilepsy. *Am J Psychiatry*. 1966;123:303–310.

93. Mark VH, Ervin FR. *Violence and the Brain*. New York: Harper & Row; 1970.

94. Bach-y-Rita G, Lion JR, Climent CE, et al. Episodic dyscontrol: a study of 130 violent patients. *Am J Psychiatry*. 1971;127:1473–1478.

95. Maletzky BM. The episodic dyscontrol syndrome. *Dis Nerv Sys*. 1973;36:178–185.

96. Elliott FA. The neurology of explosive rage. *Practitioner*. 1976;217:51–60.

97. Elliott FA. Neurological aspects of antisocial behavior. In: Reid WH, ed. *The Psychopath: A Comprehensive Study of Antisocial Disorders and Behaviors*. New York: Brunner/Mazel; 1978.

98. Elliott FA. Neurological findings in adult minimal brain dysfunction and the dyscontrol syndrome. *J Nerv Ment Dis*. 1982;170:680–687.

99. Elliott FA. Biological contributions to family violence. In: Hansen JC, ed. *Clinical Approaches to Family Violence*. Rockville, MD: Aspen Systems Corp.; 1982.

100. Jennett B, Teasdale G. *Management of Head Injuries*. Philadelphia: Davis; 1981.

101. Clark K. *Dark Ghetto*. New York: Harper & Row; 1965.

102. Ramos SM, Delany HM. Free falls from heights: A persistent urban problem. *J Natl Med Assoc*. 1986;78:111–115.

103. American Psychiatric Association. *Diagnostic and Statistical Manual of Mental Disorders*, 3rd ed. Washington, DC: American Psychiatric Association; 1979.

104. Bell CC. The need for accreditation of correctional health care facilities. *J Natl Med Assoc*. 1984;76:571–572.

105. Morrison JR, Minkoff K. Explosive personality as a sequel to the hyperactive-child syndrome. *Compreh Psychiatry*. 1975;16:343–348.

106. Hertzig ME, Birch HG. Neurologic organization in psychiatrically disturbed adolescents. *Arch Gen Psychiatry*. 1968;19:528–537.

107. Quitkin F, Rifkin A, Klein DF. Neurologic soft signs in schizophrenia and character disorders. *Arch Gen Psychiatry*. 1976;33:845–853.

108. Andrulonis PA, Glueck BC, Stroebel CF, et al. Organic brain dysfunction and the borderline syndrome. *Psychiatr Clin North Am.* 1980;4:47–66.

109. Andrulonis PA, Glueck BC, Stroebel CF, et al. Borderline personality sub-categories. *J Nerv Ment Dis.* 1982;170:670–679.

CHAPTER 12:
Coma and the Etiology of Violence, Part 2

*Have retained the original reference number from Chapter 11.

*6. Allen NH. Homicide prevention and intervention. *Suicide Life Threat Behav.* 1981;11:167–179.

*11. Taylor PJ, Gunn J. Violence and psychosis, 1: risk of violence among psychotic men. *Br Med J.* 1984;288:1945–1949.

*13. Bell CC, Thompson B, Shorter-Gooden K, et al. Prevalence of coma in black subjects. *J Natl Med Assoc.* 1985;77:391–395.

*20. Reis DJ. Central neurotransmitters in aggression. *Res Publ Assoc Res Nerv Ment Dis.* 1974;52:119–148.

*21. Goldstein M. Brain research and violent behavior. *Arch Neurol.* 1974;30:1–35.

*51. Bender L. Children and adolescents who have killed. *Am J Psychiatry.* 1959;116:510–513.

*95. Maletzky BM. The episodic dyscontrol syndrome. *Dis Nerv Sys.* 1973;36:178–185.

*97. Elliott FA Neurological aspects of antisocial behavior. In: Reid WH, ed. *The Psychopath: A Comprehensive Study of Antisocial Disorders and Behaviors.* New York: Brunner/Mazel; 1978.

*101. Clark K. *Dark Ghetto.* New York: Harper & Row; 1965.

*102. Ramos SM, Delany HM, Freefalls from heights: A persistent urban problem. *J Natl Med Assoc.* 1986;78:111–115.

110. Healy W. A review of some studies of delinquents and delinquency. *Arch Neurol Psychiatry.* 1925;14:25–30.

111. Kasanin J. Personality changes in children following cerebral trauma. *J Nerv Ment Dis.* 1929;69:385–406.

112. Lewis DO. Delinquency, psychomotor epileptic symptoms and paranoid ideation: a triad. *Am J Psychiatry.* 1976;133:1395–1398.

113. Lewis DO, Shanok SS, Cohen RJ, et al. Race bias in the diagnosis and disposition of violent adolescents. *Am J Psychiatry.* 1980;137:1211–1216.

114. Lewis DO, Pincus JH, Shanok SS, Glaser GH. Psychomotor epilepsy and violence in a group of incarcerated adolescent boys. *Am J Psychiatry.* 1982;139:882–887.

115. Lewis DO, Shanok SS, Grant M, et al. Homicidally aggressive young children: neuropsychiatric and experimental correlates. *Am J Psychiatry.* 1983;140:148–153.

116. Lewis DO, Moy E, Jackson LD, et al. Biosocial characteristics of children who later murder: a prospective study. *Am J Psychiatry.* 1985;142:1161–1167.

117. Malmquist CP. Premonitory signs of homicidal aggression in juveniles. *Am J Psychiatry.* 1971;128:461–465.

118. Inamdar SC, Lewis DO, Siomopoulos G, et al. Violent and suicidal behavior in psychotic adolescents. *Am J Psychiatry.* 1982;139:932–935.

119. Whitlock FA, Broadhurst AD. Attempted suicide and the experience of violence. *J Biosoc Sci.* 1969;1:353–368.

120. Hendin H. *Black Suicide.* New York: Harper & Row; 1971.

121. Swanson WC, Breed W. Black suicide in New Orleans. In: Schneidman ES, ed. *Suicidology: Contemporary Developments.* New York: Grune & Stratton; 1976:99–128.

122. Gunn J, Bonn J. Criminality and violence in epileptic prisoners. *Br J Psychiatry.* 1971;118:337–343.

123. Hill D. Cerebral dysrhythmia: its significance in aggressive behavior. *Proc R Soc Med.* 1944;37:317–330.

124. Hill D, Watterson D. EEG studies on psychopathic personalities. *J Neurol Psychiatry.* 1942;5:47–65.

125. Hill D. EEG in episodic psychotic and psychopathic behavior. *Electroencephalogr Clin Neurophysiol.* 1952;4:419–442.

126. Williams D. Neural factors related to habitual aggression. *Brain.* 1969;92:503–520.

127. Sayed ZA, Lewis SA, Britain RP. An electroencephalographic and psychiatric study of 32 insane murderers. *Electroencephalogr Clin Neurophysiol.* 1969;27:332–335.

128. Stafford-Clark D, Taylor FH. Clinical and EEG studies of prisoners charged with murder. *J Neurol Neurosurg Psychiatry.* 1949;12:325–330.

129. Gibbons TCN, Pond DA, Stafford-Clark D. A follow-up study of criminal psychopaths. *J Ment Sci.* 1959;105:108–115.

130. Frazier SH. Murder-single and multiple. *Res Publ Assoc Nerv Ment Dis.* 1974;52:304–312.

131. Langevin R, Bain J, Ben-Aron M, et al. Sexual aggression: constructing a predictive equation. In: Langevin R, ed. *Erotic Preference, Gender Identity, and Aggression in Men*, in press.

132. Climent CE, Ervin FR. Historical data in the evaluation of violent subjects. *Arch Gen Psychiatry.* 1972;27:621–624.

133. Lion JR, Bach-y-Rita G, Ervin FR. The self-referred violent patient. *J Am Med Assoc.* 1968;205:503–505.

134. Lion JR, Bach-y-Rita G, Ervin FR. Violent patients in the emergency room. *Am J Psychiatry*. 1969;125:1706–1710.

135. Lion JR. Conceptual issues in the use of drugs for the treatment of aggression in man. *J Nerv Ment Dis*. 1975;160:76–82.

136. Bell CC, Palmer JM. Violence among inpatients, letter to the editor. *Am J Psychiatry*. 1983;140:516–517.

137. Bell CC, Palmer JM. Survey of the demographic characteristics of patients requiring restraints in a psychiatric emergency service. *J Natl Med Assoc*. 1983;75:981–987.

138. Bell CC, Palmer JM. Security procedures in a psychiatric emergency service. *J Natl Med Assoc*. 1981;73:835–842.

139. Bell CC. Interface between psychiatry and the law on the issue of murder. *J Natl Med Assoc*. 1980;72:1093–1097.

140. ltil TM, Wadud A. Treatment of human aggression with major tranquilizers, anti-depressants, and newer psychotrophic drugs. *J Nerv Men Dis*. 1975;160:83–99.

141. Darling HF. Haloperidol in 60 criminal psychotics. *Dis Nerv Syst*. 1971;32:31–34.

142. Faretra G, Dooher L, Dowling J. Comparison of haloperidol and fluphenazine in disturbed children. *Am J Psychiatry*. 1970;126:146–149.

143. Sheard MH. Lithium in the treatment of aggression. *Nerv Ment Dis*. 1975;160:108–118.

144. Sheard MH. Effect of lithium on aggression. *Nature*. 1971;230:113–114.

145. Tupin JP, Smith DB, Clanon TL, et al. The long-term use of lithium in aggressive prisoners. *Compr Psychiatry*. 1973;14:311–317.

146. Morrison SD, Erwin CW, Gianturco DT, et al. Effect of lithium on combative behavior in humans. *Dis Nerv Syst*. 1973;34:186–189.

147. Rifkin A, Quitkin F, Carrillo C, et al. Lithium carbonate in emotionally unstable character disorder. *Arch Gen Psychiatry*. 1972;27:519–523.

148. Tunks ER, Dermer SW. Carbamazepine in the dyscontrol syndrome associated with limbic system dysfunction. *J Nerv Ment Dis*. 1977;164:56–63.

149. Stewart JT. Carbamazepine treatment of a patient with Kluver-Bucy syndrome. *J Clin Psychiatry*. 1985;46:496–497.

150. Monroe RR. Anticonvulsants in the treatment of aggression. *J Nerv Ment Dis*. 1975;160:119–126.

151. Monroe RR, Dale R. Chlordiazepoxide in the treatment of patients with "activated EEGs." *Dis Nerv Syst*. 1967;28:390–396.

152. Monroe RR, Wise SP. Combined phenothiazine, chlordiazepoxide, and primidone therapy for uncontrolled psychotic patients. *Am J Psychiatry*. 1965;122:694–698.

153. Elliott FA. Propranolol for the control of belligerent behavior following acute brain damage. *Ann Neurol*. 1977;1:489–491.

154. Yudofsky S, Williams D, Gorman J. Propranolol in the treatment of rage and violent behavior in patients with chronic brain syndromes. *Am J Psychiatry*. 1981;138:218–220.

155. Williams DT, Mehl R, Yudofsky S, et al. The effect of propranolol on uncontrolled rage outbursts in children and adolescents with organic brain dysfunction. *J Am Acad Child Psychiatry*. 1982;21:129–135.

156. Yudofsky SC, Stevens L, Silver J, et al. Propranolol in the treatment of rage and violent behavior associated with Korsakoff's psychosis. *Am J Psychiatry*. 1984;141:114–115.

157. Allen RP, Safer D, Covi L. Effects of psychostimulants on aggression. *J Nerv Ment Dis*. 1975;160:138–145.

158. Azcarate CL. Minor tranquilizers in the treatment of aggression. *J Nerv Ment Dis*. 1975;160:100–108.

159. Lion JR. The role of depression in the treatment of aggressive personality disorders. *Am J Psychiatry*. 1972;129:347–349.

160. Lion JR, Bach-y-Rita G. Group psychotherapy with violent outpatients. *Int J Group Psychother*. 1970;20:185–191.

CHAPTER 13:
Head Injury with Subsequent Intermittent, Non-schizophrenic, Psychotic Symptoms and Violence

1. American Psychiatric Association. *Diagnostic and Statistical Manual of Mental Disorders*, 3rd ed. Washington, DC: American Psychiatric Association, 1979.

2. Shukla S, Cook BL, Mukherjee S, et al. Mania following head trauma. *Am J Psychiatry*. 1987;144:93–96.

3. Riess H, Schwartz CE, Kierman GL. Manic syndrome following head injury: Another form of secondary mania. *J Clin Psychiatry*. 1987;48:29–30.

4. Krauthammer C, Kierman GL. Secondary mania. *Arch Gen Psychiatry*. 1978;35:1333–1339.

5. Bell CC, Thompson B, Shorter-Gooden K, et al. Prevalence of coma in black subjects. *J Natl Med Assoc*. 1985;77:391–395.

6. Bell CC, Mehta H. Misdiagnosis of black patients with manic depressive illness. *J Natl Med Assoc*. 1980;72:141–145.

7. Bell CC, Mehta H. The misdiagnosis of black patients with manic depressive illness: second in a series. *J Natl Med Assoc*. 1981;73:101–107.

8. Jones BE, Gray BA, Parson EB. Manic-Depressive illness among poor urban blacks. *Am J Psychiatry*. 1981;138:654–657.

9. Mukherjee S, Shukla S, Woodle J, et al. Misdiagnosis of schizophrenia in bipolar patients: a multiethnic comparison. *Am J Psychiatry*. 1983;140:1571–1574.

10. Adebimpe VR, Gigandet J, Harris E. MMPI diagnosis of black psychiatric patients. *Am J Psychiatry*. 1979;136:85–87.

11. Williams CL. Issues surrounding psychological testing of minority patients. *Hosp Com Psychiatry*. 1987;38:184–189.

12. Bell CC. Coma and the etiology of violence, part 1. *J Natl Med Assoc*. 1986;78:1167–1176.

13. Bell CC. Coma and the etiology of violence, part 2. *J Natl Med Assoc*. 1987;79:79–85.

14. Lewis DO, Pincus JH, Feldman M, et al. Psychiatric, neurological, and psychoeducational characteristics of 15 death row inmates in the United States. *Am J Psychiatry*. 1986;143:838–845.

15. Whitman S, Coonley-Hoganson R, Desai BT. Comparative head trauma experience in two socioeconomically different Chicago-area communities: a population study. *Am J Epidemiology*. 1984;119:570–580.

16. Rivara FP, Mueller BA. The epidemiology and prevention of pediatric head injury. *J Head Trauma Rehabil*. 1986;1:7–15.

17. Ramos SM, Delany HM. Free falls from heights: a persistent urban problem. *J Natl Med Assoc*. 1986;78:111–115.

18. Hawkins DF, ed. *Homicide Among Black Americans*. Lanham, MD: University Press of America; 1986.

19. Bell CC, Prothrow-Stith D, Smallwood-Murchinson C. Black-on-black homicide: the National Medical Association's responsibilities. *J Natl Med Assoc*. 1986;78:1139–1141.

20. Poussaint A. *Why Blacks Kill Blacks*. Virplanck, NY: Emmerson-Hall, 1972.

21. Bell CC. Preventing violence, editorial. *New Physician*. 1986;35:7–8.

22. Thomas CW. Pride and purpose as antidotes to black homicidal violence. *J Natl Med Assoc*. 1987;79:155–160.

23. Schorer CE. Behavioral efficacy of propranolol in black patients. *J Natl Med Assoc*. 1987;79:221–222.

CHAPTER 14:
The Need for Victimization Screening in a Black Psychiatric Population

1. Centers for Disease Control. *Homicide Surveillance: High-Risk Racial and Ethnic Groups—Blacks and Hispanics, 1970–1983*. Atlanta: Centers for Disease Control; 1986.

2. Koop CE. *Surgeon General's Workshop on Violence and Public Health: Source Book*. Washington, DC: National Center on Child Abuse and Neglect, 1985.

3. Hillard JR, Zung W, Ramm D, et al. Accidental and homicidal death in a psychiatric emergency room population. *Hosp Corn Psychiatry*. 1985;36:640–643.

4. Rounsaville B, Weissman MM. Battered women: a medical problem requiring detection. *Intl J Psychiatry Med*. 1978;8:191–202.

5. Stark E, Flitcraft A. Medical therapy as repression: the case of the battered woman. *Health Med*. 1982;Summer/Fall:29–32.

6. Hilberman E, Munson K. Sixty battered women. *Victimology*. 1978;2:460–470.

7. Post RD, Willet AB, Franks RD, et al. A preliminary report on the prevalence of domestic violence among psychiatric inpatients. *Am J Psychiatry*. 1980;137:974–975.

8. Carmen E, Rieker PP, Mills T. Victims of violence and psychiatric illness. *Am J Psychiatry*. 1984;141:378–383.

9. Jacobson A, Koehler JE, Jones-Brown C. The failure of routine assessment to detect histories of assault experienced by psychiatric patients. *Hosp Community Psychiatry*. 1987;38:386–389.

10. Barnhill LR, Squires MF, Gibson G. The epidemiology of violence in a CMHC setting: a violence epidemic? In: Hansen JC, Barnhill LR, eds. *Clinical Approaches to Family Violence*. Rockville, MD: Aspen Systems Corp.; 1982:21–33.

11. Bureau of Justice Statistics. *Criminal Victimization in the United States, 1983*. Washington, DC: US Department of Justice; 1985.

12. Kilpatrick DG, Best CL, Veronen LR, et al. Mental health correlates of criminal victimization: a random community survey. *J Consulting Clinical Psychology*. 1985;53:866–873.

CHAPTER 15:
The Need for Victimization Screening in a Poor, Outpatient Medical Population

1. Federal Bureau of Investigation. *Crime in the United States, 1986*. Washington, DC: US Department of Justice; 1987.

2. Oliver W. Black males and the tough guy image: a dysfunctional compensatory adaptation. *West J Black Studies*. 1984;8:199–203.

3. Centers for Disease Control. *Homicide Surveillance: High Risk Racial and Ethnic Groups—Blacks and Hispanics, 1970 to 1983*. Atlanta: Centers for Disease Control; 1986.

4. Illinois Coalition Against Domestic Violence: Handbook for Domestic Violence Victims. Chicago: Illinois Criminal Justice Information Authority; 1986.

5. Straus MA, Steinmetz SK, Gelles RJ. *Behind Closed Doors: Violence in the American Family*. Garden City, NY: Anchor Books; 1980.

6. Straus MA. Domestic violence and homicide antecedents. *Bull NY Acad Med*. 1986;62:446–465.

7. Stark E, Flitcraft A. Medical therapy as repression: the case of the battered woman. *Health Med.* 1982;Summer/Fall:29–32.

8. Klaus PA, Rand MR. *Bureau of Justice Statistics Special Report: Family Violence.* Washington, DC: US Department of Justice; 1984.

9. Barnhill LR. Clinical assessment of intrafamilial violence. *Hosp Community Psychiatry.* 1980;31:543–547.

10. Okun L. *Woman Abuse: Facts Replacing Myths.* Albany, NY: State University of New York Press Albany; 1986.

11. Steinmetz SK. The violent family. In: Lystad M, ed. *Violence in the Home: Interdisciplinary Perspectives.* New York: Bruner/Mazel; 1986:51–70.

12. Dietz PE. Patterns in human violence. In: Hales RE, Frances AJ, eds. *Psychiatric Update: The American Psychiatric Association Annual Review.* Vol. 6. Washington, DC: American Psychiatric Press; 1987:465–490.

13. Costantino JP, Kuller LH, Perper JA, et al. An epidemiologic study of homicides in Allegheny County, Pennsylvania. *Am J Epidemiol.* 1977;106:314–324.

14. Rose HM. *Black Homicide and the Urban Environment.* Washington, DC: Government Printing Office; 1981. US Dept of Health and Human Services, NIMH.

15. Dennis RE, Kirk A, Knuckles BN, et al. *Black Males at Risk to Low Life Expectancy: a Study of Homicide Victims and Perpetrators.* Washington, DC: Center for Studies of Minority Group Mental Health; 1981. NIMH grant 1 R01 MH36720..

16. Bell CC, Taylor-Crawford K, Jenkins EJ, Chalmers D. Need for victimization screening in a black psychiatric population. *J Natl Med Assoc.* 1988;80:41–48.

17. Bryer JB, Nelson BA, Miller JB, et al. Childhood sexual and physical abuse as factors in adult psychiatric illness. *Am J Psychiatry.* 1987;144:1426–1430.

18. Camen E, Rieker PP, Mills T. Victims of violence and psychiatric illness. *Am J Psychiatry.* 1984;141:378–383.

19. Risin LI, Koss MD. The sexual abuse of boys. *J Interpersonal Violence.* 1987;12:309–323.

20. Finkelhor D. *Sexually Victimized Children.* New York: Free Press; 1979.

21. Block CR. *Lethal Violence in Chicago Over Seventeen Years: Homicides Known to the Police, 1965–1981.* Chicago: Illinois Criminal Justice Information Authority; 1985.

22. Koop CE. *Surgeon General's Workshop on Violence and Public Health: Source Book.* Washington, DC: National Center on Child Abuse and Neglect; 1985.

23. Jacobson A, Koehler JE, Jones-Brown C. The failure of routine assessment to detect histories of assault experienced by psychiatric patients. *Hosp Community Psychiatry.* 1987;38:386–389.

24. Bell CC. Preventive strategies for dealing with violence among blacks. *Community Mental Health J.* 1987;23:217–228.

25. Kilpatrick DG, Best CL, Veronen LJ, et al. Mental health correlates of criminal victimization: a random community survey. *J Consult Clin Psychol.* 1985;53:866–873.

26. Bryer JB, Nelson BA, Miller JB, et al. Childhood sexual and physical abuse as factors in adult psychiatric illness. *Am J Psychiatry.* 1987;144:1426–1430.

27. Burgess AW, Hartman CR, McCormack A. Abused to abuser: antecedents of socially deviant behaviors. *Am J Psychiatry.* 1987;144:1431–1436.

28. Green AH. Self-destructive behavior in battered children. *Am J Psychiatry.* 1978;135:579–582.

29. Rounsaville B, Weissman MM. Battered women: a medical problem requiring detection. *Intl J Psychiatry in Medicine.* 1978;8:191–202.

CHAPTER 16:
Circumstances of Sexual and Physical Victimization of Black Psychiatric Outpatients

1. Carmen E, Rieker PP, Mills T. Victims of violence and psychiatric illness. *Am J Psychiatry.* 1984;141:378–383.

2. Jacobson A, Richardson B. Assault experiences of 100 psychiatric inpatients: evidence of the need for routine inquiry. Presented at the American Psychiatric Association Annual Meeting, Dallas, TX, May 18–24, 1985.

3. Hillard JR, Zung W, Ramm D, et al. Accidental and homicidal death in a psychiatric emergency room population. *Hosp Community Psychiatry.* 1985;36:640–643.

4. Bell CC, Taylor-Crawford K, Jenkins EJ, et al. Need for victimization screening in a black psychiatric population. *J Natl Med Assoc.* 1988;80:41–48.

5. Finkelhor D. *A Sourcebook on Child Sexual Abuse.* Beverly Hills, CA: Sage Publishing Co., Inc.; 1986.

6. Green AH. Self-destructive behavior in battered children. *Am J Psychiatry.* 1978;135:579–582.

7. Kilpatrick DG, Best CL, Veronen LJ, et al. Mental health correlates of criminal victimization: a random community survey. *J Consult Clin Psychol.* 1985;53:866–873.

8. Williams DH. The epidemiology of mental illness in Afro-Americans. *Hosp Community Psychiatry.* 1986;37:42–49.

9. Jones BE, Gray BA. Problems in diagnosing schizophrenia and affective disorders among blacks. *Hosp Community Psychiatry.* 1986;37:61–65.

CHAPER 17:
Traumatic Stress and Children

1. Shakoor B, Chalmers D. Co-victimization of African-American children who witness violence and the theoretical implications of its effect on their cognitive, emotional, and behavioral development. *J Natl Med Assoc.* 1991;83:233–238.

2. Pynoos R, Eth S. Developmental perspectives on psychic trauma on childhood. In: Figley R, ed. *Trauma and its Wake.* New York: Brunner/Mazel; 1985.

3. Bachelor I, Wicks N. *Study of Children and Youth as Witness to Homicide, City of Detroit.* Detroit: Family Bereavement Center, Frank Murphy Hall of Justice-Victim Services; 1985.

4. Dubrow NF, Garbarino J. Living in the war zone: mothers and young children in a public housing development. *J Child Welfare.* 1989;68:3–20.

5. Jenkins EJ, Thompson B. Children talk about violence: preliminary findings from a survey of black elementary children. Presented at the Association of Black Psychologists Annual Convention, Oakland, CA, 1986.

6. Widom CS. Does violence beget violence?: a critical examination of the literature. *Psychol Bull.* 1989;106:3–28.

7. Uehara E, Chalmers D, Jenkins E, et al. Youth encounters with violence: results from the Chicago Community Health Council Violence Screening Project. Unpublished; 1990.

8. Griffith EH, Bell CC. Recent trends in suicide and homicide among blacks. *J Am Med Assoc.* 1989;262:2265–2269.

9. Bell CC, Jenkins EJ. Preventing black homicide. In: Dewart J, ed. *The State of Black America, 1990.* New York: National Urban League; 1990.

10. Report of the Secretary's Task Force on Black and Minority Health, Vol. 1, Executive Summary. Washington, DC: US Department of Health and Human Services; 1985. US Dept of Health and Human Services publication PHS 0-487-637.

11. Fingerhut LA, Kleinman JC. International and interstate comparisons of homicide among young males. *J Am Med Assoc.* 1990; 263:3292–3295.

12. US headed for a homicide record, Senators say. *New York Times.* Aug. 1. 1990:B3.

13. Block CR. *Lethal Violence in Chicago over Seventeen Years: Homicides Known to the Police, 1965–1981.* Chicago: Illinois Criminal Justice Information Authority; 1985.

14. Recktenwald W, Blau R. Youth homicides up 22 percent in city. *Chicago Tribune.* Jan 28, 1990:1.

15. Kotlowitz A. Urban trauma: day-to-day violence takes a terrible toll on inner-city youth. *Wall Street J.* 1987;1:26.

16.   Pynoos R, Nader K. Psychological first aid and treatment approaches to children exposed to community violence: Research implications. *J Traumatic Stress*. 1988;1:445–473.

17.   Terr L. Consultation advised soon after child's psychic injury. *Clin Psychiatr Times*. May 1989;17(5).

18.   Hyman IA, Zelikoff W, Clarke J. Psychological and physical abuse in the schools: a paradigm for understanding post-traumatic stress disorder in children and youth. *J Traumatic Stress*. 1988;1:243–67.

19.   Gardner G. Aggression and violence: the enemies of precision learning in children. *Am J Psychiatry*. 1971;128:445–50.

20.   Dyson J. The effects of family violence on children's academic performance and behavior. *J Natl Med Assoc*. 1990;82:17–22.

21.   Pynoos RS, Nader K. Children's exposure to violence and traumatic death. *Psychiatr Ann*. 1986;334–44.

22.   Rynearson EK. Psychological effects of unnatural dying on bereavement. *Psychiatr Ann*. 1986;62:272–5.

23.   Timnick L. Children of violence. *Los Angeles Times Magazine*. Sept 3, 1989:6–15.

24.   Terr L. Children of Chowchilla: Study of psychic trauma. *Psychoan Stud Child*. 1972;34:547–623.

25.   Bandura A. *Aggression: A Social Learning Approach*. Englewood Cliffs, NJ: Prentice-Hall; 1973.

26.   National Committee for Injury Prevention and Control and Education Development Center, Inc. *Injury Prevention: Meeting the Challenge*. New York: Oxford University Press; 1989.

27.   Wilson-Brewer RI Cohen S, O'Donnell L, et al. Violence prevention for early teens: the state of the art and guidelines for future program evaluation. Working paper. Boston: Educational Development Center; 1990.

28.   Sulton AT. Shaping the Future Agenda of Urban Crime Control Policy and Research. National Symposium on Community Institutions and Inner-city Crime. Washington, DC: Police Foundation; 1987.

29.   Personal correspondence. Judith Batchelor, Family Bereavement Center, Frank Murphy Hall of Justice-Victim Services, June 19, 1990.

30.   Enstad R, lbata D. School rampage: one dies, six shot. *Chicago Tribune*. May 21,1988:1.

31.   Buursma B. School gropes for reason for slaughter. *Chicago Tribune*. Jan. 19, 1988:3.

32.   Edstrom K. Victims of violence: separate but unequal treatment. *Chicago Reporter*. Sept. 1988:2.

33.   Bell CC, Hildreth CJ, Jenkins EJ, et al. The need for victimization screening in a poor, outpatient medical population. *J Natl Med Assoc*. 1988;80:853–60.

34.   Ibid:841–8.

35. Jacobson A, Koehler JE, Jones-Brown C. The failure of routine assessment to detect histories of assault experienced by psychiatric patients. *Hosp Community Psychiatry*. 1986;56:143–6.

36. Davidson J, Smith R. Traumatic experiences in psychiatric outpatients. *J Traumatic Stress*. 1990;3:459–75.

37. Willie CV. *Black and White Families*. New York: General Hall; 1985.

38. Gary LE, Berry GL. Predicting attitudes toward substance abuse use in a black community: implications for prevention. *Community Mental Health J*. 1985;21:42–51.

39. Lee J. Rural black adolescents. In: Jones RL, ed. *Black Adolescents*. Berkeley, CA: Cobb & Henry; 1989.

CHAPTER 18:
States of Consciousness

1. Butts JD. Altered states of consciousness. *J Natl Med Assoc*. 1978;70:743–744.

2. Krippner S. Altered states of consciousness. In: White J, ed. *The Highest State of Consciousness*. Garden City, NY: Doubleday; 1972:1.

3. Dement W, Guilleminault C. Sleep disorders: the state of the art. *Hosp Pract*. 1973;8:57–71.

4. Schlauch R. Hypnopompic hallucinations and treatment with imipramine. *Am J Psychiatry*. 1979;136:219–220.

5. Bell C. The need for psychoanalysis is alive and well in community psychiatry. *J Natl Med Assoc*. 1979;71:361–368.

6. Tseng W. Psychiatric study of shamanism in Taiwan. *Arch Gen Psychiatry*. 1972;26:561–565.

7. Martin R. Modern psychiatry and the macumba ritual. *Psychiatry Ann*. 1978;8:81–89.

8. Woolfolk R. Psychophysiological correlates of meditation. *Arch Gen Psychiatry*. 1975;32:1326–1333.

9. Corby J, Roth W. Psychophysiological correlates of the practice of tantric yoga meditation. *Arch Gen Psychiatry*. 1978;35:571–577.

10. Shapiro DH, Giber D. Meditation and psychotherapeutic effects. *Arch Gen Psychiatry*. 1978;35:294–302.

11. Kennedy R. Self-induced depersonalization syndrome. *Am J Psychiatry*. 1976;133:1326–1328.

12. Shimano ET, Douglas D: On research in Zen. *Am J Psychiatry*. 1975;132:1300–1302.

13. Bucke RM. From self to cosmic consciousness. In: White J, ed. *The Highest State of Consciousness*. Garden City, NY: Doubleday; 1972:79–93.

14. Maslow A. The "core-religious" or "transcendent" experience. In: White J, ed. *The Highest State of Consciousness*. Garden City, NY: Doubleday; 1972:352–364.

CHAPTER 19:
Black Intrapsychic Survival Skills: Altering One's States of Consciousness

1. Bell CC. States of consciousness. *J Natl Med Assoc*. 1980;72:331–334.

2. Freud S. Interpretation of Dreams (1901). In: Strachey J, trans. & ed. *Complete Psychological Works*. Vols. 4 and 5. London: Hogarth Press; 1957.

3. Bell CC. The need for psychoanalysis is alive and well in community psychiatry. *J Natl Med Assoc*. 1979;71:361–368.

4. Kohut H. Introspection, empathy, and psychoanalysis. In: Ornstein P, ed. *The Search for the Self*. Vol. 1. New York: International Universities Press, 1978:205–232.

5. Kohut H, Levarie S. On enjoyment of listening to music. In: Ornstein P, ed. *The Search for the Self*. Vol. 1. New York: International Universities Press, 1978:135–158.

6. Kohut H. Thoughts on narcissism and narcissistic rage. In: Ornstein P, ed. *The Search for the Self*. Vol. 1. New York: International Universities Press, 1978:615–658.

7. Fenichel O. *The Psychoanalytic Theory of Neurosis*. New York: WW Norton, 1954:117–128.

8. Bell CC. Racism: a symptom of the narcissistic personality disorder. *J Natl Med Assoc*. 1980;72:661–665.

9. Bell CC. A social and nutritional survey on the population of the children and youth center of Meharry Medical College of North Nashville, Tennessee. *J Natl Med Assoc*. 1971;63:397–398.

10. Jackson JS, Neighbors HW. Assessing black mental health: a national survey. Presented at the American Psychiatric Association Annual Meeting, Toronto, Canada, May 1982.

11. Caplan G. Mastery of stress: psychosocial aspects. *Am J Psychiat*. 1981;138:413–420.

12. Koestler A. *The Act of Creation*. New York: Macmillan; 1964.

13. Butts JD. Altered states of consciousness. *J Natl Med Assoc*. 1978;70:743–744.

14. Shapiro DH, Giber D. Meditation and psychotherapeutic affects. *Arch Gen Psychiatry*. 1978;35:294–302.

15. Woolfolk RL. Psychophysiological correlates of mediation. *Arch Gen Psychiatry*. 1975;32:1326–1333.

16. Eyerman J. Transcendental meditation and mental retardation. *J Clin Psychiatry*. 1981;42:35–36.

17. Sow I. *Anthropological Structures of Madness in Black Africa*. New York: International Universities Press; 1980.

18. Snow LF. Folk medical beliefs and their implications for care of patients: a review based on studies among black Americans. *Ann Intern Med*. 1974;81:82–96.

19. Jordan WC. Voodoo medicine. In: Williams R, ed. *Textbook of Black-Related Disease*. New York: McGraw-Hill; 1975:715–738.

20. Wintrob RM. The influence of others: witchcraft and rootwork as explanations of behavior disturbances. *J Nerv Ment Dis*. 1973;156:318–326.

21. Martin RD. Modern psychiatry and the macumba ritual. *Psychiatr Ann*. 1978;8:81–89.

22. Golden KM. Voodoo in Africa and the United States. *Am J Psychiatry*. 1977;134:1425–1427.

23. Griffith EH, English T, Mayfield V. Possession, prayer, and testimony: therapeutic aspects of the Wednesday night meeting in a black church. *Psychiatry*. 1980;43:120–128.

24. Clissold S. *The Wisdom of the Spanish Mystics*. New York: New Directions; 1977.

CHAPTER 20:
Altered States of Consciousness Profile: An Afrocentric Intrapsychic Evaluation Tool

1. Bell CC. States of consciousness. *J Natl Med Assoc*. 1980;72:331–334.

2. Willie CV. *A New Look at Black Families*. Bayside, New York: General Hall; 1981.

3. Wintrob RM. The influence of others: witchcraft and rootwork as explanations of behavior disturbances. *J Nerv Ment Dis*. 1973;156:318–326.

4. Golden KM. Voodoo in Africa and the United States. *Am J Psychiatry*. 1977;134:1425–1427.

5. Snow LF. Traditional health beliefs and practices among lower class black Americans. *West J Med*. 1983;139:820–828.

6. Snow LF. Folk medicine beliefs and their implications for care of patients. *Ann Intern Med*. 1974;81:82–96.

7. Snow LF. Sorcerers, saints and charlatans: black folk healers in urban America. *Cult Med Psychiatry*. 1978;2:69–106.

8. Griffith EEH. The impact of culture and religion on psychiatric care. *J Natl Med Assoc*. 1982;74:1175–1179.

9. DeKnight F. *The Ebony Cook Book*. Chicago: Johnson; 1962.

10. Jones L. *Blues People*. New York: William Morrow; 1963.

11. Raskins J, Butts HF. *The Psychology of Black Language*. New York: Barnes & Noble; 1973.

12. Mbiti JS. *African Religions and Philosophy*. New York: Doubleday; 1969.

13. Sow I. *Anthropological Structures of Madness in Black Africa*. New York: International Universities Press; 1980.

14. Bell CC, Bland IJ, Houston E, Jones BE. Enhancement of knowledge and skills for the psychiatric treatment of black populations. In: Chunn JC, Dunston PJ, Ross-Sheriff F, eds. *Mental Health and People of Color*. Washington, DC: Howard University Press; 1983:205–237.

15. Bell CC. The need for psychoanalysis is alive and state may be that of being strongly attracted to the well in community psychiatry. *J Natl Med Assoc*. 1979;71:361–368.

16. Olarte SW, Lenz R. Learning to do psychoanalytic therapy with inner city population. *J Am Acad Psychoanal*. 1984;12:89–99.

17. Gale MS, Beck S, Springer K. Effects of therapists' biases on diagnosis and disposition of emergency service patients. *Hosp Community Psychiatry*. 1978;29:705–708.

18. Bell CC, Mehta H. The misdiagnosis of black patients with manic depressive illness. *J Natl Med Assoc*. 1980;72:141–145.

19. Bell, CC, Mehta H. Misdiagnosis of black patients with manic depressive illness: second in a series. *J Natl Med Assoc*. 1981;73:101–107.

20. Simon RJ, Fleiss JL, Gurland BJ, et al. Depression and schizophrenia in hospitalized black and white mental patients. *Arch Gen Psychiatry*. 1973;28:509–512.

21. Helzer JE. Bipolar affective disorder in black and white men. *Arch Gen Psychiatry*. 1975;32:1140–1143.

22. Mukherjee S, Shukla S, Woodle J, et al. Misdiagnosis of schizophrenia in bipolar patients: a multiethnic comparison. *Am J Psychiatry*. 1983;140:1571–1574.

23. Adebimpe VR, Hedlund JL, Cho DW, Wood JB. Symptomatology of depression in black and white patients. *J Natl Med Assoc*. 1982;74:185–189.

24. Adebimpe VR. Overview: white norms and psychiatric diagnosis of black patients. *Am J Psychiatry*. 1981;138:279–285.

25. Collins JL, Rickman LE, Mathura CB. Frequency of schizophrenia and depression in a black inpatient population. *J Natl Med Assoc*. 1980;72:851–856.

26. Weiner A, Liss JL, Robbins E. Psychiatric symptoms in white and black inpatients, II: follow-up study. *Compr Psychiatry*. 1978;14:483–488.

27. Cannon M, Locke B. Being black is detrimental to one's mental health: myth or reality? *Phylon*. 1977;38:408–428.

28. Thomas A, Sillen S. *Racism and Psychiatry*. New York: Brunner-Mazel; 1972.

29. Lewis DO, Shanok SS, Cohen RJ, et al. Race bias in the diagnosis and disposition of violent adolescents. *Am J Psychiatry*. 1980;137:1216–1221.

30. Gross H, Herbert MR, Kantterud GL, et al. The effects of race and sex on the variation of diagnosis and disposition in a psychiatric emergency room. *J Nerv Merit Dis*. 1969;148:638–642.

31. Jones BE, Gray BA, Parson EB. Manic-depressive illness among poor urban blacks. *Am J Psychiatry*. 1981;138:645–657.

32. Kramer M, Rosen B, Willis EM. Definitions and distributions of mental disorders in a racist society. In: Willie CV, Kramer BM, Brown BS, eds. *Racism and Mental Health*. Pittsburgh: University of Pittsburgh Press; 1973:353–459.

33. DeHoyos A, DeHoyos G. Symptomatology differentials between Negro and white schizophrenics. *Int J Soc Psychiatry*. 1965;11:245–255.

34. Vitols MM, Waters HG, Keeler MH. Hallucinations and delusions in white and Negro schizophrenics. *Am J Psychiatry*. 1963;120:472–476.

35. Bell CC, Shakoor B, Thompson B, et al. Prevalence of isolated sleep paralysis in black subjects. *J Natl Med Assoc*. 1984;76:501–508.

36. List JL, Weiner A, Robins E, et al. Psychiatric symptoms in white and black inpatients, 1: record study. *Compr Psychiatry*. 1973;14:475–481.

37. Adebimpe VR, Klein HE, Fried J. Hallucinations and delusions in black psychiatric patients. *J Natl Med Assoc*. 1981;73:517–520.

38. Adebimpe VR, Chung-Chou C, Klein HE, Lange MH. Racial and geographic differences in the psychopathology of schizophrenia. *Am J Psychiatry*. 1982;139:888–891.

39. Jones BE, Robinson W, Parson EB, Gray MA. The clinical picture of mania in manic-depressive black patients. *J Natl Med Assoc*. 1982;74:553–557.

40. Spurlock J. Black Americans. In: Gaw A, ed. *Cross-Cultural Psychiatry*. Boston: Publishing Sciences Group; 1982:163–178.

41. Yamamoto J, Steinberg A. Ethnic, racial, and social class factors in mental health. *J Natl Med Assoc*. 1981;73:231–240.

42. Bell CC, Thompson JP, Lewis D, et al. Misdiagnosis of alcohol-related organic brain syndromes in blacks: implications for treatment. In: Brisbane F, Womble M, eds. *Treatment of Black Alcoholics*. New York: Haworth Press; 1985:45–65.

43. Barnes E. Cultural retardation or shortcomings of the assessment techniques. In: Jones R, ed. *Black Psychology*. New York: Harper & Row; 1974:66–74.

44. Williams R. Abuses and misuses in testing black children. In Jones R, ed. *Black Psychology*. New York: Harper & Row; 1974:77–99.

45. Adebimpe VR, Gigandet J, Harris E. MMPI diagnosis of black psychiatric patients. *Am J Psychiatry*. 1979;136:85–87.

46. Raskin A, Crook TH, Herman KD. Psychiatric history and symptom differences in black and white depressed inpatients. *J Consult Clin Psychol*. 1975;43:73–80.

47. Pinderhughes CA. Racism and psychotherapy. In: Willie CV, Kramer BM, Brown BS. *Racism and Mental Health*. Pittsburgh: University of Pittsburgh Press; 1973:61–121.

48. Pinderhughes CA. Differential bonding: toward a psychophysiological theory of stereotyping. *Am J Psychiatry*. 1979;136:33–37.

49. Pinderhughes CA. The origins of racism. *Int J Psychiatry*. 1969;8:929–933.

50. Flaherty JA, Meagher R. Measuring racial bias in inpatient treatment. *Am J Psychiatry*. 1980;137:679–682.

51. Sabshin M, Diesenhaus H, Wilkerson R. Dimensions of institutional racism in psychiatry. *Am J Psychiatry*. 1970;127:787–793.

52. Butts H. Economic stress and mental health. *J Natl Med Assoc*. 1979;71:375–379.

53. Jones BE, Lightfoot O, Palmer D, et al. Problems of black residents in white training institutions. *Am J Psychiatry*. 1970;127:798–803.

54. Sue S, Allen D, McKinney H, Hall J. *Delivery of Community Mental Health Services to Black and White Patients*. Seattle: University of Washington Press; 1974.

55. Rosenthal D, Frank J. Fate of psychiatric clinic outpatients assigned to psychotherapy. *J Nerv Ment Dis*. 1958;127:330–343.

56. Wilder J, Coleman M. The "walk-in" psychiatric clinic: some observations and follow-up. *Int J Soc Psychiatry*. 1963;9:192–199.

57. Krebs R. Some effects of a white institution on black psychiatric outpatients. *Am J Orthopsychiatry*. 1971;41:4.

58. Comer J. What happened to minorities and the poor? *Psychiatric Ann*. 1977;7:79–96.

59. American Psychiatric Association. *Diagnostic and Statistical Manual of Mental Disorders*, 3rd ed. Washington, DC: American Psychiatric Association; 1979.

60. Johnson JT. Alcoholism: a social disease from a medical perspective. In: Williams R, ed. *Textbook of Black-Related Diseases*. New York: McGraw-Hill; 1975:639–654.

61. Viamontes J, Powell BJ. Demographic characteristics of black and white male alcoholics. *Int J Addict*. 1974;9:489–494.

62. Spitzer RL, Skodol AE, Gibbon M, Williams JB. *DSM-III Case Book*. Washington, DC: American Psychiatric Association; 1981.

63. Stone A. Conceptual ambiguity and morality in modern psychiatry, presidential address. *Am J Psychiatry*. 1980;137:887–894.

64. Bell CC. DSM-III Case Book, book review. *J Am Med Assoc*. 1981;246:2078.

65. Gaw A, ed. *Cross-Cultural Psychiatry*. Boston: Publishing Sciences Group; 1982.

66. Acosta FX, Yamamoto J, Evans LA. *Effective Psychotherapy for Low-Income and Minority Patients*. New York: Plenum Press; 1982.

67. Bradshaw W. Training psychiatrists for working with blacks in basic residency programs. *Am J Psychiatry*. 1978;135:1520–1524.

68. Griffith E, Delgado A. On the professional socialization of black psychiatric residents in psychiatry. *J Med Educ*. 1979;54:471–476.

69. Bell CC, Thompson B, Shorter-Gooden K, et al. Prevalence of episodes of coma in black subjects. *J Natl Med Assoc*. 1985;77:391–395.

70. Bell CC, Thompson B. Shorter-Gooden K, et al. States of consciousness: their relationship to black-on-black murder. Prepared for the Black Psychiatrists of America for the Black Homicide Workshop on Mental Health and Prevention, sponsored by the National Association of Social Workers and the National Institute of Mental Health, Office of Prevention and Center for the Study of Minority Group Mental Health. Washington, DC, June 14–16, 1984.

71. Griffith EEH, English T, Mayfield V. Possession, prayer, and testimony: therapeutic aspects of the Wednesday night meeting in a black church. *Psychiatry*. 1980;43:120–128.

72. Starker S. Fantasy in psychiatric patients: Exploring a myth. *Hosp Community Psychiatry*. 1979;30:25–30.

73. Bell CC. Black intrapsychic survival skills: alterations of states of consciousness. *J Natl Med Assoc*. 1982;74:1017–1020.

CHAPTER 21:
The Prevalence of Isolated Sleep Paralysis in Blacks

1. Merritt HH. *A Textbook of Neurology*. Philadelphia: Lea & Febiger; 1975.

2. Freud S. Interpretation of Dreams (1901). In: Strachey J, trans. & ed. *Complete Psychological Works*. Vols. 4, 5. London: Hogarth Press; 1957.

3. Binns E. *The Anatomy of Sleep, or, The Art of Procuring Sound and Refreshing Slumber at Will*. London: John Churchill; 1842.

4. Mitchell SW. Some disorders of sleep. *VA Med Monthly*. 1876;2:769–781.

5. Mitchell SW. Some disorders of sleep. *Am J Med Sc. C*. 1890;109–127.

6. Pfister H. Uber Storungen des Erwachens. *Berl Klin Wochenschr*. 1903;40:385–387.

7. Daniels LE. Narcolepsy. *Medicine*. 1934;13:1–122.

8. Lhermitte J, Dupont Y. Sur la cataplexie et plus specialement sur la cataplexie du reveil. *Encephale*. 1928;23:424–434.

9. Ethelberg S. Sleep paralysis or post-dormital chalastic fits in cortical lesions of the frontal pole. *Acta Psychiatr Neurol*. 1956;108 (suppl):121–130.

10. Bell CC. States of consciousness. *J Natl Med Assoc*. 1980;72:331–334.

11. Levin M. Sleep paralysis. *Curr Med Dig*. 1967;34:1229–1232.

12. Wilson SAK. The narcolepsies. *Brain*. 1928;21:63–109.

13. Yoss RE, Daly DD. Criteria for the diagnosis of the narcolepsy syndrome. *Proc Mayo Clin*. 1957;32:320–328.

14. Levin M. The pathogenesis of narcolepsy with a consideration of sleep paralysis and localized sleep. *J Neurol Psychopathol*. 1933;14:1–13.

15. Goode GB. Sleep paralysis. *Arch Neurol*. 1962;6:228–234.

16. Levin M. Premature waking and postdormital paralysis. *J Nerv Ment Dis*. 1957;125:140–141.

17. Lichtenstein BW, Rosenblum AH. Sleep paralysis. *J Nerv Ment Dis*. 1942;95:153–155.

18. Vander Heide C, Weinberg J. Sleep paralysis and combat fatigue. *Psychosomat Med*. 1945;7:330–334.

19. Schneck JM. Sleep paralysis. *Psychosomatics*. 1961;2:360–361.

20. Schneck JM. Sleep paralysis without narcolepsy or cataplexy. *J Am Med Assoc*. 1960;173:1129–1130.

21. Schneck JM. Sleep paralysis: a new evaluation. *Dis Nerv Sys*. 1957;18:144–146.

22. Schneck JM. Personality components in patients with sleep paralysis. *Psychoanal Q*. 1969;43:343–348.

23. Everett HC. Sleep paralysis in medical students. *J Nerv Ment Dis*. 1963;136:283–287.

24. Roth B, Bruthoua S, Perkova L. Familial sleep paralysis. *Schweiz Arch Neurol Neurochir Psychiatr*. 1968;102:321–330.

25. Hobson JA, McCarley RW, Wyzinski PW. Sleep cycle oscillation: reciprocal discharge by two brainstem neuronal groups. *Science*. 1975;189:55–58.

26. McCarley RW, Hobson JA. Neuronal excitability modulation over the sleep cycle: a structural and mathematical model. *Science*. 1975;189:58–60.

27. Hishikawa Y. Sleep paralysis. In: Guilleminault C, Dement WC, Passovant P, eds. *Narcolepsy: Proceedings of the First International Symposium on Narcolepsy*. New York: Spectrum; 1976:97–124.

28. Redmond DE, Huang YH, Snyder DR, et al. Behavioral effects of stimulation of the locus coeruleus in the stumptail monkey (*Macaca arctoides*). *Brain Res*. 1976;166:502–510.

29. Curtis J, Detert R. *How to Relax: A Holistic Approach*. Palo Alto, CA: Mayfield; 1981:35.

30. Bell CC, Thompson B, Shorter-Gooden K, et al. Altered states of consciousness: their relationship to black on-black murder. Presented at the Black Homicide Workshop, Conference on Mental Health and Mental Illness Prevention, National Association of Social Workers, Washington, DC, June 14–16, 1984.

31. Bell CC. Racism: a symptom of the narcissistic personality disorder. *J Natl Med Assoc*. 1980;72:661–665.

32. Bell CC. Black intrapsychic survival skills: Alterations of states of consciousness. *J Natl Med Assoc*. 1982;74:1017–1020.

33. Bell CC. Racism, survival fatigue, and stress related essential hypertension. Presented at the conference, "Culture and the Human Biologic Nature: The Impact of Racism on Essential Hypertension," Wayne State University, Detroit, MI, July 23, 1983.

34. Fenichel O. *The Psychoanalytic Theory of Neurosis*. New York: WW Norton; 1945:117.

35. Schneck JM. Sleep paralysis. *Am J Psychiatry*. 1952;108:921–923.

36. Payn SB: A psychoanalytic approach to sleep paralysis. *J Nerv Ment Dis*. 1965;140:427–433.

37. Levin M. Sleep, cataplexy, and fatigue as manifestations of Pavlovian inhibition. *Am J Psychother*. 1961;15:122–137.

38. Grier WH, Cobbs PM. *Black Rage*. New York: Basic Books; 1968.

39. Rofe Y, Lewin I. Daydreaming in a war environment. *J Ment Imagery*. 1980;4:57–75.

40. Bell CC. Simultaneous treatment of hypertension and opiate withdrawal using an alpha-2 adrenergic agonist. *J Natl Med Assoc*. 1983;75:89–93.

41. Akimoto H, Honda Y, Takahashi Y. Pharmacotherapy in narcolepsy. *Dis Nerv Syst*. 1960;21:1–3.

42. Drachman DA, Kapem S. Sleep disturbance. *J Am Med Assoc*. 1981;246:163–164.

43. Schauch R. Hypnopompic hallucinations and treatment with imipramine. *Am J Psychiatry*. 1979;136:219–220.

44. Rickels K. Nonbenzodiazepine anxiolytics: clinical usefulness. *J Clin Psychiatry*. 1983;44:38–43.

45. Gershon S, Eison AS. Anxiolytic profiles. *J Clin Psychiatry*. 1983;44:45–46.

46. Redmond DE. New and old evidence for the involvement of a brain norepinephrine system in anxiety. In: Fann WE, Karacan 1, Porkney AD, et al., eds. *Phenomenology and Treatment of Anxiety*. New York: Spectrum; 1979.

47. Nardi JJ. Treating sleep paralysis with hypnosis. *Int J Clin Experimental Hypnosis*. 1981;29:358–365.

48. Ostrow DG, Okonek A, Gibbons R, et al. Biologic markers and antidepressant response. *J Clin Psychiatry*. 1983;44(9):10–13.

49. Wolff PH. Ethnic differences in alcohol sensitivity. *Science*. 1972;175:449–450.

50. Ewing JA, Rouse BA, Pellizzari ED. Alcohol sensitivity and ethnic background. *Am J Psychiatry*. 1974;131:206–210.

51. De Hoyos A, De Hoyos G. Symptomatology differentials between Negro and white schizophrenics. *Int J Soc Psychiatry*. 1965;11:245–255.

52. Vitols MM, Waters HG, Keeler MH. Hallucinations and delusions in white and Negro schizophrenics. *Am J Psychiatry*. 1963;120:472–476.

53. Bell CC, Mehta H. The misdiagnosis of black patients with manic depressive illness. *J Natl Med Assoc*. 1980;72:141–145.

54. Bell CC, Mehta H. Misdiagnosis of black patients with manic depressive illness: second in a series. *J Natl Med Assoc*. 1981;73:101–107.

55. Shapiro B, Spitz H. Problems in the differential diagnosis of narcolepsy versus schizophrenia. *Am J Psychiatry*. 1976;133:1321–132.

CHAPTER 22:
Further Studies on the Prevalence of Isolated Sleep Paralysis in Black Subjects

1. Bell CC, Shakoor B, Thompson B, et al. Prevalence of isolated sleep paralysis in black subjects. *J Natl Med Assoc*. 1984;76:501–508.

2. Bell CC. States of consciousness. *J Natl Med Assoc*. 1980;72:331–334.

3. Goode GB. Sleep paralysis. *Arch Neurol*. 1962;6:228–234.

4. Everett HC. Sleep paralysis in medical students. *J Nerv Ment Dis*. 1963;136:283–287.

5. Hufford D. *The Terror that Comes in the Night*. Pennsylvania: University of Pennsylvania Press; 1982:23.

6. Charney DS, Heninger GR, Breier A. Noradrenergic function in panic anxiety. *Arch Gen Psychiatry*. 1984;41:751–763.

7. Charney DS, Heninger GR. Noradrenergic function and the mechanism of action of antianxiety treatment. *Arch Gen Psychiatry*. 1985;42:473–481.

8. Vander Heide C, Weinberg J. Sleep paralysis and combat fatigue. *Psychosom Med*. 1945;7:330–334.

9. Roth B, Bruthoua S, Perkova L. Familial sleep paralysis. *Schweiz Arch Neurol Neurochir Psychiatry*. 1968;102:321–330.

10. American Psychiatric Association. *Diagnostic and Statistical Manual*. 3rd ed. Washington, DC: American Psychiatric Association Press; 1980.

11. Pierce C. Acceptance speech for the E. Y. Williams Senior Scholar of Distinction Award. Presented at the National Medical Association Annual E. Y. Williams Awards Breakfast, Las Vegas, NV, July 24, 1985.

12. Hyatt HM. *Hoodoo-Conjuration-Witchcraft-Rootwork*. Cambridge, MD: Western; 1978:3994–4003.

13. Gibson GS, Gibbons A. Hypertension among blacks: an annotated bibliography. *Hypertension*. 1982;4:7–28.

14. Marks I, Ladner M. Anxiety state (anxiety neurosis): a review. *J Nerv Ment Dis*. 1973;150:3–18.

15. Weissman MM, Meyers JK, Harding PS. Psychiatric disorders in a US urban community: 1975–1976. *Am J Psychiatry.* 1978;135:459–462.

16. Uhlenhuth EH, Balter MB, Mellinger GD, et al. Symptom checklist syndromes in the general population: correlations with psychotherapeutic drug use. *Arch Gen Psychiatry.* 1983;40:1167–1173.

17. Noyes R, Clancy J, Crowe R, et al. The family prevalence of anxiety neurosis. *Arch Gen Psychiatry.* 1978;35:1057–1059.

18. Crowe RR, Noyes R, Pauls DL, et al. A family study of panic disorder. *Arch Gen Psychiatry.* 1983;40:1065–1069.

19. Harris EL, Noyes R, Crowe RR, et al. Family study of agoraphobia. *Arch Gen Psychiatry.* 1983;40:1061–1064.

20. Pauls DL, Noyes R, Crowe RR. The familial prevalence in second-degree relatives of patients with anxiety neurosis (panic disorder). *J Affective Disord.* 1979;1:279–285.

21. Adams JR, Wahby VS, Giller EL. EEG of panic disorder and narcolepsy. Presented at the American Psychiatric Association Annual Meeting, Dallas, TX, May 21, 1985.

22. Ettedgui E, Bridges M. Post-traumatic stress disorder. *Psychiatr Clin North Am.* 1985;8:89–103.

23. Burstein A. Treatment of post-traumatic stress disorder with imipramine. *Psychosomatics.* 1984;25:681–687.

24. Falcon S, Ryan C, Chamberlain K, et al. Tricyclics: possible treatment for post-traumatic stress disorder. *J Clin Psychiatry.* 1985;46:385–389.

25. Hishikawa Y. Sleep paralysis. In: Guilleminault C, Dement WC, Passovant P, eds. *Narcolepsy: Proceedings of the First International Symposium on Narcolepsy.* New York: Spectrum; 1976:97–124.

26. Akimoto H, Honda Y, Takahashi Y. Pharmacotherapy in narcolepsy. *Dis Nerv Syst.* 1960;21:1–3.

27. Drachman DA, Kapem S. Sleep disturbance. *J Am Med Assoc.* 1981;246:163–164.

28. Schauch R. Hypnopompic hallucinations and treatment with imipramine. *Am J Psychiatry.* 1979;136:219–220.

29. Kolb LC, Burris BC, Griffith S. Propranolol and clonidine in treatment of the chronic post-traumatic stress disorders of war. In: Van der Kolb BA, ed. *Post-Traumatic Stress Disorder: Psychological and Biological Sequelae.* Washington, DC: American Psychiatric Press; 1984.

CHAPTER 23:
The Relationship between Isolated Sleep Paralysis, Panic Disorder, and Hypertension

1. Bell CC, Shakoor B, Thompson B, et al. Prevalence of isolated sleep paralysis in black subjects. *J Natl Med Assoc.* 1984;76:501–508.

2. Bell CC, Dixie-Bell DD, Thompson B. Further studies on the prevalence of isolated sleep paralysis in black subjects. *J Natl Med Assoc.* 1986;78:649–659.

3. Bell CC. States of consciousness. *J Natl Med Assoc.* 1980;72:331–334.

4. Charney DS, Redmond DE. Neurobiological mechanisms in human anxiety. *Neuropharmacology.* 1983;22:1531–1536.

5. Charney DS, Heninger GR, Redmond DE. Yohimbine-induced anxiety and increased noradrenergic function in humans: Effects of diazepam and clonidine. *Life Sci.* 1983;33:19–29.

6. Charney DS, Heninger GR, Breier A. Noradrenergic function in panic anxiety. *Arch Gen Psychiatry.* 1984;41:751–763.

7. Nesse RM, Cameron OG, Curtis GC, et al. Adrenergic function in patients with panic anxiety. *Arch Gen Psychiatry.* 1984;41:771–776.

8. Liebowitz MR, Fyer AJ, McGrath P, et al. Clonidine treatment of panic disorder. *Psychopharmacology.* 1981;17:122–123.

9. Grant SJ, Huang YH, Redmond DE. Benzodiazepines attenuate single-unit activity in the locus coeruleus. *Life Sci.* 1980;27:2231–2236.

10. Hoehn-Saric R, Merchant AF, Keyser ML, et al. Effects of clonidine on anxiety disorders. *Arch Gen Psychiatry.* 1981;38:1278–1282.

11. Ko GN, Elsvorth JD, Roth RH, et al. Panic-induced elevation of plasma MHPG levels in phobic-anxious patients. *Arch Gen Psychiatry.* 1983;40:425–430.

12. Ward DE, Gunn CG. Locus coeruleus complex: Differential modulation of depressor mechanisms. *Brain Res.* 1976;107:407–411.

13. Bell CC. Simultaneous treatment of hypertension and opiate withdrawal using an alpha-2 adrenergic agonist. *J Natl Med Assoc.* 1983;75:89–93.

14. Chesney MA, Rosenman RH, ads. *Anger and Hostility in Cardiovascular and Behavioral Disorders.* New York: Hemisphere Publishing; 1985.

15. Bell CC. Black intrapsychic survival skills: Alteration of state of consciousness. *J Natl Med Assoc.* 1982;74:1017–1020.

16. Uhde TW, Boulenger J, Roy-Byrne PP, et al. Longitudinal course of panic disorder: Clinical and biological considerations. *Prog Neuropsychopharmacol Biol Psychiatry.* 1985;9:39–51.

17. Finlay-Jones R, Brown GW. Types of stressful life event and the onset of anxiety and depressive disorders. *Psychol Med.* 1981;11:803–815.

18. Faravelli C, Webb T, Ambonetti A, et al. Prevalence of traumatic early life events in 31 agoraphobic patients with panic attacks. *Am J Psychiatry*. 1985;142:1493-1494.

19. Coryell W, Noyes R, Clancy J. Excess mortality in panic disorder. *Arch Gen Psychiatry*. 1982;39:701-703.

20. Noyes R, Clancy J, Hoenk PR, et al. Anxiety neurosis and physical illness. *Comp Psychiatry*. 1978;19:407-413.

21. Katon W. Panic disorder and somatization. *Am J Med*. 1984;77:101-106.

22. Noyes R, Clancy J, Hoenk PR, et al. The prognosis of anxiety neurosis. *Arch Gen Psychiatry*. 1980;37:173-178.

23. Shear MK, Kligfield R, Harshfield G, et al. Cardiac rate and rhythm in panic patients. *Am J Psychiatry*. 1987;144:633-637.

24. Warheit GJ, Holzer CE, Arey SA. Race and mental health: an epidemiologic update. *J Health Soc Behav*. 1975;16:243-256.

25. American Psychiatric Association. *Diagnostic and Statistical Manual of Mental Disorders*. 3rd ed. Washington, DC: American Psychiatric Association Press; 1980.

26. Pollack MH, Rosenbaum JF. Management of antidepressant-induced side effects: A practical guide for the clinician. *J Clin Psychiatry*. 1987;48:3-8.

27. Ohaeri JU, Odejide AO, lkuesan BA, et al. The pattern of isolated sleep paralysis among Nigerian medical students. *J Natl Med Assoc.*, in press.

28. Von Korff M, Shapiro S, Birke JD, et al. Anxiety and depression in primary care clinic. *Arch Gen Psychiatry*. 1987;44:152-156.

29. Katon W, Vitaliano PP, Russo J, et al. Panic disorder: Epidemiology in primary care. *J Fam Pract*. 1986;23:233-239.

CHAPTER 24:
The Prevalence of Coma in Black Subjects

1. Bell CC. States of consciousness. *J Natl Med Assoc*. 1980;72:331-334.

2. Bell CC, Shakoor B, Thompson B, et al. Prevalence of isolated sleep paralysis in black subjects. *J Natl Med Assoc*. 1984;76:501-508.

3. Bell CC. Black intrapsychic survival skills: alterations of states of consciousness. *J Natl Med Assoc*. 1982;74:1017-1020.

4. Hanley J. The signature of post-concussion syndrome in the sleep tracing. *Neuropsychiatric Bull*. 1983;8:1-3.

5. Merritt HH. *A Textbook of Neurology*. Philadelphia: Lea & Febiger; 1975:341-342.

6. Jennett B, Teasdale G. *Management of Head Injuries*. Philadelphia: FA Davis; 1981:289.

7. Gronwall D, Wrightson P. Delayed recovery of intellectual function after minor head injury. *Lancet*. 1974;2:605-609.

8. Strub RL, Black FW. *Organic Brain Syndromes: An Introduction to Neurobehavioral Disorders*. Philadelphia: FA Davis; 1981:275.

9. Lewis DO, Shanok SS, Cohen RJ, et al. Race bias in the diagnosis and disposition of violent adolescents. *Am J Psychiatry*. 1980;137:1216–1221.

10. Desai BT, Whitman S, Coonley-Hoganson R, et al. Urban head injury: a clinical series. *J Natl Med Assoc*. 1983;75:875–881.

11. Staples R. *Black Masculinity*. San Francisco: Black Scholar Press; 1982:68.

12. Bach-y-Rita G, Lion JR, Climent C, et al. Episodic dyscontrol: a study of 130 violent prisoners. *Am J Psychiatry*. 1971;127:1473–1478.

13. Jason J, Flock M, Tyler CW. Epidemiologic characteristics of primary homicide in the United States. *Am J Epidemiol*. 1983;117:419–428.

14. Rose HM. *Black Homicide and the Urban Environment*. Washington, DC: US Government Printing Office; 1981.

5. Dennis RE, Kirk A, Knuckles BN, et al. *Black Males at Risk to Low Life Expectancy: A Study of Homicide Victims and Perpetrators*. Washington, DC: Center for Studies of Minority Group Mental Health; 1981. NIMH grant 1 R01 MH36720.

16. Bell CC. Racism, narcissism, and integrity. *J Natl Med Assoc*. 1978;70:89–92.

17. Bell CC. Racism: a symptom of the narcissistic personality disorder. *J Natl Med Assoc*. 1980;72:661–665.

18. Barber JB, Webster JC. Head injuries: a review of 150 cases. *J Natl Med Assoc*. 1974;66:201–204.

19. Elliott FA. The neurology of explosive rage: the dyscontrol syndrome. *Practitioner*. 1976;217:51–60.

CHAPTER 25:
The Misdiagnosis of Black Patients with Manic Depressive Illness, Part 1

1. Thomas A, Sillen S. *Racism and Psychiatry*. New York: Brunner/Mazel; 1972:128.

2. Malzberg B: Mental disorders in the US. In: Deutsch A, Fishman H, eds. *Encyclopedia of Mental Health*. Vol. 3. New York: Franklin Watts Inc.; 1963:1051–1066.

3. Prange A, Vitols M. Cultural aspects of the relatively low incidence of depression in Southern Negroes. *Internat J Social Psychiatry*. 1962;8:104–112.

4. Jaco G. *Social Epidemiology of Mental Disorders*. New York: Russell Sage Foundation; 1960.

5. Johnson G, Gershon S, Hekimian L. Controlled evaluation of lithium and chlorpromazine in the treatment of manic states: an interim report. *Compr Psychiatry*. 1968;9:563–573.

6. Faris R, Dunham W. *Mental Disorders in Urban Areas*. Chicago: University of Chicago Press; 1939.

7. Frumkin RM. Race and major mental disorders. *J Negro Educ.* 1954;23:97-98.

8. Taube C. Admission rates to state and county mental hospitals by age, sex, and color, United States, 1969. *National Institute of Mental Health (Rockville, MD): Statistical Note 41*; 1971:1-7.

9. Simon R, Fleiss J. Depression and schizophrenia in hospitalized patients. *Arch Gen Psychiatry.* 1973;28:509-512.

10. Helzer J. Bipolar affective disorder in black and white men. *Arch Gen Psychiatry.* 1975;32:1140-1143.

11. Cannon M, Locke B. Being black is detrimental to one's mental health: myth or reality? *Phylon.* 1977;38:408-428.

12. Bell C. The role of psychiatric emergency services in aiding community alternatives to hospitalization in an inner-city population. *J Natl Med Assoc.* 1978;70:931-935.

13. Taylor M, Abrams R: The phenomenology of mania. *Arch Gen Psychiatry.* 1973;29:520-522.

14. Kolb L. *Noyes' Modern Clinical Psychiatry*. 7th ed. Philadelphia: WB Saunders, 1968:336.

CHAPTER 26:
The Misdiagnosis of Black Patients with Manic Depressive Illness, Part 2

1. Prange A, Vitols M. Cultural aspects of the relatively low incidence of depression in Southern Negroes. *Internatl J Social Psychiatry.* 1962;8:104-112.

2. Jaco G. *Social Epidemiology of Mental Disorders*. New York: Russell Sage Foundation; 1960.

3. Johnson G, Gershon S, Hekimian L. Controlled evaluation of lithium and chlorpromazine in the treatment of manic states: an interim report. *Compr Psychiatry.* 1968;9:563-573.

4. Cannon M, Locke B. Being black is detrimental to one's mental health: myth or reality? *Phylon.* 1977;38:408-428.

5. Malzberg B. Mental disorders in the US. In: Deutsch A, Fishman H, eds. *Encyclopedia of Mental Health*. Vol. 3. New York: Franklin Watts Inc.; 1963:1051-1066.

6. Faris R, Dunham W. *Mental Disorders in Urban Areas*. Chicago: University of Chicago Press; 1939.

7. Frumkin RM. Race and major mental disorders. *J Negro Educ.* 1954;23:97-98.

8. Taube C. Admission rates to state and county mental hospitals by age, sex, and color, United States, 1969. *National Institute of Mental Health (Rockville, MD): Statistical Note 41*; 1971:1–7.

9. Simon R, Fleiss J. Depression and schizophrenia in black increases the likelihood of misdiagnosis and of hospitalized patients. *Arch Gen Psychiatry.* 1973;28:509–512.

10. Thomas A, Sillen S. *Racism and Psychiatry.* New York: Brunner/Mazel; 1972:128.

11. Bell C, Mehta H. The misdiagnosis of black patients manic depressive illness. *J Natl Med Assoc.* 1980;72:141–145.

12. Bell C. The role of psychiatric emergency services in aiding community alternatives to hospitalization in an inner-city population. *J Natl Med Assoc.* 1978;70:931–935.

13. Garvey M, Tuason V. Mania misdiagnosed as schizophrenia. *J Clin Psychiatry.* 1980;41:75–78.

14. Winokur G, Clayton P, Reich T. *Manic Depressive Illness.* St. Louis: CV Mosby; 1969.

15. Corange A, Levine P. Age of onset of bipolar affective illness. *Arch Gen Psychiatry.* 1978;35:1345–1348.

16. Helzer J. Bipolar affective disorder in black and white men. *Arch Gen Psychiatry.* 1975;32:1140–1143.

17. Kendel R, Cooper J, Goulay A. The diagnostic criteria of American and British psychiatrists. *Arch Gen Psychiatry.* 1971;25:123–130.

18. Taylor M, Abrams R. The phenomenology of mania. *Arch Gen Psychiatry.* 1973;29:520–522.

19. Langsley D, Robinowitz C. Psychiatric manpower: an overview. *Hosp Comm Psychiatry.* 1979:30:749–755.

20. Spar J, Ford C, Liston E. Bipolar affective disorder in aged patients. *J Clin Psychiatry.* 1979;40:504–507.

Suggested Reading: Jones BE, Gray BA, Parson EB. Manic depressive illness among poor urban blacks. Presented at the American Psychiatric Association Annual Meeting, San Francisco, CA, May 8, 1980.

CHAPTER 28:
The Need for Minority Curriculum Content in Psychiatric Training

1. Chunn JC, Dunston PJ, Ross-Sheriff F, eds. *Mental Health and People of Color.* Washington, DC: Howard University Press; 1984.

2. Thomas A, Sillen A. *Racism and Psychiatry.* New York: Brunner-Mazel; 1972.

3. Coombs N. *The Black Experience in America*. New York: Twayne; 1972.

4. Pinderhughes CA. The origins of racism. *Int J Psychiatry*. 1969;8:929–933.

5. Pinderhughes CA. Differential bonding: toward a psycho-physiological theory of stereotyping. *Am J Psychiatry*. 1979;136:33–37.

6. Allport GW. *The Nature of Prejudice*. Garden City, NY: Doubleday Anchor; 1958.

7. Willie CV. *A New Look at Black Families*. Bayside, NY: General Hall; 1981.

8. Bell CC, Thompson B, Shorter-Gooden K, et al. Altered states of consciousness profile: an Afrocentric intrapsychic evaluation tool. *J Natl Med Assoc*. 1985;77:715–728.

9. Bell CC, Thompson JP, Lewis D, et al. Misdiagnosis of alcohol-related organic brain syndromes: Implications for treatment. In: Brisbane FL, Womble M, ads. *Treatment of the Black Alcoholic*. NY: Haworth Press; 1985:45–65.

10. Bell CC. Impaired black health professionals: vulnerabilities and treatment approaches. *J Natl Med Assoc*. 1986;78:925–930.

11. Bell CC. Black intrapsychic survival skills: alterations of states of consciousness. *J Natl Med Assoc*. 1982;74:1017–1020.

12. Bell CC, Prothrow-Stith D, Smallwood-Murchison C. Black- on-black homicide: the National Medical Association's responsibilities. *J Natl Med Assoc*. 1986;12:1139–1141.

13. Griffith E, Delgado A. On the professional socialization of black psychiatric residents in psychiatry. *J Med Educ*. 1979;54:471–476.

14. Jones BE, Lightfoot O, Palmer D, et al. Problems of black residents in white training institutions *Am J Psychiatry*. 1970;127:798–803.

CHAPTER 29:
Impaired Black Health Professionals: Vulnerabilities and Treatment Approaches

1. Blackwell JE. *Mainstreaming Outsiders: The Production of Black Professionals*. New York: General Hall; 1981.

2. Delgado AK. On being black. In: Acosta FX, Yamamoto J, Evans LA, eds. *Effective Psychotherapy for Low-Income and Minority Patients*. New York: Plenum Press; 1982:109–116.

3. Pierce CM. Offensive mechanisms: the vehicle for microaggression. In: Barabour FB, ed. *The Black 70s*. Boston: Porter Sargent; 1970.

4. Sabshin M, Diesenhaus H, Wilkerson R. Dimensions of institutional racism in psychiatry. *Am J Psychiatry*. 1970;127:787–793.

5. Bell CC. Racism, narcissism, and integrity. *J Natl Med Assoc*. 1978;70:89–92.

6. Bell CC. Racism: a symptom of the narcissistic personality disorder. *J Natl Med Assoc.* 1980;72:661–665.

7. Hughes L. *The Panther and the Lash-Poems of Our Times.* New York: Alfred Knopf; 1967:4.

8. Shea S, Fullilove M. Entry of black and other minority students into US medical schools. *N Engl J Med.* 1985;313:933–940.

9. Keith SN, Bell RM, Swanson AG, Williams AP. Effects of affirmative action in medical schools. *N Engl J Med.* 1985;313:1519–1525.

10. Bullock SC, Houston E. Perceptions of racism by black medical students in predominately white medical schools. Presented at the American Psychiatric Association Annual Meeting, New Orleans, LA, May 14, 1981.

11. Bell CC, Thompson JP, Lewis D, et al. Misdiagnosis of alcohol-related organic brain syndromes: implications for treatment. In: Brisbane FL, Womble M, eds. *Treatment of Black Alcoholics.* New York: Haworth Press; 1985:45–66.

12. Bell CC. Statistics on black populations, letters. *J Natl Med Assoc.* 1982;74:829–830.

13. Bell CC, Thompson B, Shorter-Gooden K, et al. Altered states of consciousness profile: an Afrocentric intrapsychic evaluation tool. *J Natl Med Assoc.* 1985;77:715–728.

14. Carter JH. Frequent mistakes made with black patients in psychotherapy. *J Natl Med Assoc.* 1979;71:1007–1009.

15. Jones BE, Gray BA. Black and white psychiatrists: therapy with blacks. *J Natl Med Assoc.* 1985;77:19–25.

16. Brantley T. Racism and its impact on psychotherapy. *Am J Psychiatry.* 1985;140:1605–1608.

17. Bradshaw W. Training psychiatrists for working with blacks in basic residency programs. *Am J Psychiatry.* 1978;135:1520–1524.

18. Pinderhughes C. Racism and psychotherapy. In: Willie C, Solomon P, Brown B, ed. *Racism and Mental Health.* Pittsburgh: University of Pittsburgh Press; 1973:61–121.

19. Thomas A, Sillen S. *Racism and Psychiatry.* New York: Brunner/Mazel; 1972.

20. Bell CC, Bland I, Houston E, Jones BE. Enhancement of knowledge and skills for the psychiatric treatment of black populations. In: Chunn JC, Dunston PJ, Ross-Sheriff F, eds. *Mental Health and People of Color.* Washington, DC: Howard University Press; 1983:205–237.

21. Baker FM, Black suicide attempters in 1980: a preventive focus. *Gen Hosp Psychiatry.* 1984;6:131–137.

22. Poussaint AF. Black suicide. In: Williams RA, ed. *Textbook of Black-Related Diseases.* New York: McGraw-Hill; 1975:707–714.

23. Prudhomme C. The problem of suicide in the American Negro. *Psychol Rev.* 1938;25:372–391.

24. Clark KB. *Dark Ghetto.* New York: Harper & Row; 1965.

25. Spurlock J. Survival, guilt, and the Afro-American of achievement. *J Natl Med Assoc.* 1985;77:29–32.

26. Norris DM, Bell AM. Success: pychological conflict for black Americans. Presented at the American Psychiatric Association Annual Meeting, Dallas, TX, May 22, 1985.

27. Davis R. Black suicide in the seventies: current trends. *Suicide Life Threat Behav.* 1979;9:131–140.

28. Gary LE. Suicide and support systems in the black community: its implications for the black community. Presented at "A Challenge to Live: Symposium on Black Suicide," Chicago, IL, April 22–23, 1980.

29. Durkheim E. In: Spaulding JA, Simpson G, trans. *Suicide: A Study in Sociology.* New York: Free Press; 1951.

30. Powell GJ. A six-city study of school desegregation and self-concept among Afro-Am Junior high school students: a preliminary study with implications for mental health. In: Bass BA, Wyatt GE, Powell GJ, eds. *The Afro-American Family.* New York: Grune & Stratton; 1982:265–316.

31. Griffith EEH, Delgado A. On the professional socialization of black residents in psychiatry. *J Med Ed.* 1979;54:471–476.

32. Gary LE, Berry GL. Predicting attitudes toward substance abuse use in a black community: implications for prevention. *Community Ment Health J.* 1985;21:42–51.

33. Swanson W, Breed W. Black suicide in New Orleans. Shneidman, ES, ed. *Suicidology: Contemporary Developments.* New York: Grune & Stratton; 1976:99–130.

34. Jones BE, Lightfoot OB, Palmer D, et al. Problems of black psychiatric residents in white training institutes. *Am J Psychiatry.* 1970;127:98–103.

35. Collins JL. The impaired physician. *J Natl Med Assoc.* 1982;74:221–223.

CHAPTER 31:
Treatment Issues for African-American Men

1. Jones BE, Gray BA. Black males and psychotherapy: theoretical issues. *Am J Psychother.* 1983;37:77–85.

2. Pinderhughes CA. Racism and psychotherapy. In: Willie CV, Kramer BM, Brown BS, eds. *Racism and Mental Health.* Pittsburgh, PA: University of Pittsburgh Press; 1973:61–121.

3. Adams WA. The Negro patient in psychiatric treatment. *Am J Orthopsychiatry.* 1950;20:305–310.

4. Frank JD. Adjustment problems of selected Negro soldiers. *J Mental and Nervous Diseases.* 1947;105:647.

5. St. Clair HR. Psychiatric interview experiences with Negroes. *Am J Psychiatry* 1951;108:113–119.

6. Baker FM. Psychiatric treatment of older African Americans. *Hosp Community Psychiatry.* 1994;45:32–37.

7. Calnek M. Racial factors in the countertransference: the black therapist and the black client. *Am J Orthopsychiatry.* 1970;40:39–46.

8. Carter JH. Frequent mistakes made with black patients in psychotherapy. *J Natl Med Assoc.* 1979;71:1007–1009.

9. Wood WD, Sherrets SD. Requests for outpatient mental health services: a comparison of whites and blacks. *Compr Psychiatry.* 1984;25:329–334.

10. Siegel JM. A brief review of the effects of race in clinical service interactions. *Am J Orthopsychiatry.* 1974;4:555–562.

11. Yamamoto J, James QC, Palley N. Cultural problems in psychiatric therapy. *Arch Gen Psychiatry.* 1968;19:45–49.

12. Mayo JA. Utilization of a community mental health center by blacks: admission to inpatient status. *J Nerv Ment Dis* 1974;158:202–207.

13. Sue S, McKinney H, Allen D, Hall J. Delivery of community mental health services to black and white clients. *J Consult Clin Psychol* 1974;42:794–801.

14. Flaskerud JH, Hu L. Racial/ethnic identity and amount and type of psychiatric treatment. *Am J Psychiatry.* 1992;149:379–384.

15. Bell CC, Bland IJ, Houston E, Jones BE. Enhancement of knowledge and skills for the psychiatric treatment of black populations. In: Chunn JC, Dunston PJ, Ross-Sheriff F, eds. *Mental Health and People of Color.* Washington, DC: Howard University Press; 1983:205–237.

16. Kupers T. *Public Therapy: The Practice of Psychotherapy in the Public Mental Health Clinic.* New York, NY: Free Press; 1981.

17. Jones BE, Gray BA, Jospitre J. Survey of psychotherapy with black men. *Am J Psychiatry.* 1982;139:1174–1177.

18. Jones BE, Gray BA. Black and white psychiatrists: therapy with Blacks. *J Natl Med Assoc.* 1985;77:19–25.

19. Turner S, Armstrong S. Cross-racial psychotherapy-what the therapists say. *Psychotherapy: Theory, Research and Practice.* 1981;18:375–378.

20. Jones BE, Gray BA. Similarities and differences in black men and women in psychotherapy. *J Natl Med Assoc.* 1984;76:21–27.

21. Neighbors HW, Jackson JS, Bowman PJ, Gurin G. Stress, coping, and black mental health: preliminary findings of a national study. *Prevention in Human Services.* 1983;2:5–29.

22. Grier WH, Cobbs PM. *Black Rage.* New York, NY: Basic Books; 1968.

23. Griffith EEH, Griffith EJ. Racism, psychological injury, and compensatory damages. *Hosp Community Psychiatry.* 1986;37:71–75.

24. Pierce CM. Stress in the workplace. In: Conner-Edwards AF, Spurlock J, eds. *Black Families in Crisis.* New York, NY: Brunner/Mazel; 1988:27–33.

25. Pierce CM. Public health and human rights: racism, torture and terrorism. Presented at the American Psychiatric Association Annual Meeting, Washington, DC, May 4,1992.

26. Brantly T. Racism and its impact on psychotherapy. *Am J Psychiatry.* 1983;140:1605–1608.

27. Bell CC. Finding a way through the maze of racism. *Emerge.* September 1994:80.

28. Jenkins EJ, Bell CC. Violence exposure, psychological distress and high risk behaviors among inner-city high school students. In: Friedman S, ed. *Anxiety Disorders in African-Americans.* New York, NY: Springer Publishing; 1994:76–88.

29. Carter RT. *The Influence of Race and Racial Identity in Psychotherapy.* New York, NY: Wiley & Sons; 1995.

CHAPTER 32:
Racism, Narcissism, and Integrity

1. Kohut H. *The Analysis of the Self.* New York: International Universities Press; 1971.

2. Masterson JF. *Treatment of the Borderline Adolescent: A Developmental Approach.* New York: John Wiley; 1972.

3. Kernberg O. Borderline personality organization. *J Am Psychoanal Assoc.* 1967;15:641–685.

4. Fannon F. *Black Skin, White Masks.* New York: Grove Press; 1967:93.

5. Hughes L. *The Panther and the Lash Poems of Our Times.* New York: AA Knopf; 1967:14.

6. Grier WH, Cobbs PM. *The Jesus Bag.* New York: Bantam Books, 1971.

7. Kohut H. Forms and transformations of narcissism. *J Am Psychoanal Assoc.* 1966;14:264–268.

8. Clark KB. *Dark Ghetto.* New York: Harper & Row; 1965.

9. Schulke F, ed. *Martin Luther King, Jr.: A Documentary—Montgomery to Memphis.* New York: WW Norton; 1976:222–224.

CHAPTER 33:
Racism: A Symptom of the Narcissistic Personality Disorder

1. Allport GW. *The Nature of Prejudice.* New York: Doubleday; 1958:388.

2. Adorno T, et al. *The Authoritarian Personality.* New York: Harper; 1950:118.

3. LaPiere R. The individual and his society: disagreements between sociology and psychoanalysis. In: Schoeck H. *Psychiatry and Responsibility.* Princeton, NJ: D Von Nostrand; 1962:68–82.

4. Allport G. *The Person in Psychology.* Boston: Beacon Press; 1968.

5. Grier W, Cobbs P. *Black Rage.* New York: Basic Books; 1968.

6. Kovel J. *White Racism: A Psycho-history.* New York: Vintage Books; 1970:3.

7. Fannon F. *The Wretched of the Earth.* New York, Grove Press; 1967.

8. Thomas A, Sillen S. *Racism and Psychiatry.* New York: Brunner/Mazel; 1972.

9. Kohut H. Forms and transformations of narcissism. *J Am Psychoanal Assoc.* 1966;14:243–272.

10. Kohut H. *Analysis of the Self.* New York: International Universities Press; 1971.

11. Masterson JF. *Treatment of the Borderline Adolescent: A Developmental Approach.* New York: John Wiley; 1972.

12. Kernberg O. Borderline personality organization. *J Am Psychoanal Assoc.* 1976;15:641–685.

13. Bell C. Racism, narcissism, and integrity. *J Natl Med Assoc.* 1978;70:89–92.

14. Kohut H. Thoughts on Narcissism and Narcissistic Rage. In: *The Psychoanalytic Study of the Child,* Vol. 27. New York: NY Times Book Co.; 1972:380, 386, 390, 412.

15. Hood E. Black women, white women: separate paths to liberation. *The Black Scholar.* 1978;9:45–56.

16. Wolfe L. Why some people can't love. *Psychology Today.* 1978;12:54–59.

1 7. Davis A. Rape, racism, and the capitalist setting. *The Black Scholar.* 1978;9:26.

18. Fox R. Narcissistic rage and the problem of combat aggression. *Arch Gen Psychiatry.* 1974;31:807–811.

19. Kohut H. Creativeness, charisma, group psychology: reflections on the self-analysis of Freud. *Psychol Issues.* 1976;9:400, 417.

20. Barber J. President's inaugural address: health status of the black community. *J Natl Med Assoc.* 1979;71:87.

21. Bookert C. Address of the retiring president: equal opportunity for all. *J Natl Med Assoc.* 1979;71:86.

22. Clark KB. *Dark Ghetto.* New York, Harper & Row; 1965:11.

CHAPTER 34:
Endurance, Strength, and Coordination Exercises that do not Cause Cardiovascular or Respiratory Stress

1. Morehouse L, Rasch P. *Scientific Basis of Athletic Training*. Philadelphia: WB Saunders; 1958:123–129.
2. Huang WS. *Fundamentals of Tai Chi Chuan*. Hong Kong: South Sky Book; 1974:438–454.
3. Academy of Traditional Chinese Medicine. *An Outline of Chinese Acupuncture*. Peking: Foreign Languages Press; 1975:226–268.
4. Mann F. *Acupuncture*. New York: Vintage Books; 1973:195–225.
5. Newland A, Loh W. *Acupuncture Anesthesia*. La Porte, Indiana: Century Medical Publications; 1975:59–95.
6. Cahn AM, Carayon P, Hill C, et al. *Acupuncture in Gastroscopy*. Lancet. 1978;8057(1):182–183.
7. Needling the ear for cerebral palsy. *Medical World News*. November 28, 1977:59.
8. AMA group finds chinese medicine excels in some areas, medical news. *J Am Med Assoc*. 1974;229(13):1703.
9. Acupuncture may relieve Meniere's and other diseases. *Hospital Tribune*. October 4, 1976; 26.
10. Kurland H. Treatment of headache pain with auto-acupressure. *Dis Nerv Syst*. 1976;37(3):127–129.
11. Shiffrin W, Bailey SL. *Acupressure*. Canoga Park, CA: Major Books; 1976:22–107.
12. Namikoshi T. *Shiatsu*. San Francisco: Japan Publications Inc.; 1972:62–81.
13. Smith D. *East/West Exercise Book*. New York: McGraw-Hill; 1976:7–10.
14. Greist J, Klein M, Eischens R, et al. Antidepressant running. *Behav Med*. 1978;5:19–24.
15. Spino M. *Beyond Jogging*. Millbrae, CA: Celestial Arts; 1976:11–17.
16. Rieker H. *The Yoga of Light*. Los Angeles: Dawn Horse Press; 1974:33–41.
17. Kingsland K, Kingsland V. *Complete Hatha Yoga*. New York: Arco; 1976:34–75.
18. Liu D. *Taoist Health Exercise Book*. New York: Link Books; 1974:21–86.
19. Siou L. *Chi Kung*. Rutland, VT: Tuttle; 1975:3–47.
20. Lee Y. *Tai Chi for Health*. Hong Kong: Unicorn Press; 1968:27–31.
21. Cheng M, Smith R. *T'ai-Chi*. Rutland, VT: Tuttle; 1967:5–11.
22. Horwitz T, Kimmelman S, Lui H. *Tai Chi Ch'uan*. Chicago: Chicago Review Press; 1976:27–37.

23. Chen Y. *T'ai-Chi Ch'uan: Its Effects and Practical Applications*. Hong Kong: Unicorn Press; 1971:10–14.

24. Acupuncture and psychiatry in China. Presented at the American Psychiatric Association Convention, Toronto, Canada, May 5, 1977.

25. Davis L, ed. *Christopher's Textbook of Surgery*. 9th ed. Philadelphia: WB Saunders; 1968:1236–1238.

26. Guyton A. *Textbook of Medical Physiology*. Philadelphia: WB Saunders; 1967:976.

27. Ramazzini B. Diseases of runners; diseases of workers. *MD*. 1977;21:41–42.

28. Sports medicine. *MD*. 1977;21:79–91.

29. Wallnofer H, Rottausher A. *Chinese Folk Medicine*. New York: Signet; 1972:139–142.

30. Medeiros E. *The Complete History and Philosophy of Kung Fu*. Rutland, VT: Tuttle; 1974:62.

31. Tohei K. *This is Akido*. Tokyo: Japan Publications; 1968:178–179.

32. Grant J, Basmajian J. *Grant's Method of Anatomy*. Baltimore: Williams and Wilkins; 1965:320.

33. Benson H, Dryer T, Hartley L. Decreased volume O_2 consumption during exercise with elicitation of the relaxation response. *J Hum Stress*. 1978;4:38–42.

34. Rama, S, Ajaya, S. *Emotion to Enlightenment*. Glenview, IL: Himalayan International Institute of Yoga Science and Philosophy, 1976.

CHAPTER 35:
Psychoneuroendocrinology, Biorhythms, and Chinese Medicine

1. Krieger DT, Allen W. Relationship of bioassayable and immunoassayable plasma ACTH and cortisol concentrations in normal subjects and in patients with Cushing's disease. *J Clin Endocrinol Metabol*. 1975;40:675–687.

2. Jusko WJ, Slaunwhite WR, Aceto T. Partial pharmacodynamic model for the circadian episodic secretion of cortisol in man. *J Clin Endocrinol Metabol*. 1975;40:278–289.

3. Gutai JP, Meyer WJ, Kowarski AA, et al. Twenty-four-hour integrated concentrations of progesterone, 17-hydroxyprogesterone and cortisol in normal male subjects. *J Clin Endocrinol Metabol*. 1977;44:116–120.

4. Tanaka K, Nicholson WE, Orth DN. Diurnal rhythm and disappearance half-time of endogenous plasma immunoreactive 6-MSH (LPH) and ACTH in man. *J Clin Endocrinol Metabol*. 1978;46:883–890.

5. Luce GG. *Biological Rhythms in Human and Animal Physiology*. New York: Dover; 1971:52.

6. Snyder SH. The opiate receptor and morphine-like peptides in the brain. *Am J Psychiatry.* 1978;135:645–652.

7. Nakao K, Nakai Y, Jingami H, et al. Substantial rise of plasma 6-endorphin levels after insulin-induced hypoglycemia in human subjects. *J Clin Endocrinol Metabol.* 1979;49:838–841.

8. Guyton AC. *Textbook of Medical Physiology.* Philadelphia: WB Saunders; 1966:1057.

9. Ettiti P, Brown G. Psychoneuroendocrinology of affective disorders: an overview. *Am J Psychiatry.* 1977;134:493–501.

10. Caplan RD, Cobb S, French JR. White collar workload and cortisol: disruption of circadian rhythm by job stress? *J Psychosom Res.* 1979;23:181–192.

11. Quigley ME, Yen SC. A mid-day surge in cortisol levels. *J Clin Endocrinol Metabol.* 1979;49:945–947.

12. Rastogi GK, Dash RJ, Sharma BR, et al. Circadian responsiveness of the hypothalamic-pituitary axis. *J Clin Endocrinol Metabol.* 1976;42:798–803.

13. Mann F. *Acupuncture: The Ancient Chinese Art of Healing and How it Works Scientifically.* New York: Vintage Books; 1973:1, 106.

14. Bell C. Endurance, strength, and coordination exercises without cardiovascular or respiratory stress. *J Natl Med Assoc.* 1979;71:265–270.

15. Brandenberger G, Follenius M. Influence on timing and intensity of muscular exercise on temporal patterns of plasma cortisol levels. *J Clin Endocrinol Metabol.* 1975;40:845–849.

16. Sutton JR, Casey JH. The adrenocortical response to competitive athletics in veteran athletes. *J Clin Endocrinol Metabol.* 1975;40:135–138.

17. Newmark SR, Himatongkam T, Martin R, et al. Adrenocortical response to marathon running. *J Clin Endocrinol Metabol.* 1976;42:393–394.

18. Benefits from acupuncture are primarily physiologic. *Clin Psychiatry News.* 1978;6:61.

Index